The Silent CANINE K9 Warriors

CANINE
The Silent K9 Warriors

Maj General
BS Panwar AVSM, SM, PhD (Retd)
Indian Army

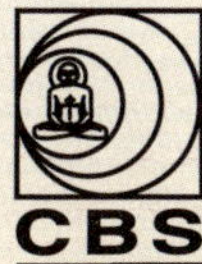

CBS Publishers & Distributors Pvt Ltd

New Delhi • Bengaluru • Chennai • Kochi • Kolkata • Mumbai
Hyderabad • Nagpur • Patna • Pune • Vijayawada

Disclaimer

Science and technology are constantly changing fields. New research and experience broaden the scope of information and knowledge. The author has tried his best in giving information available to him while preparing the material for this book. Although, all efforts have been made to ensure optimum accuracy of the material, yet it is quite possible some errors might have been left uncorrected. The publisher, the printer and the author will not be held responsible for any inadvertent errors, or inaccuracies.

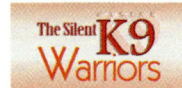

ISBN: 978-81-239-2870-8

First Edition: 2016

Published by Satish Kumar Jain and produced by Varun Jain for
CBS Publishers & Distributors Pvt Ltd
4819/XI Prahlad Street, 24 Ansari Road, Daryaganj, New Delhi 110 002, India.
Ph: 23289259, 23266861, 23266867 Website: www.cbspd.com
Fax: 011-23243014 e-mail: delhi@cbspd.com; cbspubs@airtelmail.in.
Corporate Office: 204 FIE, Industrial Area, Patparganj, Delhi 110 092
Ph: 4934 4934 Fax: 4934 4935 e-mail: publishing@cbspd.com; publicity@cbspd.com

Branches

- **Bengaluru:** Seema House 2975, 17th Cross, K.R. Road, Banasankari 2nd Stage, Bengaluru 560 070, Karnataka
  Ph: +91-80-26771678/79 Fax: +91-80-26771680 e-mail: bangalore@cbspd.com
- **Chennai:** 7, Subbaraya Street, Shenoy Nagar, Chennai 600 030, Tamil Nadu
  Ph: +91-44-26680620, 26681266 Fax: +91-44-42032115 e-mail: chennai@cbspd.com
- **Kochi:** Ashana House, No. 39/1904, AM Thomas Road, Valanjambalam, Ernakulam 682 018, Kochi, Kerala
  Ph: +91-484-4059061-62-64-65 Fax: +91-484-4059065 e-mail: kochi@cbspd.com
- **Kolkata:** 6/B, Ground Floor, Rameswar Shaw Road, Kolkata-700 014, West Bengal
  Ph: +91-33-22891126, 22891127, 22891128 e-mail: kolkata@cbspd.com
- **Mumbai:** 83-C, Dr E Moses Road, Worli, Mumbai-400018, Maharashtra
  Ph: +91-22-24902340/41 Fax: +91-22-24902342 e-mail: mumbai@cbspd.com

Representatives

- **Hyderabad** 0-9885175004
- **Nagpur** 0-9021734563
- **Patna** 0-9334159340
- **Pune** 0-9623451994
- **Vijayawada** 0-9000660880

Printed at: Magic International Pvt. Ltd., Greater Noida

Foreword

The importance of dogs in various wars, low intensity conflicts, counterinsurgency and anti-terrorism efforts has been felt time and again. These canines, also referred as war dogs or military working dogs, have proven their worth as silent warriors and saviours from times immemorial. The heroic deeds of these important auxiliary of troops have made themselves indispensable during peace and war. The last decade has witnessed a sharp rise in the demand of working dogs of various specialties in armies world over. As technology and world situations change, the dog and handler teams will continue the transformation process and give commanders the full-spectrum capabilities needed to be combat multipliers on the battlefield as well as persuasive force protection and anti-terrorism assets.

In India, right from the deployment of tracker dogs by Indian Army in December 1959 till present days, the valiant army dogs are being extensively employed in tracking saboteurs, guarding vital installations, to undertake explosive and mine detection, augmenting infantry patrol, saving valuable lives in avalanche disasters and other natural calamities. The K9 heroes have rendered yeoman service and proved their worth as force multipliers and a valuable factor. In recognition of exemplary performance, the army dogs and their handlers have been bestowed with honours and awards which speak volumes about the quality of services being rendered by them. Specially trained dogs have also been successfully utilized in high-risk personnel security missions, narcotic detection missions and on international borders to assist in law and order operations. The canine can easily detect what his handler cannot see, hear or smell. The controllable aggressive behaviour of these dogs, coupled with the physical and psychological effects they create, makes him and his handler an impressive and unmatchable team. There has been a great need of a book on the heroism of military dogs, so as to generate more awareness about the invaluable services rendered by the silent warriors during peace and war. The learned author, having vast experience, has made an excellent effort to highlight various facets of 'military working dogs'. Further, the available textual evidences have been researched, collated appropriately signifying the acts of bravery shown by these dogs and their handlers over a period of time with an outstanding coverage of the employment of dogs in the military around the world. This book will be a point of reference when seeking precedent or researching new ideas. To make the book more informative and an interesting reading, the learned author has included a chapter "Dogs in Mythology, Art and Culture".

I congratulate the author for bringing out such an excellent book which, I feel, is a valuable outcome of his sustained endeavour.

Lt Gen **Jagvinder Singh**

Director General, RVS
Army Headquarters

to

the cherished memory of
my respected parents

Late Shri Dhan Singh
and
Late Smt Chandan Kaur

as they continue to
bless me from heaven

Preface

A very common and apt adage says it all ..."A dog is a man's best friend". Through the ages, dogs have served as faithful companions to humans irrespective of being rich or poor. The natural gifts of smell, ferocity, speed coupled with dog's sixth sense, and a desire to please his master have been extensively used by man to fit into his designs. The concept of war dogs is as old as war itself. Primitive man used dog to guard his family, his belongings and himself. He took his dog into battle with him when rival tribes clashed. As such, "when we go to war, they go to war" and the hair raising tales of dogs in various wars speak volumes on their bravery, devotion and faithfulness even endangering their own lives. During Napoleonic War in 1805, Moustache, a black poodle of French Grenadiers Regiment, became a legend at the Battle of Austerlitz (a village in the then Austrian Empire, modern-day Slavkov U Brna in the Czeck Republic), when he saw a young ensign bearing the regimental colours, mortally wounded and surrounded by the enemy, attempted to save his regimental flag by wrapping round his body in his dying effort. Moustache understood what for the soldier gave his life, he successfully unfolded the strand with his teeth and paws and carried the flag in his mouth to lines. Moustache was awarded a medal of gallantry and his name was placed on the regimental books as a full-fledged soldier drawing rations and pay. This dog was entitled to wear a tri-coloured collar with a silver medal, engraved on one side "Moustache, a French dog, a brave fighter entitled to respect".

During World War I, Stubby, a bull terrier, mascot of 102nd Infantry, part of the US Army's 26th "Yankee Division", became a legend for his heroism of highest calibre by giving advance alerts of gas attacks during the battle of Chemin des Dames, France, fought between American Expeditionary Forces and German Army in May, 1918. He was awarded a gold medal and honourary rank of Sergeant by General John J Pershing, Commander of American Forces in Europe. During World War II, Chips, a Sentry dog of 3rd American Division, attacked an enemy machine gun nest in a combat situation in Sicily in July, 1943, ousted four Italian soldiers out of pillbox and did not allow them to move till their capture by his unit. He was honoured and a feature film made on his heroism.

A study revealed that during the Korean War, wherever military working dogs were deployed, troop's casualty was significantly reduced and 26th Infantry Dog Platoon received a citation for its outstanding service. Similarly, in Vietnam War, over 9000 handlers and 4000 military working dogs were employed that reportedly saved 10,000 lives. During this war, 500 dogs and 294 handlers were killed and Staff Sergeant Robert W Hartsock, a dog handler, was conferred the prestigious "Congressional Medal of Honour" posthumously for exemplary heroism and bravery. The performance of Indian Army dog Alex in tracking down the culprits successfully on a two-day-old scent, who attempted to assassinate the King of Bhutan in July, 1965, became a legend and the heroic deed of Army Dog Sundri led to award of coveted gallantry medal "Shaurya Chakra" to her handler ALD/ADT Gurbachan Singh. Similarly, the performance of Army dog Ashok at Zozila pass in

November, 1986, became the talk of glory when a huge avalanche rolled down the pass and many buried in deep snow could be saved due to his bravery and professional competence. The story goes on unabated in more recent Gulf War and Afghanistan War.

While serving in Army, I was responsible for organizing the canine resources in consonance with the requirement of strategic and tactical employment of Army dogs to meet the military objectives. My interaction with people at large in various sphere of society gave me feeling that they are generally aware about the pet dogs but do not know much about the war dogs, working as 'silent K9 warriors'. Hence, my humble effort to disseminate knowledge in this regard has culminated in publication of this book. I have focused on the ever-changing scenario of battlefields, counter-insurgency and anti-terrorism operations necessitating enhanced role of war dogs. Readers would also interestingly know more about various breeds, dog's character and personality, canine olfaction and sixth sense, management practices and an insight into the basic and specialized training of K9 heroes. "New Horizons", as discussed in Chapter 13, depicts the vast potential of military working dogs as a force multiplier and anti-terrorism asset to meet the end state objectives. Mesmerising telltales of "Dogs in Mythology, Art and Culture" narrated in Chapter 22, focus on the social traditions, taboos, ethnic and cultural ties, to make readers aware about less known aspect of man's best friend. The hallmark Chapter 21, "War Dog Memorials", would make the readers consciously realize that man also owes respect and remembrance to his faithful companion and best friend.

It has been my sincere endeavour to highlight the gallant acts of war dogs and their handlers, "made for each other duo," along with other related aspects that would enrich not only the military personnel but all canine lovers and people at large. In this book the readers will be able to visualize and appreciate the difficult tasks, inhospitable terrain, uncongenial environment coupled with constant threat to life of the dog and handler team under which they operate without caring for adversities, yet perform the challenging tasks to the highest degree of perfection that make the 'silent K9 warriors' indispensible.

Maj General
BS Panwar AVSM, SM, PHD (RETD)

Acknowledgements

I wish to convey my gratitude to Lt General VG Patankar (Retd), PVSM, UYSM, VSM, former Quarter Master General, Indian Army, and the then Colonel Commandant, Remount Veterinary Corps, for motivating me to write a book on military working dogs. Soon after my retirement on 1st October, 2005, I did remember his learned advice and decided to undertake this herculean task, duly inspired with the vision of General Patankar for which I shall always remain grateful to him. I sincerely thank Lt General Jagvinder Singh, Director General Remount Veterinary Services, for his kind cooperation, valuable suggestions and writing the Foreword to my book. I also thank him for all the kind gestures and positivity whenever I approached him for consultation or assistance during his tenure as Commandant, RVC Centre and College. I wish to convey my heartfelt thanks to Colonel Raj Pal (Retd) and his son Saurabh, for the generous support and appropriate advice regarding the contents and layout of text. My thanks are due to Colonel JS Maan and Lt Colonel Sukhbir Singh, for being very positive and helpful whenever consulted. I also take this opportunity to convey my thanks to Brigadier Deepak Badial (Retd), Brigadier Raja Ram Yadav (Retd) and Brigadier PR Venkatesh, for their help and encouraging conversation whenever I met them at various social platforms and interacted about my dream project.

I would like to thank my daughter Ms Monika Varma for her valuable suggestions, constant encouragement and editorial assistance with lots of love and blessings. A special thank goes to my beloved wife Reeta for her sustained inspiration, unstinted support and unsolicited tolerance towards my obsession in writing this book.

While compiling this book, I have consulted various texts/reference books, journals and other published/unpublished literature, released text material and released photographs on web world pertaining to the subject matter and the same wherever quoted/reproduced is hereby acknowledged gratefully. Finally, I would like to acknowledge all the assistance from various sources I have had while compiling this book and all textual references as mentioned in the bibliography or elsewhere in the text are duly acknowledged.

Maj General

BS Panwar AVSM, SM, PHD (RETD)

Contents

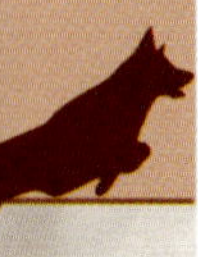

Part 2

Part 1

1. Introduction
2. Evolution of War Dog
3. History of War Dogs
4. War Dogs in the Napoleonic and Pre-World War Era
5. War Dogs of World War I
6. War Dogs in Sino-Japanese War
7. War Dogs of World War II
8. War Dogs in Korean and Vietnam Wars
9. War Dogs in Recent Wars and Conflicts
10. Indian Army Dogs
11. Dogs in Disaster Management
12. Dogs in the UN Peacekeeping Missions
13. New Horizons
14. Breeds of Modern War Dogs
15. Canine Olfaction, Character and Personality
16. Specialities and Training of Working Dogs

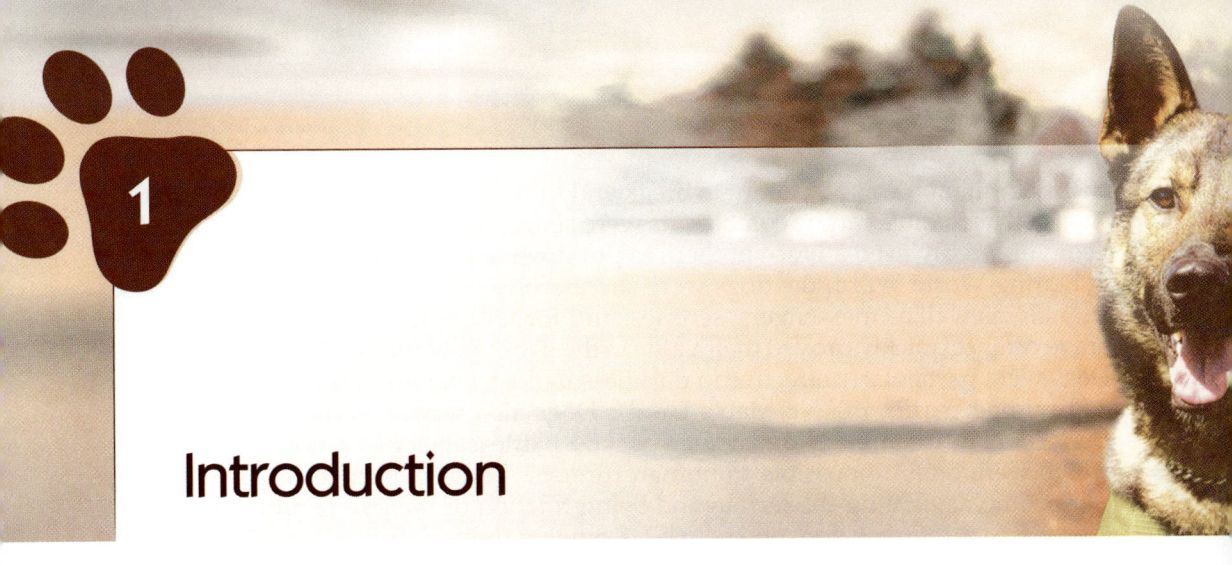

1 Introduction

"All knowledge, the totality of all questions and answers, is contained in the dog."

... Franz Kafka—Investigations of the dog

The importance of war dogs in war and peace has been recognized time and again. The heroic deeds of these true friends of mankind have made themselves very important asset of the soldiers. Right from the domestication and use of dogs as human companions, the concept of war dogs kept on evolving simultaneously. It was realized that dogs have high potential of boosting the war efforts and the same has been successfully utilized by the various armies around the world. The highly intelligent dogs and their motivated handlers are very agile and can effectively be employed expertly at short notice in all types of terrain and geographical conditions. They are of immense value in support operations and act as combat multiplier in battle field. Their versatility allows for effective transformation at all echelons from readiness for deployment to operations on the ground in the battlefield.

Archeologists believe that humans have been using dogs in warfare since the animals were first domesticated more than 27,000 years ago. The first textual evidence of the use of war dogs in battle, is around 600 BC when, the first ruler, Alyattes, of the ancient Kingdom of Lydia (modern day Turkey) reportedly made his soldiers let loose packs of dogs on Cimmerian troops (ancient Indo-European people). The Lydian attack dogs proved particularly effective against enemy cavalry. Around the same time, Magnesian, a Greek toponym, derived from the tribal name *magnetes*, from Anatolia used their war dogs in conjunction with their mounted warriors against their enemy. Magnesian riders released their hounds on the enemy phalanxes to soften them up before the cavalry charge in a war against the Ephesians. Subsequently, the Roman routinely deployed their war dogs in various battles and for this purpose, the *Canis Molossus* or Molossian breed was specially bred just for combat as it was the legion's preferred breed of fighting dog. Spanish conquistadores in the New World made brutally effective use of fighting dogs in the late Middle Ages against Native Americans. They used mixed breed of Deer Hound and Mastiff and festooned them with padded armour and spiked collars. The Aboriginal Native American warriors were terrified of these enormous fighting animals. Furthermore, in order to precipitate a total route, the Spaniards used to release the beasts once an

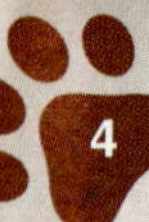

enemy formation was just about to break and these dogs were known to devour the enemy. The Spain's canine combatants were so fearful that the conqueror Ponce De Leon reportedly used a brace of them to put down a slave rebellion in Puerto Rico.

During World War I, the dogs were successfully used on the battlefield as pack animals, as well as messengers, sentries, and for killing rats in the trenches. These brave canines quickly proved their value in the trenches of the Western Front. Trench Dogs were particularly effective in darkness to detect enemy reconnaissance teams and raiding parties in "No Man's Land". Dogs also served as messengers on the front lines in the muddy and crater pocked battlescapes of France and Flanders which were often impossible to human runners. These messenger dogs had a far easier time navigating the terrain and being fraction of the size of a human being, they were hard targets for snipers to hit. Knowing their usefulness, the British army established a dog training centre in Scotland to prepare large number of messenger carriers for the trenches. It is also believed that Germany reportedly used more than 30,000 war dogs during this war whereas the French sent 20,000 to the front line in battlefield.

World War II, witnessed the biggest surge in use of working dogs to support military operations and their heroism contributed significantly to the war efforts. These silent warriors were used not only in new innovative ways but also sometimes in cruel ways. Soon after entering the great war, USA, Britain and other allies gave a call to their respective citizens to volunteer their pets to help defeat the Axis and a large number of dogs were inducted into the service. The US military alone, deployed more than 10,000 specially trained canines as sentries, scouts, messengers, mine detectors, search and rescue dogs, etc. All other allies also deployed a large number of dogs in their war against the Axis. In the Soviet Union, during the initial weeks of the Nazi invasion, Russian troops used dogs to destroy enemy tanks. Dog handlers with the Red Army spent weeks conditioning their animals to dart under German Panzers when released onto the battlefield. The dogs would carry mines that would be magnetically detonated when the charges came in contact with the steel hulls. The explosion would knock out the tank but also kill the dog in the process. Indeed, it was cruel. These dogs although trained to run beneath the tanks, yet many times they simply leaped into friendly trenches amid the noise of battle, thereby killing Soviet troops instead of the enemy.

During Malayan Emergency from 1948 to 1960, British Army developed the concept of Tracker and Patrol Dogs in the jungles of Malaysia, as such, they may be credited as the initiators of the modern war dog. Similarly, in Northern Ireland, from August, 1969 to July, 2007, they demonstrated the concept of Search and Tracker Dogs for the detection of explosive and firearms during "Operation Banner". These training methodologies were subsequently finetuned with appropriate modifications in other countries.

Between the years 1964 and 1973, America had deployed an estimated 4,000 war dogs and 10,000 handlers to help defend South Vietnam from invasion by North Vietnam. During the ground war, Veterinarians and Veterinary Technicians were also deployed throughout South Vietnam to help manage the diets and medical health of the war dogs. The success of the war dogs and handlers walking point, tracking, guarding, patrolling, and protecting American lives and military assets, ultimately reduced the enemy's capacity for surprise attacks. As a result, the enemy placed a price tag on the heads of the war dog teams and hunted them with extreme prejudice. In 1973, when the United States and its allies ceased combat operations and withdrew the last of its ground combat forces from South Vietnam, several thousand surviving war dogs were created surplus because their masters were ordered out of South Vietnam. In 1975, South Vietnam fell to North Vietnam and the war officially ended. The war dogs were classified as equipment and several thousand Military Working Dogs (MWDs) were left behind after the war which was the the "saddest chapter" in MWDs history. Their final fate was either to be transferred to the South Vietnam Army or to be euthanized after each war dog unit was methodically and strategically deactivated throughout South Vietnam. Sadly, thousands of Military Working Dogs were left on the shores of enemies to unknown fate as troops sailed home after the conflicts. Later on, the herculean efforts of WW II Marine War Dog Platoon Leader and Veterinarian, Dr William Putney and the help of the US Congressman Roscoe Bartlett of Maryland, changed the tide in favour of war dog adoption law in the year 2000. This issue has also highlightened the fact that present generation may not accept any such policy in which a Military Dog serving in combat overseas will be left behind or destroyed due to quarantine restrictions preventing its return. It is strongly felt that we should take care of the brave MWDs who make it home, ensure they can enjoy their retirement and we also remember those dogs that lost their lives keeping other soldiers safe. These dogs are very special for those men and women who have been fighting for their country and have seen these animals giving their life for their comrades. They are very special and should be treated accordingly

In 2012, the Senate passed landmark piece of legislation in the USA, called the "Canine members of the Armed Forces Act". The Act, which was also called Senate Bill 2134 and House Bill 4103, was important to Military Working Dog (MWD) rights for three reasons:

- The act would require retired MWDs to be transported to the 341 Training Squadron at the Lackland Air Force Base in San Antonio, Texas, or another suitable location where the dogs can be placed up for adoption.
- The act would require the establishment of a system for the veterinary care of retired Military Working Dogs.
- The act would name MWDs official members of the US Armed Forces, allowing dogs those perform great acts of courage or merit during deployments to be recognized and decorated for their service.

In this context, the US House of Representatives passed House Bill 4103 in the spring of 2012 and the Senate following suit, approved the bill. However, as the canine members of the Armed Forces Act became attached to the larger National Defence Authorisation Act of 2013, a key part of the legislation was noticeably omitted. While retired MWDs are now guaranteed transportation and veterinary medical care so they can have the chance of a good home after returning to the US from their deployments, the last part of the act which would require MWDs to be classified as service members and decorated in a way that reflects their service and sacrifice was left out. So while MWDs often go through rigorous training, detect deadly explosives, parachute into enemy territory, guard against attacks, dodge bullets and risk their lives right alongside their human handlers, these dogs are not given the same recognition as other soldiers, simply because they walk on four legs instead of two.

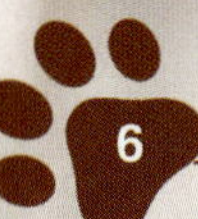

The vast majority of Military Working Dogs, around the world are German Shepherd, Belgian Malinois and Labrador breeds since these are aggressive, smart, loyal and athletic. We want a high-strung dog with aggressive tendencies because that's what the mission demands. It is interesting to note that before 11th September, 2001, the USA trained about 200 working dogs a year for the Defence Department. Now that the number has gone up to more than 500, with the vast majority of dogs being trained as sentries and bomb-sniffers. Presently, more than 2,700 such dogs are protecting the US Army's interest around the world. The increased reliance on these aptly recognized "force multipliers" for safeguarding military bases, tracking infiltrators and antinational elements, search and rescue work, detection of bombs and explosives, disaster management-related relief work, sanitization of specific areas and assisting infantry patrols in counter insurgency as well as antiterrorist operations, etc. have made war dogs, the essential component of force deployment in various theatres of conflict. With an acute sense of smell five to ten times stronger than a human's, dogs are able to detect minute traces of explosives or drugs and alert their handlers of their presence. They also have the ability to inflict fear in an aggressor in a unique way that a human cannot affect.

The canine warriors are continuously serving in their transforming role as per the likes of their masters and mission demands. Similarly, dog training and employment techniques are being refined to have a highly sophisticated and versatile dog as the extension of human's own senses. It has been proved time and again that even the most complex machines are unable to duplicate the operational effectiveness of a properly trained dog and its handler. A study has brought out that during Korean War, the total number of casualties were reduced by more than 65%, wherever Military Working Dogs worked on the front line. During Vietnam War, approximately thousands of Sentry and Scout dogs were used by American troops to safeguard critical installations such as ports and airfields. At the end of the war, it was realized that more than ten thousand lives and immense property were saved as a result of the services rendered by these dogs. A new dimension in utilization of dogs also came in sight when dog teams were trained as Marijuana Detector to assist military police in suppressing illicit drug traffic, which proved to be a great success. Subsequent efforts in this direction made it possible to train an intelligent and strong dog to detect specific drugs and explosives. The optimal utilization of war dogs to work as extension of soldier's sense, force multipliers and anti-terrorist asset has paid rich dividends in various conflicts and wars ranging from Afghanistan to Africa and Balkans to Iraq. Throughout the course of the long war in Afghanistan, the US Army and Coalition troops have relied on thousands of Military Working Dogs to help keep them safe, and make their jobs easier. The dogs are trained to detect explosives, to find illegal drugs, to search for missing comrades and to target enemy combatants. They are not only active on the front lines, but also behind the lines to serve as therapy dogs, service dogs, and loyal companions.

Italy deployed its Carabineer units on peacekeeping missions, including Kosovo, Afghanistan and Iraq and many Italian dogs have seen operational action in such places. The Army Group Cinofilo (Dog Battalion) was established on July 1, 2002 in Grosseto. The battalion is unique, with its own command and organized specifically to ensure both the breeding of dogs and the training of combinations in different specializations. The group is responsible for both the training and operational employment of Military Dogs. Its core task is developing dogs for use with Italian forces abroad, but they may be employed in Italian territory for strategic objectives such as searching for weapons, ammunition and explosives. In 2003, twelve Carabineer were killed in a suicide bombing on their base in Nasiriyah, near Basra, southern Iraq, constituting the largest Italian military loss of life in a single action since World War II. Many dogs received awards for their bravery and lifesaving skills.

In South America, military and paramilitary forces use dogs in the fight against major crime as well as in the role of traditional Military Working Dog (MWD). Patrol Dogs are used to track down guerrilla insurgents such as the Colombian FARC group (Fight against Revolutionary Armed Forces of Colombia), who at one point controlled up to 40 per cent of Colombia.

The Canine Training Centre Military (CICAM for its Spanish acronym) has trained canines in various disciplines such as narcotics detection, explosive detection, foreign currency detection, search and rescue and perimeter patrol dogs for the army, air force and navy, as well as for the administrative security department, the technical research unit, the national penitentiary institute and the special administrative unit of civil aeronautics. MWDs trained in multiple techniques to counter the actions of terrorists have had excellent results. Dogs have successfully detected landmines, explosive devices, captured terrorists and helped in the confiscation of many shipments of drugs. The CICAM is now developing an ambitious project for advanced MWD training to enable a dog to alert on the presence of a narco-terrorist sniper or a remote device operator at a great distance.

In Israel, independent canine Special Forces (*sayeret*) unit (OKETZ) was founded in 1939 as part of the Haganah and used for perimeter security of villages under threat from their Arab neighbours. In 1948, following the establishment of the state, the unit joined the Israel Defence Forces (IDF) and set up its base in Kiryat Haim. In 1954, the unit was disbanded. In 1974, Yossi Labock, who was its first commander raised a new unit. The unit specializes in training and handling dogs for military applications. Originally, OKETZ trained dogs to attack kidnappers, however, dogs are now trained for various specialized tasks. OKETZ are often assigned to other units in the case of a particular need for their specialist skills. Soldiers of this unit are required to pass gruelling stamina tests followed by full combat basic training, just like their infantry counterparts. The unit specializes in training and handling dogs for military applications. Each dog is trained for a particular specialty such as, Attack Dogs, Tracker, Search and Rescue and Explosive Detection. Attack Dogs were used extensively in Lebanon as they are trained to operate in urban areas, as well as in rural and bush land. Trackers are utilized for manhunts and detecting breaches at the borders, search for guns and ammunitions. Explosive Detection Dogs sniff out hidden explosives and Search and Rescue Dogs to find people in collapsed buildings, etc. OKETZ units prefer Malinois over German Shepherds and Rottweilers which were formerly employed because they are of the perfect size to be picked up by their handler while still being able to attack an enemy. Their coats are short and generally fair in colour making them less prone to heatstroke. OKETZ is one of the highly regarded units and few infantry commanders would not even think about embarking on a mission without their support. The unit's slogan "At the front," perfectly describes the role handlers and their dogs play during a mission. In 1988, the unit participated in IDF operations in southern Lebanon launched to destroy the cave-based headquarters of the Organization Popular Front for the Liberation of Palestine in a mountainous area 20 kilometres south of Beirut. Golani Brigade Soldiers, Naval Commandos and a number of OKETZ Dogs participated in the "Operation, Blue and Brown". The operation's multi-goal was first, to kill Ahmed Jibril, the head terrorist leader of the PFLP-GC (Popular Front for the Liberation of Palestine-General Command), and secondly to force out his headquarters deep inside Lebanon. Most of the PFLP-GC headquarters were located in caves situated on high buffs off the Lebanon's coast. IDF staff decided that it would be impossible to take them out by air assault; hence ground assault was the only way. Several units were involved in the raids: Shayetet 13 (Navy Commandos), Sayeret Golany (Special Forces) and Palga Terror's Dogs, from Unit 7142. The plan called for Flotilla 13 to clear the beach, and for the Sayerets to get the Palga Terror Unit close enough to the targets, so that they could release their dogs which were carrying packs containing C4 remote control explosives. The dogs were to enter the caves and explode killing all the terrorists inside, but like everything else, in Blue and Brown Operation, the dogs did not do exactly what they were supposed to. Some didn't go where they were directed whereas in some the explosives went off prematurely and some didn't explode at all. The terrorists killed four OKETZ of the Rottweilers, immediately. During the second Lebanon War, OKETZ accompanied Golani and Paratrooper units inside southern Lebanon for searching Hizbullah underground bunker systems, locating weaponry and terrorists. Since 2002, soldiers and dogs from OKETZ have been able to prevent at least 200 suicide attacks in the central region. In 2006, alone OKETZ participated in more than 4,000 Operations and saved many lives. Soldiers grow up with their dogs, and undergo eighteen months of training together, before being deployed in the field. After six years of service, the dogs are retired and placed in the hands of former members of the unit, who are queuing up to take care of them.

In Brazil, the Army began to officially use MWDs in the 1960s. Military Working Dogs are used at security points and sensitive areas, on vital escort tasks, guarding of prisoners and searching for drugs and explosives. The units dealing with dogs are called Seccoes de Caes-de-Guerra. The Military Police (MP) is also a preventive state police force responsible for maintaining public order within the states and the federal districts and is subordinate to the state government in this regard whereas the investigation of crime is handled by the civil police forces of the various states. Brazilian MP uses various breeds of dogs including German Shepherds, Malinois, Rottweilers, Labradors and Blood Hounds and is responsible for the breeding and selection of dogs within the Brazilian Military. The Reproduction Centre for Dogs-Of-War is located in Brasília.

In South Africa, Military Working Dogs are used by the South West African Specialist Unit (SWASPES). The Koevoet Dog Section within this unit, based at Otavi, has been an elite Counter Insurgency Team (COIN) deployed to combat the terrorist threat from 1979 to 1989. In addition, dog squads exist in specialist infantry units also. However, most of the other African Nations do not use MWDs in great numbers. This may be partially due to their general distrust of dogs, religious beliefs or cultural attitudes. Erstwhile Colonial powers comprised Europeans, British, French, German and Belgian, used MWDs for sentry and guard work from the time of their settlement in that continent. They proved a useful force multiplier in those days as many Natives were afraid of these dogs, which were trained to bark and bite the locals. Presently, MWDs are also employed by the United Nations' forces and operating throughout the continent. The French use them in base security roles in their African Protectorates. In Somalia in 1993, MWDs were used by the several UN Forces in the Explosive Detection Dog (EDD) role.

In China, the concept of working dogs dates way back to the times when they were used to crawl into tunnels under the palace for sentry duty and one bark from the dog meant an intruder was approaching. Smaller breeds were used for security and hunting small game. The large war dogs were popular in China, in medieval times but these breeds died out over a period. The Kunming Dog of China, which resembles to an extent with German Shepherd, was created in the 1950s when the Military Dog Training Centre was founded. This centre was shut down in the 1960s, during the Cultural Revolution, and was not reopened until the early 1990s. Before that, some military units had been breeding and training large dogs for security and other military tasks.

Presently, China employs tactical dogs in their army and also in police forces all over the country. These dogs are trained for various roles such as patrolling, scouting, sentry, drug and explosives detection and peacekeeping duties like tracking criminals, etc. The Military Dog Training Centre is located in Beijing and it also acts as a breeding facility for future military canines. Besides using the standard working breeds like the German Shepherd and Belgian Shepherd, Kunming Dog is quickly becoming popular in the dog enthusiast community. Although Chinese are known for eating dog meat, yet the handlers are very attached to their canine partners and the dogs are treated well. Over the last decade, China has increased its force of Military Working Dogs considerably and now has about 10,000 large dogs being used for security, rescue, and detection of explosives and drugs. Paramilitary police units and disaster relief organizations that specialize in rescue operations also use many of these dogs.

In Sri Lanka, Army has been widely using dogs for detection of mines and other explosives in the north and east and optimally utilized their keen senses of smelling in the Eelam War. The Sri Lankan Army employs 75 dogs, for detecting mines, explosives and warning soldiers against ambush. One of its much-loved brave Tracker Dog, Snowy, a golden Labrador of 4 Commando Regiment, was severely injured in grenade attack during a search operation in Kambilioya, Welioya on 15th March, 2008. The brave dog subsequently died and was fondly remembered on 24 May, 2011. A memoir was published under the heading "Much-Loved Snowy, after tireless tasks in humanitarian operations bids farewell to Army". Snowy was honoured with a 'Rana Wickrema Padakkama' (Heroic deeds) medal recognizing his daunting services on the battlefront. The Regimental Headquarters of Commando Regiment at Ganemulla, condoled his death and conducted a befitting funeral and wished him to attain Nirvana.

In India, Army dogs have been used successfully during war and peace. These brave canines along with their handlers proved their mettle in war, low intensity conflicts, counter insurgency operations and natural calamities like earthquakes, avalanches, cloud bursts, tsunami, etc. These dogs are more than companions of soldiers and help in efficient functioning of field forces in various security related tasks with phenomenal capabilities and unprecedented excellence. The performance of these courageous and reliable auxiliaries in various specialized fields as tracking saboteurs, guarding vital installations, explosive and mine detection, narcotic detection, augmenting infantry patrols and saving the precious lives in avalanche disasters, earthquakes and other natural calamities, has been exemplary. The yeoman service as a valuable factor to the forces engaged in fighting enemy threats, militancy and terrorism has won not only the heart of the soldiers but also the prestigious Army medals for Gallantry and Distinguished Services which speaks volumes about their heroism. As technology and conflict situations are continuously changing, the war dog teams also continue the transformation process and give the full-spectrum capabilities needed to be force multipliers on the battlefield as well as persuasive force protection and antiterrorism assets. The contribution of these dogs in counter insurgency and anti-terrorism is highly significant leading to many-fold success in Army's efforts to contain the militancy and terrorism in areas of responsibility. The dogs have proved lifesavers for the troops in many instances, as the reconnaissance patrols led by the dog team forewarn about the buried explosives, mines and hidden militants in vulnerable area before harm is caused to the troops, as a result, units deployed in such areas utilize the services of army dogs optimally. Further, India has the unblemished record of utilizing dogs for guarding Prisoners of War (POW) camp having more than 90,000 prisoners after Indo-Pak war from 3–16 December, 1971. The dogs proved their mettle as force multipliers while guarding the POW.

Man's best friend has always been steady and true by soldiers' sides for ages. Dogs are not dependent on a power source, they do not rust up when operating in jungle conditions, nor do they seize up in a sandstorm and when all these attributes are put in one package, the value of war dog becomes self-explanatory. Even in today's 21st century Army, where some soldiers are now trained to hit their target from the opposite hemisphere with unmanned aircraft, there's still a place for this fundamental relationship between canines and their handlers in military occupational specialty. As working dogs become increasingly important to the military missions, they also need to be protected from enemy threats.

It has been proven that dogs can help service personnel cope with the stresses of being in a combat zone. Therapy dogs were deployed with 528th Medical in Northern Iraq, for the purpose of distressing soldiers. These dogs meet soldiers for a good old game of ball and provide affection and comfort to them with the hope that it will reduce their adverse reactions to stress. Research indicates that interaction with therapy dogs can temporarily affect the release of various neurotransmitters in the brain; levels of oxytocin (linked with bonding) and dopamine (involved in the reward-motivation system) are increased, while cortisol levels (an immunosuppressant associated with stress) are decreased thereby reducing the stress level.

Dogs also share the same risks as the ground troops, suffering injuries and also death on the battlefields. While the Military Working Dogs and their handlers work day and night to support troops in battlefield, Army Veterinarians posted around the world ensure their good health and fitness for duty. Telemedicine, so popular in the civilian health realm, is being used to provide expert consultation for Military Working Dogs as the emphasis is to ensure that dogs continue to stay in the field and be treated in the theatre.

There has been a great need of a book on the heroism of war dogs having useful information on unique canine traits, breed characteristics, specialized training and management practices, etc. for the awareness of one and all. Collating and documenting the various distinguished acts of war dogs will generate more knowhow at all levels about the varied spectrum of invaluable services being rendered by these valuable assets. In this book, I have focused on the role of "The

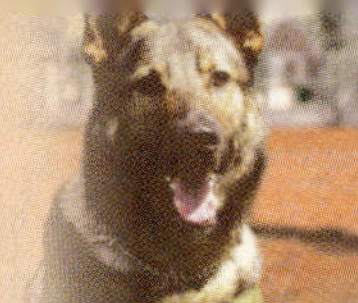

Silent K9 Warriors" in the Armed Forces of countries predominantly involved in counter insurgency operations and fighting terrorism either on their soil or on foreign soil. I sincerely tried to keep the book as comprehensive as possible yet some specifics, techniques and names might have been deliberately omitted due to security concerns.

There is a saying that "History is the Past" and so is applicable to the statistics given in this book which may also become yesterday's news since at the time of publication of this book, new events might have occurred.

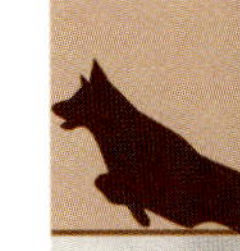

2

Evolution of War Dog

"He is your friend, your partner, your defender, your dog. You are his life, his love, his leader. He will be yours, faithful and true, to the last beat of his heart. You owe it to him to be worthy of such devotion."

... Unknown

Origin of life is considered to be 15 billion years ago and the dog is presumed to have entered ecological system of men's universal companions of Mesolithic hunters and gatherers at the end of Paleolithic and beginning of Neolithic age (10,000 BC to 1710 BC). Hence, the domestication of the dog occurred tens of millennia ago. Naturalists began debating the origins of the domestic dog, *Canis familiaris* and after centuries of study, modern scientists have declared the domestic dog's genomic ancestor to be the wolf, *Canis lupus*, not the fox or jackal, though these animals are fellow members of the *Canidae* family. There is less scientific consensus as to how this animal, once feral, became "man's best friend," though a few theories predominate. Juliet Clutton-Brock explains the process of domestication in her contribution to *The Domestic Dog*. Archaeological research of Middle Pleistocene (ca. 781,000 to 126,000 years ago) communities has uncovered the bones of early hominids and wolves in close proximity. Once rivals competing over the same food source, this evidence of shared space indicates that wolves and early hominids began to cooperate as a practical survival mechanism. Wolves may have wandered into hominid camps searching for scraps of meat and lingered out of convenience. Hominid hunters may have killed wolves for food and captured wolf pups, more docile than the adults, to eat later when they were fully grown with more meat on their bones. Some of these pups seem to have escaped this fate, perhaps due to a fondness that developed out of extended physical closeness, becoming companions and hunting partners rather than a meal for their captors. Whether the former or latter or both theories are true, the cooperation between hominids and wolf led to the development of a tamed wolf, which would eventually evolve into the domestic dog. The evolutionary change is evident in canid bones that date to the end of the last Ice Age (ca. 14,000 to 10,000 years ago). The discovery of multiple human-canid burial sites from this period in Jordan, Palestine, and Iraq, in which the canid bones are measurably distinct from early wolf bones confirms the completion of domestication. The fact that owner and animal shared a single grave signals the social significance and not just the practicality of keeping dogs as companions in the community. Domestication is not simply a biological process but a cultural one as well. The wolf became a dog by isolation from its wild ancestors and immersion in human hunter–gatherer societies, adapting traits suitable to life among humans rather than wild animals. The dog proved a useful companion among hunter–gatherers, since it could search out, track down, and occasionally capture the prey. Humans eventually abandoned this nomadic hunting lifestyle and settled into stationary communities based on farming and agriculture and the help of dogs was no longer required to kill animals for food, instead, they protected them. Shepherd dogs, animals that have evolved to be so tame that they have lost the urge to hunt, guard sheep from predators such as coyotes and wolves, the dog's direct genomic predecessor. In agricultural societies, particular breeds such as Shepherd and herding dogs play the role of farmhand, saving their human companions' time and effort.

The Saluki also known as the Persian Grey Hound is one of the oldest known breeds of domesticated dog. There are petro glyphs and rock arts in Golpaygan and Khomein in central Iran that shows Saluki-like Hounds and falcons accompanying hunters chasing preys (ca. 8000–10,000 BCE). Also on the potteries found in Susa, Iran (ca. 4200 BCE) are images of Saluki-like Hounds chasing ibex or lying next to pools and from the period of the Middle Kingdom onwards, Saluki-like animals appear on the ancient Egyptian tombs of 2134 BCE. Modern science tells us the origins of all dogs is in the east in China, but we do not know where the origin of the Saluki is located. All along the Silk Road his presence was known for almost as long as the dog has been domesticated, a testimony to his function as a hunter and his beauty as a companion. His image is found in many cultures. Recent excavations of the Sumerian empire, estimated at 7000–6000 BC have Saluki-like finds. Saluki-like images have been found on the Egyptian tombs of 2100 BC. The nomadic tribes spread the breed across the Middle East from Persia and Egypt, to as far east as Afghanistan, India and as far south as Sudan. The Saluki is a Sight Hound and historically travelled throughout Iran and through Silk Road with caravans and nomadic tribes over an area stretching from the Sahara to the Caspian Sea and China. They have been used to hunt quarry such as gazelles, hares and ibex. They exist in two varieties, smooth and feathered and are an independent breed that needs patient training. Salukis are considered to be one of the oldest dog breeds in existence and the name Saluki has many theories. Linguistics agrees that the word Saluki in Arabic is an adjective referring to where an individual was from. Sir Terence Clark, a British retired diplomat and writer, reports on four possible locations for the place Saluq including today's Yemen, Iraq and Turkey. Also there are two more places with similar names in northwest Iran near the other four locations mentioned above. In Persian, the dog is referred to as Tazi, which means to run, and in Kurdish areas also word Tazi is used for dog. The breed is still held in high regard throughout the Middle East, and has been hunting dogs for nobles and rulers around the region.

Cultivators of Indus Valley were well-known for their Pariah Dogs. These dogs are naturally gifted with highly developed senses of smell, hearing, vision and also sixth sense, which helped dogs in hunting skill to kill their prey for their own survival prior to their domestication. These senses coupled with other identifiable traits in dogs such as speed, stamina, ferocity, faithfulness and willingness to do task to please their masters were subsequently exploited optimally by the man for his own benefit. Hence, primitive man first used dogs to guard his premise, family, and his belongings and subsequently he took the dogs into battlefield with him when rival tribe clashed. The changing role of dogs from hunter–gatherer to farmhand in agricultural societies clearly proves that the domestic dog adapts to fit the role demanded by humans.

The Indian Pariah Dog belongs to the aboriginal landrace, or naturally selected "breed" of the Indian subcontinent. It is also called the Indian Native Dog and is nowadays referred to as the INDog by experts and enthusiasts. The term "Pariah Dog" is not derogatory in the canine context and refers to a class of primitive dogs of a specific appearance known as the "long-term pariah morph".

The Indian Native Dog (INDog) is an ancient autochthonous (landrace) type of dog that is found all over India, Pakistan, Bangladesh and even beyond South Asia. It was featured on National Geographic Channel's film, 'Search for the First Dog' along with the other related ancient types such as the Canaan Dog of Israel and the Australian Dingo. This is the original breed of the country, found free-living as a commensal of man all over the Indian subcontinent. Where not mixed with the blood of European dogs or other breeds and types, it is similar in appearance all across the entire country. The type represents one of the few remaining examples of mankind's original domestic dog and its physical features are the same as those of the dogs whose fossil remains have been found in various parts of the world, from very early remains in Israel and China to later ones such as those found in the volcanic lava at Pompeii, near Naples in Italy. In India these were the hunting partners and companion animals of the Aboriginals. They are still found with the aboriginal communities who live in forested areas. Since these dogs have never been selectively bred, their appearance, physical features and mental characteristics come from the process of natural selection alone. The INDog has not been recognized by any kennel club although similar ancient or 'primitive' dogs have been recognized such as Azawakh and Basenji both of which are also Sight Hound and Pariah. However, INDog has been recognized by the Primitive and Aboriginal Dog Society (PADS), a worldwide grouping of enthusiasts based in the USA.

From 500 BC onwards, Afghans, Pathans, Mongols, Persians, and the Arabs came to India through the Khyber Pass and they brought with them their companion dogs of many breeds like the Saluki, Sloughi and Grey Hound. Dogs of these breeds were also exchanged as gifts between the Indian, Persian, and Turkish kingdoms during that period. Selectively these dogs were bred in India to hunt and to withstand the weather and other qualities. Over a period of time, these dogs took on the names of the areas in which they lived. The Caravan Hound, Mudhol Hound, Rampur Grey Hound, probably owe their ancestry to these dogs. Chatrapathi Shivaji's loyal dogs were entombed near his own tomb at Raigadh. The dogs depicted bear a close resemblance to the Mudhol Hound. There is also the story of the Hounds belonging to Shahuji Maharaj who fought and killed a tiger that attacked the king.

The Indian Mastiff, is also of ancient origin, and considered to be the direct offspring of the Alaunt and Hyrcania dogs of Ancient Persia, as well as the legendary Assyrian Molossus, brought in the Indian subcontinent by the Indo-Aryan invaders. There is evidence that India had such Mastiff type dogs long before the arrival of the British, and are mentioned in the literature of Alexander the Great and Aristotle. Through early contacts between the Persian and Assyrian empires, and the Indus Valley civilization, it is possible that the large Mastiff type dogs of India and those of the Persians/Assyrians, have influenced each other. Similarly, The Rampur Hound is a member of the big Sight Hound family and is often described as a smooth haired Sight Hound substantially built to cover great distances at high speed, and thus capable of great endurance. His Royal Highness Ahmed Ali Khan Bahadur of Rampur, India, bred these dogs by combining the blood lines of very powerful but ferocious Tazi, brought in by the Afghans, and the English Grey Hound that was more obedient but less resistant to the varying climatic conditions. He gave the name 'Rampur Hound' to the dogs he bred. The Rampur Hound far exceeded his expectations as it got its looks and stalwart character from Tazi and Afghan ancestors and speed from the English Grey Hound. Here was a dog that would seldom back down in confrontations, and could more or less keep up with the fastest prey. It was the favoured Hound of the Maharajahs for jackal control, and was also used to hunt lions, tigers, leopards, and panthers. It was considered a test of courage for a single hound to take down a golden jackal. Another breed of Indian Hound Rajapalayam, as Sight Hound, was the companion of the royalty and aristocracy in Southern India, particularly in the town Rajapalayam, from where it gets its name. Rajapalayam Hounds were primarily bred and used by Nayak dynasty of Tamil Nadu (1529 AD until 1736 AD). It is speculated by some researchers that the Rajapalayam may have been one of the dogs used in the breeding of the modern Dalmatian. It is believed that the Rajapalayam dogs were used during the Carnatic Wars (1744–1763) and in Polygar War (1799–1805) against the British cavalry as they are fast, strong and aggressive in attacking the opponents. There is also folktale that four Rajapalayam dogs once saved the life of their master fighting against a tiger and killing it bravely near forest in Virudhunagar district of Tamil Nadu, India. This breed looks like a miniature Great Dane, with its powerful, muscular, and heavy build and often used for hunting wild boars and hares.

Throughout the histories of warfare from the days of the Egyptians, the Greeks, the Persian and the conquests of the Roman Empire most of the world's armies have used dogs as mascots and also to boost the war efforts. The war dogs have participated in active service at the sides of their masters and played the role of heroes, by showing bravery under fire, saving lives even by sacrificing their own and bringing comfort to the injured and infirm. Textual evidence indicates valuable contribution of dogs in ancient warfare; for example, Alexander and his soldiers stared in wonder at fearful combats of beasts during the Indian campaign in 326 BC and told strange stories of dogs that were not afraid to fight with lions. The Teutones warriors with armed women and wolf-like dogs defended their camp against Marius' legionaries at Vercellae in 102 BC. During the Hyrcanian revolt against the Parthians in 59 AD, Hyrcanian, Caspian and Tapurian warriors were accompanied with armored Hyrcanian war dogs. In AD 685, the defeated Saxons were tracked with the help of dogs after the battle of Dunnichen Moss.

One large, ancient breed influenced the use of war dogs throughout history and is commonly considered to be the ancestor of today's mastiff-type dogs, often referred to as Molossus Dogs or Molossers. These dogs were used for hunting in ancient Assyria, as well as for military purposes and protection. The ancient Mastiffs were later imported from Assyria, Egypt and Asia Minor by other countries. Xerxes I of Persia led predatory wars, taking large war dogs with him, to enlarge the borders of his empire. When Sir Peers Legh was wounded in the Battle of Agincourt in 1415, his Mastiff stood over and protected him for many hours. Large Mastiff breeds have been used by the military for thousands of years in combat and also to haul supplies.

Once the Mastiff reached the Roman Empire, it was bred to suit special purposes, which was the first step in the development of 'breeds' within a species. With the passage of time, the Romans developed one breed that closely resembles the Swiss Mountain Dog of today and also took their Mastiffs into Gaul, now known as France. The Roman army had whole companies composed entirely of dogs. They wore spiked collars around their neck and ankles, made more dangerous by the large curved knives protruding from the collars. Sometimes, they were starved before battle, and then unleashed on an unsuspecting enemy. The dogs guarded the mountain passes where a few hundred years later the St Bernard would be found. Today, St Bernards are used in Chile by the Mountain Regiment for both search and rescue and patrol work. These early Mastiffs also contributed to French breeds like the Dogue de Bordeaux and, in Italy, the Neapolitan Mastiff. In Spain, very near the homeland of the Great Pyrenees, the Spanish Mastiff was developed. To the north, in Belgium, the feared tracker, St Hubert's Hound, the ancestor of today's Blood Hound, was developed from the descendants of fierce hunting dogs. From the Alps, the Mastiff is thought to have been adopted by the Germanic peoples and then to have travelled to Great Britain with Angles and Saxons. The Great Dane is known as the Deutsche Dogge (or German Mastiff).

In 43 AD, the Roman conquest of Britain made Britannia a Roman province. At that time in Britain there were giant, wide-mouthed dogs, which the Romans called Pugnaces Britanniae, that surpassed their Molossus dogs. A Procurator Cynegii was stationed in Venta Belgarum (now Winchester) and made responsible for selecting these dogs, which were exported to Rome for contests in the amphitheatre and for use by the Roman army. The Pugnaces Britanniae were dogs well-respected by royalty and warriors. They were given as gifts to men of honour, and many warriors and chiefs took the name as a title to show their loyalty and courage. The Romans used them against many enemies, including Celtic tribes, Greeks and fellow Romans. Hounds were the traditional guardian animals of roads and crossways and are believed to protect and guide lost souls in the other world. The Irish Wolf Hound was used to hunt wolves and deer but it was also used as a war dog to attack men on horseback and knock them from their saddles.

During Middle Ages, in the early part of 14th century, dogs were used to guard convoys and caravans. Spanish conquistadors used trained Grey Hounds against Native Americans in their subjugation of New World in 16th century. The Army of Fredrick the Great used dogs as messengers during seven years war from 1756 to 1763 in Europe. During Napoleonic era 1799 to 1815, dogs were used as sentries at the gates of Alexandria in Egypt for early warning to troops against attack by the enemy forces. Dogs were used to guard naval installations in France till 1770. Americans used Cuban bred Blood Hounds during the Seminole War of 1835 and in 1842 dogs were used in Florida and Louisiana to trap Red Indians and runaway slaves in the swamps. Similarly, during the Civil War from 1861 to 1865, in the United States, dogs were used as messengers, guards and mascots. In 1898, during the Spanish-American war, dogs were used as scouts in the jungles of Cuba. At the beginning of the 20th century, like many European, Italy began using war dogs not only in combat but also in diverse and complex tasks such as healthcare. They were used in World War I as sentinels in the Balkans and Tripoli.

The Rottweiler, or Metzgerhund (Butcher's dog), a medium- to largesiged breed originated in Germany as a herding dog. Rottweilers worked as draught dogs, pulling carts to carry meat and other products to market. The breed is an ancient one, whose history stretches back again to the Roman Empire. The principal ancestor of the first Rottweilers during this time was supposed to be the Roman droving dog. In those times, the legions travelled with their meat on the hoof and required the assistance of working dogs to herd the cattle. The Army took note of these local dogs on its travels as one of its often travelled routes was through Wurttemberg on to the small market town of Rottweil. The Rottweiler was officially recognized in 1910 as a police dog in Germany. Later, during World Wars I and II, Rottweilers were put into service in various roles, including messenger, draught and guard dogs. Currently, they are often used in search and rescue, assistance guide dogs for the blind, guard and police dogs in addition to their traditional roles. The Israeli Army considered using them strapped with explosives as suicide dogs as recently as the late 1980s. They are still used by several European military units.

Several breeds of Spitz group, commonly called Huskies were used by the military as Sled Dog. Actually, the word 'husky' is a corruption of the derogative term 'Eskie' applied to the Inuit tribes discovered by Europeans who made early expeditions into their lands. The Siberian Husky, Samoyed, and Alaskan Malamute are the breeds that are considered direct descendent of the original sled dog. Siberian Huskies also served in the United States Army's Arctic Search and Rescue Unit of the Air Transport Command during World War II. The Blood Hound (also known as the St Hubert Hound, first bred in 1000 AD by monks at the St Hubert monastery in Belgium) is a large breed of dog famed for its ability to follow old scents over great distances. The combination of keen nose and powerful drive to track give it its place as top Scent Hound. The breed is used to track escaped prisoners and missing persons, as well as for military use.

The Belgian Shepherd Dog (Malinois) is one of four types considered to be varieties of a single breed rather than as a separate breed. In Belgium, Germany, the Netherlands and other European countries, as well as in the United States, Canada and Australia, the Malinois is bred primarily as a working dog for personal protection, detection police work and search and rescue. The United States' Secret Service uses the breed exclusively. OKETZ units of the Israel Defense Forces also use these dogs extensively. OKETZ favours the slighter build of the Malinois to the German Shepherd and Rottweiler, which were employed formerly. The German Shepherd (also known as an Alsatian), is a relatively new breed whose origins dates to 1899 in Germany. It is a breed of large-sized dog, a part of the herding group, developed originally for herding sheep. German Shepherds are very popular selection as working dogs. Initially, these dogs were especially well-known for their police work, where they were used for tracking criminals, patrolling troubled areas, detection and holding of suspects. However, by now a large number of German Shepherds have been used by the military and presently this breed is one of the most preferred one in armies world over. This is one of the most widely used breeds in variety of scent work roles such as search and rescue, cadaver searching, narcotics detection, explosives detection, accelerant detection and mine detection, etc. because of their keen sense of smell and their ability to work without distraction.

It was the German Army who established the first organized Military School for training war dogs at Lechernich, near Berlin in 1885 and wrote the first training manual. Dogs played a vital part in World War I throughout the Western Front. It is estimated that by 1918, Germany had employed 30,000 dogs whereas Britain, France and Belgium employed over 20,000 and Italy 3000. America, at first, did not use dogs except a few hundred from the allies for specific missions. Later, after a chance stowaway, the USA produced the most decorated and highly ranked service dog "Sergeant Stubby". Lots of dog breeds were used during World War I, but the most popular type of dogs were medium-sized, intelligent and trainable breeds. Particularly two breeds were used because of their superior strength, agility, territorial nature and trainability, i.e. Doberman Pinschers and German Shepherds (GSDs), both native to Germany. Dobermans were used because they are both highly intelligent and easily trainable, and possess excellent guarding abilities. Being of light frame and extremely agile, their dark coat allowed them to slip undetected through terrain without alerting the enemy whereas German Shepherds were used because of their strength, intelligence and trainability, being eager to please their masters.

Other dog breeds associated with WW I were smaller breeds such as Terriers, who were most often employed as 'Ratters', dogs trained to hunt and kill rats in the trenches. The Airedale, a breed of the terrier type that originated in Airedale, a geographic area in Yorkshire, England, was also extensively used in World War I to carry messages to soldiers behind enemy lines and to transport mail. They were also used by the Red Cross to find wounded soldiers on the battlefield.

The Labrador Retriever, also known as simply Labrador or Lab, is one of several kinds of retrievers, a type of gun dog, recognized by the American Kennel Club, Australia, Canada, New Zealand, the United Kingdom, and the United States. The foundational breed of what is now the Labrador Retriever was known as the St John's Dog, or Lesser Newfoundland. When the dogs were later brought to England, they were named after the geographic area known as "the Labrador". It is a favourite assistance dog breed in these and other countries, Labradors are frequently trained to aid people who are blind and people with autism, act as therapy dogs, and perform screening and detection work for law enforcement and other official agencies. They are prized as sporting and waterfowl hunting dogs. The first written reference to the breed was in 1814 ("Instructions to Young Sportsmen" by Colonel Peter Hawker). The first St John's dog was said to be brought to England in or around 1820, however, the breed's reputation had spread to England long before. There is a story that the Earl of Malmesbury saw a St John's Dog on a fishing boat and immediately made arrangements with traders to have some of these dogs exported to England. These ancestors of the first Labradors so impressed the Earl with their skill and ability for retrieving anything within the water and on shore that he devoted his entire kennel to develop and stabilize this breed. By 1870, the name Labrador Retriever became common in England. The breed was recognized by The Kennel Club in 1903. The first American Kennel Club (AKC) registration was in 1917. Labradors acquired popularity as hunting dogs during the 1920s and especially after World War II. They gained wide recognition in the USA, being the combination of the best traits of the two favourite breeds, i.e. Game Finders and Water Dogs. Outside North America and Western Europe, the Labrador arrived subsequently as household pets of diplomats and others in the foreign ministry. Further, improved access to overseas dog shows and bloodliness is said to have helped dissemination of this breed world over.

Labradors are even-tempered and well-behaved around young children and the elderly. They are athletic, playful, and the most popular breed of dog by registered ownership in America. The predominate canine selected by the US Military during the Vietnam War was the German Shepherd, which was utilized in the roles of Scout Dogs, Sentry Dogs and Mine Detection Dogs. The US Navy used Water Dogs to detect enemy under water divers in South Vietnam. The Labrador Retriever was the military's choice for their Combat Tracker Teams (CTTs) which consisted of one Labrador and four men: the handler, an observer, a security man, and the team leader. Labradors were selected by the military for tracking because of their distinct smelling qualities, and were utilized to locate the wounded US servicemen, enemy patrols, and downed allied airmen in Vietnam. These dogs received their combat training at the British Army's Jungle Warfare School in Malaysia. Today, Labradors are used by armies world over as Military Working Dogs for variety of roles.

ROLES AND FUNCTIONS OF WAR DOGS

Military dogs in World War I were positioned in a variety of roles, depending on their size, intelligence and training. Generally, the roles fell into the category of Sentry Dogs, Scout Dogs, Casualty Dogs, Explosive Dogs, Ratters and Mascot Dogs.

Sentry Dogs: These dogs were used for patrolling using a short leash and a firm hand. They were trained to accompany usually one specific guard and were taught to give a warning signal such as a growl, bark or snarl to indicate when an unknown or a suspect presence was in the secure area such as a camp or military base. Dobermans were generally used as Sentry Dogs.

Scout Dogs: These dogs were of a quiet, disciplined and of highly trainable type. Their role was to move ahead of soldiers on foot patrolling the terrain so as to detect enemy scent up to 1000 yards away, sooner than any man could. Instead of barking and thus drawing attention, the dogs would stiffen, raise its shackles and point its tail, which indicated that the enemy was encroaching upon the terrain. Scout dogs were widely used because they were highly efficient in avoiding detection of the column by the enemy.

Casualty Dogs: Such dogs were also called 'Mercy' dogs and were considered as vital in World War I. Originally trained in the late 1800s by the Germans and known as 'Sanitatshunde' in Germany. These dogs were trained to find the wounded and dying on battlefields and were equipped with medical supplies to aid those suffering. Those soldiers who could help themselves to supplies would attend to their own wounds, whilst other more seriously wounded soldiers would seek the company of a Mercy dog to wait with them whilst they died. These dogs were later used across Europe.

Messenger Dogs: They proved to be as reliable as soldiers in the vulnerable job of running messages. The complexities of trench warfare meant that communication was always a problem. Field communication systems were crude and there was always the very real possibility that vital messages from the front would never get back to Headquarters or vice versa. Human runners were potentially large targets, weighed down by their uniforms and chance of such runner getting through the enemy's fire was considerably less in the heat of a battle. As such, the dogs were the obvious solution to this pressing problem. A trained dog was faster than a human runner, presented less of a target to a sniper and could travel over any terrain. Above all, well trained dogs proved to be extremely reliable in this arduous task. A dog training school was established in Scotland, and a trained dog from this school got through over 4000 metres, on a "very difficult terrain" on the Western Front, with an important message to a Brigade Headquarters, in less than sixty minutes when all other methods of communicating with the Headquarters had failed.

Mascot Dogs: These dogs were of great psychological comfort to soldiers trapped in the horrors of trench warfare. He did take away, even if for a short time, the horrors they lived through. It is said that Adolf Hitler kept a dog with him in the German trenches. For many soldiers on any of the sides that fought in the trenches, a dog must have reminded them of home comforts. There are two types of military mascots: (a) Those who appear as part of the regiment's official history and are part of the order of battle with service rank and number. 'Official' British Army mascots were entitled to the services of the Royal Army Veterinary Corps as well as quartering and feeding at public expense. (b) There are also mascots whose costs are borne by the regiment or unit itself. The Irish Wolf Hound, for example, is the mascot of the Irish Guards. The first one was given to the regiment in 1902 and they were kept as pets until they became the official mascots in 1961. Although fearsome looking, Wolf Hounds are generally good natured and well-behaved, and thus make perfect regimental mascots. The Irish Guards is the only Guards regiment, presently permitted to have their mascot lead them on parade.

The heroic and hair raising tales of legendary Mascot Dogs in war speak volumes on their bravery, devotion and faithfulness for their masters. Dog named Magrita, a humanitarian dog served with Zouaves of the Guard and carried bandages in a sack hung around his neck and offered the bandages as first aid to the wounded soldiers in the battlefield. Similarly, who would easily believe that Moffino, a companion dog of an Italian corporal, was supposed to have been lost while crossing the Berezina River, travelled from Russia to Italy to reunite with his master a year later at Milan.

Russians utilized Ambulance Dogs in 1904 during Russo-Japanese War. A large number of dogs were used to carry ammunition bags and also as couriers under the line of enemy fire. They even used Sled Dogs to pull light guns, men and supplies. White Samoyeds were used to pull white clad marksmen on sled close to enemy line and in one sector, a team of Sled dogs carried 1239 wounded men from the battlefield and hauled 327 tons of ammunition within five working days. During this period French also used dogs extensively as ammunition carriers.

During World War I, "Stubby" became the most decorated dog in war, wining several medals and even the honorary rank of Sergeant. In 1921, General Blackjack Pershing, the supreme commander of American forces during the war, pinned Stubby with a "Gold Hero Dog Medal" that was commissioned by the Humane Education Society, the forerunner of current Humane Society. He became lifetime member of the Red Cross and YMCA. During the Italian-German invasion of Yugoslavia in 1941, Italians used dogs to guard prisoners of war and vital assets, such as railheads and bridges in the country. During World War II, a trained Sentry Dog named "Chips," employed with a unit of 3rd American Division, single handedly attacked an enemy machine gun nest manned by four soldiers in a combat situation in Sicily and was awarded "Silver Star and Purple Heart".

British Army used "Para Dogs" to support their troops in locating mines and booby traps after parachuting in to the enemy territory. One of such dog named "Bing" also known as "Brian" proved his mettle in saving the lives of troops at numerous occasions and was awarded the "PDSA Dickin Medal" which is awarded to bravest of the brave animal and is considered as an animal version of "Victoria Cross". Similarly, German Shepherd "Crumstone Irma, aka Irma," assisted in the rescue of 191 people trapped under blitzed buildings while serving with London's Civil Defence Services during World War II and was known for her ability to tell if buried victims were dead or alive. Irma was awarded the "PDSA Dickin Medal" in 1945, and is buried at the PDSA Animal Cemetery, Ilford, which is considered a great honour.

Scout Dogs proved their mettle in combat patrol during Korean War, and owing to outstanding performance, their handlers were awarded three Silver Stars, Six Bronze Stars for valour and thirty-five Bronze Stars for meritorious service whereas the 26th Infantry Scout Dog Platoon of the US Army, received a citation for its distinguished services. One Scout Dog named "York" of this unit completed 148 combat patrols and the last one on the day Armistice was signed. A large number of Military Working Dogs (MWDs) served with American troops and their coalition army troops in the Vietnam War. They earned tremendous respect for their work and reportedly saved ten thousand lives. During this war, 500 dogs and 294 dog handlers were killed. Staff Sergeant Robert W Hartsock, a dog handler of the US Army, was awarded the "Congressional Medal of Honor" posthumously for exemplary heroism and bravery.

The performance of Indian Army dog "Alex" in tracking down the culprits who attempted to assassinate the King of Bhutan in July 1965 on a two days old scent has become a legend. Similarly, Army dog Sundri displayed undeterred tracking potential in dark night bearing inhospitable terrain and adverse climatic conditions. The bravery and swift action by the dog and handler successfully led to the location where the terrorists had cut the cables of highly sensitive signal receiver station of Army in Northern Sector. In recognition of the gallant act of the team of Sundri and Gurbachan, "Shaurya Chakra" was awarded to the handler L/Dfr Gurbachan Singh. The performance of Army dog "Ashok" became the talk of glory at Zozila pass in India during November, 1986, when a huge avalanche rolled down the pass and many were buried alive. This Avalanche Rescue Dog and his handler searched and saved many live personnel enabling their timely rescue. Several casualties buried in deep snow were also detected and the duo continued working relentlessly till wounded. These tales speak volumes about the heroism of these silent warriors and their handlers.

Military dogs also proved their mettle in Gulf war and Afghanistan war. American marines started deployment of military dogs with just nine bomb-sniffing dogs in Afghanistan in 2007 and by the end of 2011, the number of dogs deployed by them grew to 650 which depicts not only the potential of these dogs as a valuable factor in military efforts of forces deployed in the theatre but also utmost faithfulness to their masters. One such dog of the slain US Navy, SEAL remained loyal even in death, refusing to walk away from his master's cask who was killed when a US helicopter was shot down by Taliban insurgents on 6th Aug, 2011. British Army also considered essential to induct its Military Dog Regiment comprising specialist Military Working Dogs with primary role to support their lead Brigade in war zone in 2010.

The gallant acts of these silent warriors, have earned great admiration and love for Military Working Dogs and their handlers at all levels. However, their efforts have escaped public attention owing to the lack of dedicated memorials on their sacrifices in war. The good news is that this recognition is slowly on the increase and many memorials have now been made in various countries and more memorials are expected to spring up around the world in due course of time. The distinguished and yeoman service rendered by war dogs have earned them not only applause but gallantry and distinguished services medals too. A most appropriate tribute to these warriors will be to make aware the people at large about the brave dogs of war and notable gallant acts of their equally courageous handlers, a made for each other duo and inseparable team. The acts of their courage and faithfulness will make a reader to visualize and appreciate the difficult tasks, inhospitable terrain, uncongenial environment coupled with constant threat to lives of the dog and handlers while the duo perform the challenging tasks to the highest degree of perfection under trying circumstances.

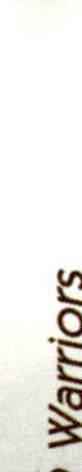

Hence, it may be concluded that evolution and transformation of war dogs is linked with the human development. As the concept and dimension of war change with the time, the role of dogs in the war also get transformed as per the requirement of the mission. War dogs have always been with the warriors and will continue to be with them in battlefield as well as in counter insurgency and anti-terrorism efforts.

3

History of War Dogs

"Histories are, more, full of examples of the fidelity of dogs than of friends."

... Alexander Pope

The history of war dogs is as old as war itself, as such, "when we go to war, they go to war". For centuries ago it has been realized that dogs can be suitably trained for military purposes. The ancient Greek and Roman artworks depict Mastiff-like animals employed as Attack Dogs. It was initially during the days of the Roman Empire, that entire formations of Attack Dogs, frequently equipped with armour or spiked collars were sent into battle against the enemy as a recognized and effective instruments of offensive warfare. The Hounds were used as war dogs to haul men off horseback and out of chariots. Assyrians, Persians, and Babylonians also used Mastiffs wearing spiked collars and armour against their enemies in the forward line of battle. Hammurabi, the sixth king of Babylon who reigned from 1792 to 1750 BC, equipped his soldiers with huge war dogs. In Egypt, murals dating back to perhaps 4000 BC commemorate the fighting spirit of dogs in battle. They show vicious animals unleashed by their soldier-masters and leaping upon their feeble enemies.Those days, dogs were trained to attack the enemies' legs, causing them to lower their shields so that they become more vulnerable. Pugnaces Britanniae (Latin) or War Dog of Britannia, now an extinct breed of dog and progenitor to the English Mastiff was exclusively bred for combat dogs. In the fourth century BC, there was a Greek state called Epirus, where the rulers called themselves 'Molossians'. History suggests that when Roman forces over-ran Epirus, the dogs of great size and power were plundered in the fighting arena.

During 7th century BC, in the archaic period in Greece from 800 BC to 480 BC, Magnesian horsemen were known to be accompanied each by a war dog and a spear-bearing attendant in the war waged by the Ephesians again Magnesia on the Maeander in Ionia. The dogs were released first to break the enemy ranks, followed by an assault of spears, then a cavalry charge. An epitaph records the burial of a Magnesian horseman named Hippaemon with his dog Lethargos, his horse, and his spearman. The earliest use of war dogs in a battle recorded in classical sources was by Alyattes of Lydia against the Cimmerians around 600 BC. The Lydian dogs killed some invaders and routed others. Often war dogs would be sent into battle with large protective spiked metal collars and coats of mail armour. The Greeks and Romans cultivated several kinds of dog, which were used in chase of the wolf and wild boar, in pursuit of the stag or roe deer, as guardians of the flock, and also as watch dogs in fortresses and citadels. The Greeks appear to have had Grey Hounds, and wolf-like hounds with erect ears. The citadel of Corinth was guarded externally by an advanced post of fifty dogs, which, on one occasion, during the drunken somnolence of the garrison, had to defend the place against the attack of an enemy. Forty-nine out of the fifty dogs lost their lives after a valiant resistance, and the survivor, whose name was Soter, retreated to the citadel. The soldiers, alarmed by him, roused themselves to action and repelled the enemy. The dog was rewarded by the grateful senate with a silver collar, inscribed, 'Soter, defender and preserver of Corinth.' A marble monument was also erected to commemorate the names and glorious achievement of the fifty canine heroes. It is generally believed that Romans were the first to train Molossus dogs, who were huge Mastiff-like Hounds able to knock a man off a galloping horse. The Mastiff dogs descend from the "Roman Canis Pugnaces" and both the "Cane Corso (light version) and Neapolitan Mastiff (heavy version)" are the rightful heirs to this legendary war dog. Cambyses II, the king of kings of Persia, at the battle of Pelusium in 525 BC applied a psychological tactic against the Egyptians by arraying dogs and other animals in the front line to effectively take advantage of the Egyptian religious reverence for animals. The Persian phrase sag-e karzari means canine warrior.

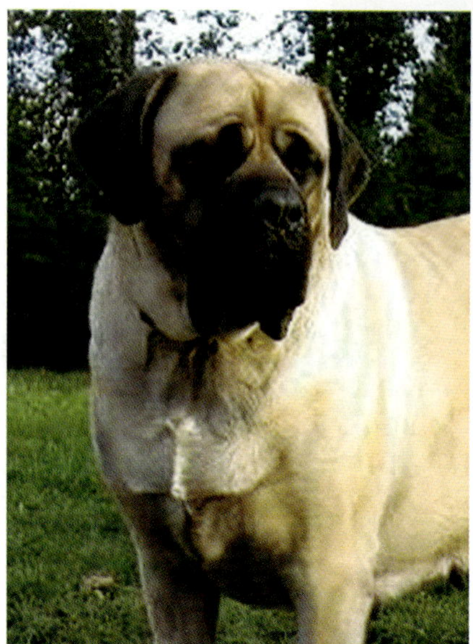

Molossus Dog

At the battle of Marathon in 490 BC a dog followed his hoplite master, (citizen-soldiers of Ancient Greek city-states, who were primarily armed with spears and shields), into battle against the Persians and has been memorialized in a mural Dogs were highly prized among the Persian aristocracy. The Persian phrase sage-e karzari means canine warriors.

In 385 BC, during the siege of Mantineia, fighting dogs cut off enemy reinforcement. A dog belonging to Darius III (336–30 BC) supposedly refused to leave Darius' corpse after he had been struck down by Bessus. Xerxes I of Persia was accompanied by vast packs of hounds while invading Greece in 480 BC. One of the Persian satraps (Governors) of Babylon assigned the revenues derived from four large villages in that province to the care of his hounds. Alexander the Great, who dominated, conquered, and created one of the largest empires in ancient history, as documented from July 356 BC to June 323 BC, had dog by his side named Peritas, a Molossian dog. Alexander was 11 years old when he got Peritas and he was very fond of this dog. The name Peritas seemed to have come from Macedonian word for January. Peritas accompanied Alexander during his military exploits. The greatest loyalty of Peritas was in the story of how he saved Alexander the Great in Mallian Campaign from November 326 BC to February 325 BC against the Mallis of eastern Punjab in India. While fighting, Alexander was trapped behind the Mallian fortification and his soldiers were momentarily unable to rescue him. Leonnatus, who was fighting fiercely, heard Peritas hawl and bark from behind him. Without looking back, Leonnatus shouted "Go Peritas! Run Alexander". The courageous dog ran through the soldiers fighting and leapt at the group of Mallians who had just wounded Alexander with a javelin. Peritas killed several men giving time to the Alexander's soldiers to save him and also stopped Mallians from slaughtering Alexander. The brave dog was also mortally wounded with a javelin as well. With Peritas's last strength he laid his head on the wounded king's lap and died gazing into his master's eyes. The name of this dog lives on forever since Alexander founded a city, as the spoils of the war, and gave it the name Peritas. According to Pliny the Elder, a Roman author as well as naval and army commander of the early Roman Empire, it was perhaps the king Pyrrhus of Epirus (NW Greece), who delighted Alexander by giving him a dog which had attacked and beaten both a lion and an elephant. There is also the story of Alexander meeting Sopeithes, a ruler of an area probably around Jech Doab in Punjab, India (now in Pakistan), Sopeithes gave Alexander one hundred and fifty dogs known for their fearsome strength and courage and also organized a lion fight with dogs to demonstrate their heroism.

The Roman Consul Marcus Pomponius Matho, leading the Roman legions through the island of Sardinia, where the inhabitants led guerrilla warfare against the invaders, used dogs from Italy to hunt out the natives who tried to hide in the caves in 231 BC. Hammurbi equipped his warriors with huge fighting dogs in 210 BC. Bituito, the king of Arvernii in 120 BC, attacked a small force of Romans led by the Consul Fabius, using all the dogs he had in his Army. Textual evidence exist of the participation of Pharaoh's dogs in the New Kingdom Egyptian battles, Asian Greek battles and use of wolf-like dogs by Teutones warriors with armed women to defend their camp against Marius' legionaries at Vercellae in 102 BC. The gallant acts of these dogs speak volumes about the role of dogs in ancient wars. Gratius Falsius, an ancient Roman author and historian, wrote in the year 8 AD of a large exhibition of dog fights in the ancient Roman amphitheatres between the Pugnaces Britanniae from Britannia and the Molossus from Epirus. The exhibition reflected the wide-mouthed dogs from Britain were far superior to the ancient Greek Molossus.

The ancient Roman historian Strabo reported in 38 AD that large British dogs which were bred in their homeland of Britannia to hunt dangerous game, were used as war dogs. In 43 AD, the Roman conquest of Britain made Britannia, a Roman province. At that time, in Britain there were giant, wide-mouthed dogs, which the Romans called Pugnaces

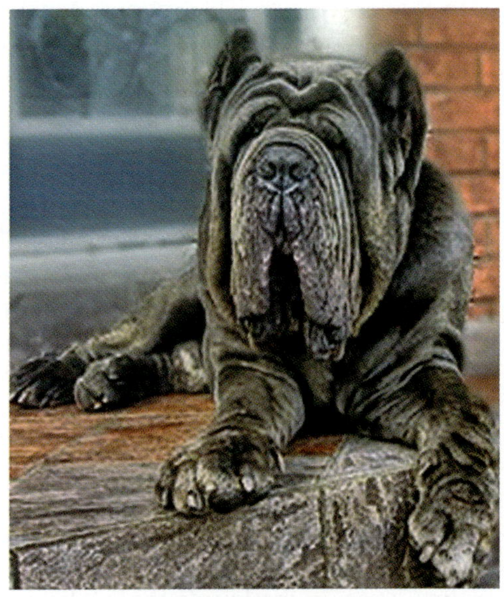

Pugnasis Britannia

Britanniae, that surpassed their Molossus dogs. A Procurator Cynegii, was stationed in Venta Belgarum responsible for selecting these dogs for exporting to Rome for contests in the amphitheatre and for integration into the military of ancient Rome as war dogs. The references by Roman writers to the Canis Pugnaces of Roman Britain, also suggest a dog of a large and heavy type with light brown eyes, truncated muzzle, loose skin above the brows, a broad back, great stature, and muscular legs.

Hyrcanian war dogs with armour were used by Hyrcanian, Caspian and Tapurian warriors during Hyrcanian revolt against the Parthians in 59 AD. Atilla, King of the Huns from 433 AD until his death in 453 AD, used giant Molossian dogs (precursors of the Mastiff) and Talbots (ancestors of the Blood Hound) in his campaigns. The defeated Saxons were tracked by dogs after the battle of Dunnichen Moss in 685 AD.

After the fall of Rome in 476 CE, armies across the globe continued using war dogs, but no longer limited their service to fighting. They were trained as Guard Dogs, Sentries, Messengers and Draught Dogs. Medieval knights draped their faithful hounds in chain mail and plunged into battle with the dogs by their side. At death, the knights, who loved the dogs dearly, had an image of these faithful hounds inscribed on their tombs, linking the two forever. William the Conqueror, the first Norman King of England, reigning from 1066 until his death in 1087, used St Hubert Hounds (Blood Hounds) to support his troops as well as to run down opponents. His St Hubert Hounds guarded and defended his Army's camps and followed remaining enemies to the end of trail. Edward Longshanks, the king Edward I of England from 1272 to 1307, employed dogs to defend the English Crown. He used armoured dogs to defend caravans, attack enemies and Blood Hounds on his borders with Scotland to track down the notorious "Moss Troopers". Longshanks established Tracker Dogs in various districts to assist the Crown forces along the border. In 1508, Spanish conquistadors took dogs to the New World and used Mastiffs and other large breed dogs against Native Americans. King Henry VIII of England, presented 400 battle Mastiffs, with iron collars, to Charles V of Spain, then at war with France in 1518. The Spanish Mastiffs were set on the French dogs at the siege of Valencia and drove them from the field. So heroic was their conduct that Charles held all the dogs up as an example of honour and courage. In 1599, Queen Elizabeth dispatched the Earl of Essex, Ireland, with an army of 22,000 men, including a large force of 800 Blood Hounds, to put down the Irish chieftain rebellion. The French Navy used attack dogs in St Malo France to guard naval dock installations from early 14th century till 1770, when they were abolished after a young naval officer was unfortunately killed by one of the dogs.

Prince Rupert of the Rhine (1619–1682), nephew of the ill-fated Charles I of England, was taken prisoner at the Battle of Lemgo in 1638 and confined at Lintz until 1641. During this hiatus, Lord Arundell, English ambassador to Vienna, gave him a white Poodle named "Boy". It was curious to observe that Prince Rupert personally took interest to teach discipline to Boy. This Poodle was Prince Rupert's constant companion until the dog's death at the Battle of Marston Moor on 2nd July 1644. Boy was the subject of hilarious roundhead satire as narrated by Anne Osborne in "Rupert of the Rhine, Anecdotes in the life of Prince Rupert—dog lover", Tail-Wagger Magazine, June, 1950. ("Boy was reputed to know many tricks. At "Charles", he jumped for joy, he slept in Prince Rupert's bed, Boy had more haircuts than his master, he sat in the king's chair, played with his children, enjoyed a sung Mass, lay

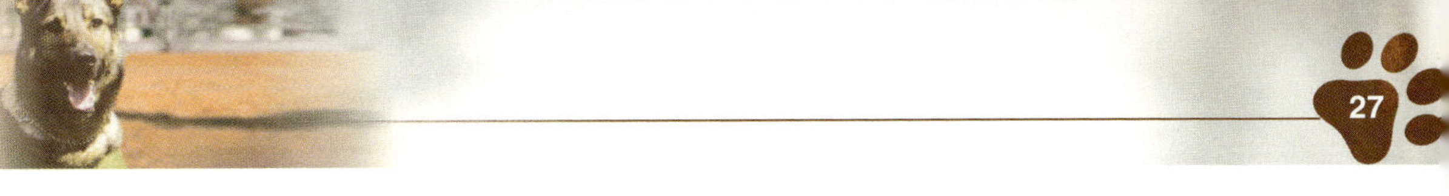

with his paw on young Prince Charles' foot, and Charles I fed him choice morsels of roast beef and breast of capon from the table, he could go invisible and that's how he spied and delved into necromancy").

During Medieval Times, dog handlers were called fewterers and were responsible for their lord's war and hunting dogs. Large Mastiff-type breeds were trained to attack humans and Hound breeds were used as tracker dogs. Use of dogs to guard convoys and caravans was quite prevalent during this period. The dogs were used as messengers by the Army of Fredrick the Great during seven years war from 1756 to 1763. In 1799, Napoleon positioned a large numbers of fighting dogs in front of his reserves and also ordered his troops to station dogs as guardians while occupying Egypt. He used dogs as sentries at the gates of Alexandria in Egypt, for early warning to his troops against attack by the enemy forces.

As Europeans expanded into the New World, so did their dogs. Perhaps the first war dogs in America were those used especially by the Spaniards against Aboriginal Americans, who in turn used dogs for their own purposes, such as guarding the camp or for early warning. Many of the United States' founders saw the effectiveness of dogs in battle and used them whenever they could. Native Aboriginal Americans used dogs for pack and sentry work. The first recorded use of dogs by the United States Army was in 1835 during the Second Seminole War. Thirty-three Cuban-bred Blood Hounds were bought at a cost of several thousand dollars and five handlers were used by the US Army to track the Seminoles and the runaway slaves harbouring in the swamps of western Florida and Louisiana. During the Civil War in United States from 1861 to 1865, dogs were used as messengers, guards and as mascots. As per a heart warming story, a woman named Mrs Pfieff left her home in Illinois to find the remains of her husband Lt Louis Pfieff of the 3rd Illinois Infantry, who had died on the battlefield of Shiloh. When she arrived, no one knew for certain the final resting place of her beloved husband. She was undeterred and trekked through the battlefield for clues. Her perseverance was rewarded when she saw her husband's faithful dog, whom he had brought along with him, walking towards her. She embraced the dog who led her and she, knowing the dog's devotion, followed. The dog took her to an unmarked grave of her late husband. She learned later that the dog had stood by the grave for 12 days.

Dogs were used as scouts for Teddy Roosevelt's Rough Riders' horseback patrols in the dense jungles of Cuba, during the Spanish-American War in 1898. Each of these 'War Dogs' were trained as point scouts. Ambushes by the enemy became near impossible and the lessons learned in Cuba by the US Corps were later proven in many Pacific Island jungles conflict against Japan during World War II and much later in Vietnam. During World War I, America did not have a war dog policy. However, the attack upon Pearl Harbour and the sudden entry of the United States into World War II, greatly stimulated interest in the use of dogs. 25 Marine War Dogs gave their lives liberating Guam in 1944 and many more served as Sentries, Messengers, and Scouts, exploring caves, detecting mines and booby traps, and bringing vital information across the battlefield. A statue was erected in their honour and the inscription on the statue perhaps sums up the efforts of war dogs throughout history. "Given in their memory and on behalf of the surviving men of the 2nd and 3rd Marine War Dogs Platoons, many of whom owe their lives to the bravery and sacrifice of these gallant animals..." Always Faithful "was inspired by the spirit of these heroic dogs who are the embodiment of love and devotion." Presently, USA is the world's largest user of modern military dogs.

Japan has a long history of employing dogs. The Akita dog of Japan is said to have guarded Samurai homes and used in the field to carry loads. One of the earliest examples of using dogs in war, is tracking down Russian prisoners of war in the Russo-Japanese War in 1894–1895. Japanese Military Dogs were used in Manchuria in 1931 as Messenger and Guard dogs. During World War II, dogs were used in sentry roles, and it is believed that attempts were made to train Suicide Dogs who would run towards enemy-emplacements prior to exploding with a timed fuse. Today the Japanese Self Defence Force (JSDF) employs MWDs in the Air Force Branch to guard bases.

Many of the Military Working Dogs that we use today can have their lineages traced back to Germany and the war dogs of that nation. The Sanitatshunde "sanitary dogs," as the Germans referred to these canine Red Cross workers also called Ambulance Dogs were trained to find the wounded among the battlefield casualties that lay littered across a no man's land. These dogs were trained to go out into that legendary zone, with water or alcohol packs in saddle bags strapped to their bodies, to offer the injured what was often some small comfort before the men died. More important, the dogs were sent out to identify the location of the wounded, most often at night, and return with some token, a cap, a helmet, or other identifier, and then lead a handler to the site of the wounded man so that he could be recovered. The German Army established the first organized Military School for training War Dogs at Lechernich, near Berlin in 1885 and wrote the first dog training manual.

During World War I, the Germans used possibly 30,000 dogs, the French 20,000, and the Italians 3,000. The other allied forces used thousands more. The French employed chiens de brie, large sheep dogs, in sentry duties. In Belgium, draught dogs towed gun carriages. Italians used a large number of dogs in Alpine areas, climbing narrow paths where horses or mules could not venture. Kilo for kilo, a dog can pull a greater weight than a horse. The US did not use war dogs but borrowed some from their allies.

By the beginning of World War II, the Germans upped the ante, training more than 200,000 dogs for a variety of roles, such as guarding airfields, railway heads and logistical areas against sabotage and commando-style attacks. In the USA, about 10,000 dogs were trained for the Army, Navy, Marine Corps and Coast Guard. The Soviet Army trained and used 68,000 dogs in different disciplines including Anti-Tank Mine Dogs. The French started World War II with considerable numbers of war dogs, however, due to France's quick defeat they did not get a chance to prove themselves. British Army also used a large number of dogs as guard, mine detection and parachute dogs. A large number of mascots and other war dogs trained and utilised for specific tasks were deployed by the armies of various countries and the allied forces used approximately 250,000 dogs in their war efforts.

During offensive operations ranging from World War II to the present Gulf conflicts and Afghanistan war against terrorism, Mine Detection Dogs (MDDs) were employed prior to zero hour at the forefront, clearing a path with other engineering assets for the main forces to exploit 'Those that hold the lead' is a motto seen on many MWD handlers' t-shirts. The double meaning of the word 'lead' is apt, as MWD handlers are frequently at the forefront of operations.

MODERN WAR DOGS

The appearance of the ancient warrior with his war dog has not been altered greatly over time. The ancient soldier was lightly armed and clad for speed of movement on the battlefield. The war dog wore a light protective jacket made up of leather with spikes and matching collar for throat protection at most.

Today, both Dog and man are more valued in society and greater protection is afforded to both. War Dogs do wear bulletproof vests and rubber booties for protection. Communication devices and video systems can be attached to the dogs, so that handlers cannot only see and command dogs in the heat of battle but also allow them to be recalled to safety if required. The dog handler is also better clad for battle than ever before, with communications, modern weapons with laser and night vision capabilities, individual night-viewing devices and tactical protective body armour. Handlers also possess a rich knowledge of medical and first aid treatments to immediately aid their canine partners if needed in battle. Along with wearing advanced equipment, war dogs today are also multiskilled in battlefield functions. Many are dual-roled to attack or detect specialist substances. It might have been imagined earlier that with the increased complexity of military operations, the value of War Dogs will slowly decline but the reverse is true. Dogs still possess many advantages over modern technology and their use is expected to continue well into the future. Dogs are an invaluable aid to ground troops in jungle warfare as was demonstrated by the British in the Malayan Campaign and again in Borneo. Additionally, Tracker Dogs were used by the US and Australian forces in Vietnam and by Australian peacekeeper troops in East Timor. Over open country or in urban areas, in pursuit of intruders, detecting enemy forces on patrol or locating terrorist ammunitions dumps, dogs have been successfully used in Kenya, Cyprus, Hong Kong, Bosnia, Kosovo, Northern Ireland, the Middle East, Asia, Iraq and Afghanistan and many other countries.

CHRONOLOGY OF MILITARY DOG HISTORY

628 BC:	The Lydians deploy a separate battalion of fighting dogs against Cimmerians.
525 BC:	Cambyses II, The Persian king use huge fighting dogs against Egyptian spearmen and archers.
490 BC:	***Hoplites,*** the citizen-soldiers of Ancient Greek city-states use dogs against Persians in the battle of Marathon, a brave fighting dog was immortalized in a mural.
480 BC:	Xerxex I of Persia use fighting dogs against Greece.
385 BC:	Siege of Mantineia: fighting dogs cut off enemy reinforcements.
326 BC:	Alexender was saved by his Molossus dog, Peritas, in great Mallian campaign in east Punjab in India.
231 BC:	Roman Consul Marcus Pomponius Matho use fighting dogs against natives of Sardina.
210 BC:	Hammurabi equips his warriors with huge dogs.
102 BC:	Teutones warriors use Large Kimber Dogs led by armed women to defend their laagers against Marius legionaries at the battle of Vercellae.
AD-08:	Large exhibition of dog fights between Britanniae and Molossus dogs held in ancient Roman amphitheatres.

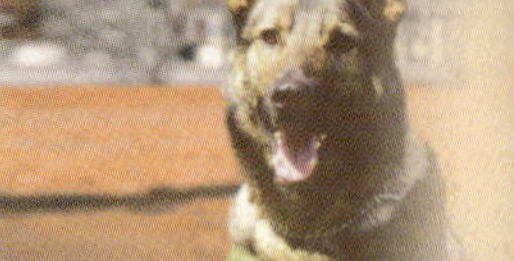

AD-43:	Rome invades Britannia. Giant fighting dogs called Pugnaces Britanniae are discovered and exported for integration into the military of ancient Rome.
AD-59:	Use of Hyrcanian war dogs with armour by Hyrcanian, Caspian and Tapurian warriors during Hyrcanian revolt against the Parthians.
101:	The Romans employ one fighting dog company per legion.
433:	Atilla, King of the Huns from 433 AD until his death in 453 AD, uses giant Molossian dogs, precursors of the Mastiff, and Talbots, ancestors of the Blood Hound, in his campaigns.
685:	The defeated Saxons were tracked by dogs after the battle of Dunnichen Moss.
1066:	William the Conqueror, the first Norman King of England, reigning from 1066 uses St Hubert Hounds (Blood Hounds) to support his troops as well as to run down opponents until his death in 1087.
1272:	The King Edward I of England employs dogs to defend the English Crown till 1307.
1508:	Spanish conquistadors took dogs to the New World and used Mastiffs and other large breeds dogs against Native Americans.
1518:	Henry VIII exports 400 Mastiffs to support Spain.
1599:	Elizabeth I sends 800 fighting dogs to fight in the Desmond Rebellions.
1756–1763:	The dogs were used as messengers by the Army of Fredrick the Great during seven years war.
1799:	Napoleon assembles a large number of fighting dogs in front of his reserves.
1835:	The first recorded use of dogs by the United States Army during the Second Seminole War.
1898:	Dogs were used as scouts for Teddy Roosevelt's Rough Riders' horseback patrols in the dense jungles of Cuba, during the Spanish-American War.
1915:	The Belgian army use carabineers, strong-muscled dogs called Bouvier des Flandres, to haul heavy cannons to the front.
1914–1918:	Dogs used by international forces to deliver vital messages in World War I.
1941–1945:	The Soviet Union uses dogs strapped with explosives to destroy invading German tanks in the World War II and other international forces use dogs to boost war efforts.
1950–1953:	Dogs were used in Korean War.
1966–1973:	Over 4,000 US war dogs serve in the Vietnam War and estimated to have saved over 10,000 human lives.
1990-1991:	A large number of Military Working Dogs were used in Gulf War by the USA and other allies.
2001 to present:	Military Working Dogs are being used by the USA and all participating countries in Afghanistan war against terrorism.

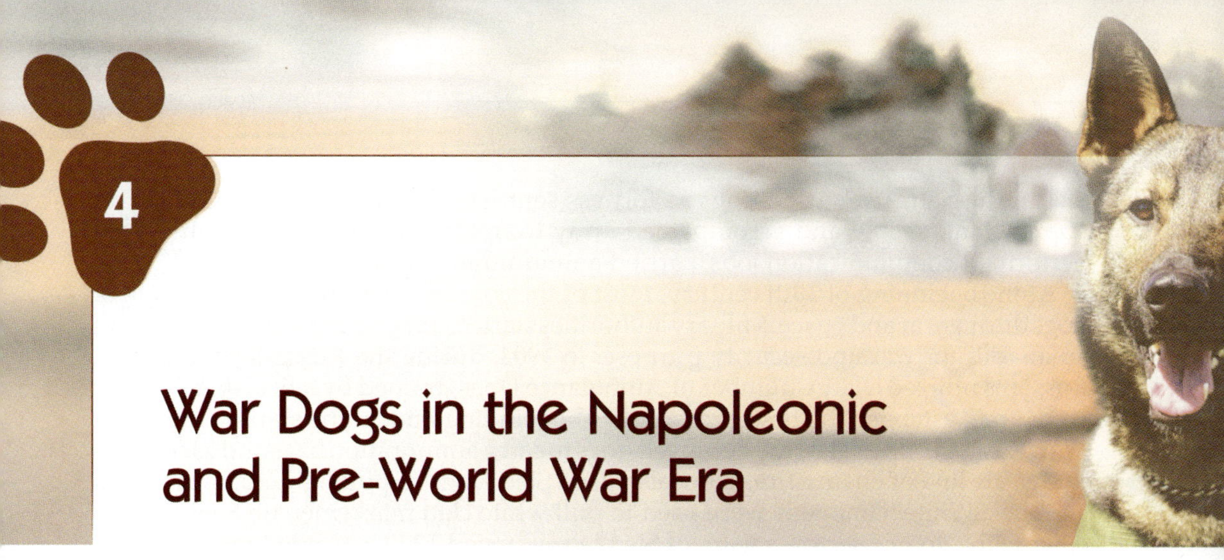

4

War Dogs in the Napoleonic and Pre-World War Era

"Heaven goes by favor. If it went by merit, you would stay out and your dog would go in."

... Mark Twain

Ancient literature mentions about the dogs accompanying their masters during the Napoleonic Wars from 1803 to 1815. A frequently cited example of War Dogs and their loyalty is, Napoleon's writing in his memoirs, "I walked over the battlefield and among the slain, a killed Poodle bestowing a last lick upon his dead friend's face, a Grenadier in the battle of Marengo, never had anything on any battlefield caused me a like emotion." The Battle of Marengo was fought on 14th June, 1800 between French forces under Napoleon Bonaparte and Austrian forces near the city of Alessandria, in Piedmont, Italy. The French overcame General Michael Von Melas's surprise attack near the end of the day, driving the Austrians out of Italy, and enhancing Napoleon's political position in Paris as First Consul of France. Today, many of us think of the French Poodle as the epitome of the spoiled, prissy canine, but Poodles have a long history as Military Working Dogs. Another instance, Petit Jean, a drummer boy was accompanied by his pet Barbuche in one of the Italian campaigns. Petit Jean died in the battle but his dog Barbuche made exemplary efforts to defend his dying master and lost one of his front legs. Subsequently, Barbuche was adopted by Seargeant Fougasse and he spent his remainder life with him. The Italian campaigns of the French Revolutionary wars (1792–1802) were a series of conflicts fought principally in Northern Italy between the French Revolutionary Army and a coalition of Austria, Russia, Piedmont-Sardinia and a number of other Italian states. Further, who would easily believe that Moffino, the companion dog of an Italian corporal, supposed to have been lost while crossing the Berezina River, travelled from Russia to Italy to reunite with his master a year later at Milan. The Battle of Berezina (or Beresina) took place from 26th to 29th November, 1812, between the French Army of Napoleon, retreating after his invasion of Russia and crossing the Berezina (near Borisov, Belarus), and the Russian Armies under General Mikhail Kutuzov, Peter Wittgenstein and Admiral Pavel Chichagov. The battle ended with a mixed outcome. The French suffered very heavy losses but managed to cross the river and avoided being trapped. Since then "Berezina" has been used in French as a synonym for "disaster."

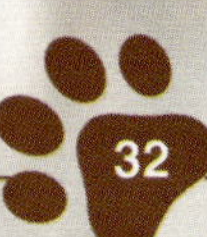

The Russian Army used dogs as fortress sentries who warned the guards of an approaching enemy and accompanied army troops during their campaigns. Dogs performed communication jobs, carried ammunition and delivered first aid.

At the beginning of 19th century, most of the countries had realized the value of dogs during war and peace. Military authorities started considering them as important auxiliaries for war and security purpose. In 1904, during the Russo-Japanese War, Russians utilized a large number of Ambulance Dogs, trained by a British, who later went on to establish the first Army Dog School in England, at the start of The Great War. Russian Imperial Army deployed dogs to carry ammunition bags and as couriers under the line of enemy fire. They also used Sled Dogs to pull light guns, men and supplies. White Samoyeds were used to pull white clad marksmen on Sled close to enemy line. In one sector, a team of Sled Dogs carried 1239 wounded men from the battlefield and hauled 327 tons of ammunition within five working days.

During Balbon upheaval in 1910, the Bulgarians used their Sheep Dogs as sentries. During the same period, Italians used their Mar Emma Sheep Dogs in Tripoli as sentry where they were picketed in sand dugouts, a few hundred yards ahead of the troops facing the enemy. British used War Dogs in the Abor Expedition in India. The Abors were an Assam tribe inhabiting a tract of hill country on the northeast frontier of India, first visited by the English in 1826. Much of the area was terra incognita and problems arose connected with the Indo-Chinese and Indo-Tibetan borders. It was the killing of the British Assistant Political Officer, Mr Williamson, and his colleague Dr Gregorson by the Abors in 1911 while they were touring the Tibetan border area, which led to the deployment of the punitive expeditionary force from October, 1911 to April, 1912. A large number of these tribals were brutually killed and their villages burned so as to teach them lesson. More details about the dogs in World War I and subsequent wars/conflicts will be covered later in respective chapters.

Although all the Mascot Dogs those participated in various wars during the Napoleonic period and prior to World war I were great heroes, yet it is not feasible to describe all of them in this text. A few of their representatives having textual evidence and considered famous Mascot Dogs of that era are described here:

JACK

One of the better-known Civil War Dogs was Jack, who served as the mascot for the 102nd Pennsylvania Infantry. Jack's regiment was made up mostly of firemen who had already adopted a brown-and-white bull terrier. One day before the war, a stray Bulldog wandered into the firehouse of the Niagara Volunteer Company on Penn Avenue in Pittsburgh. Although mistreated by some of the firemen at first, "Jack" won the hearts of all those rough men when he whipped a much larger stray dog in a fight to the finish. He went on to answer every fire call. When Lincoln's call for volunteers went out, he was enlisted along with most of the companies in the Washington Infantry in August 1861. Since he was really smart, it didn't take Jack long to learn what all the different bugle calls meant. He was very gentle and obedient with the men of his regiment, but he supposedly hated rebels, and he wouldn't have anything to do with them, even when they offered him yummy food. The first job of new regiment was to defend Washington DC, which they did until March, 1862. After that, they fought in many battles, including Yorktown, Williamsburg, Fair Oaks, Malvern Hill, Antietam, Fredericksburg, Gettysburg, Rappahannock, Wilderness, Spotsylvania, Petersburg, Sailor's Creek, and Appomattox.

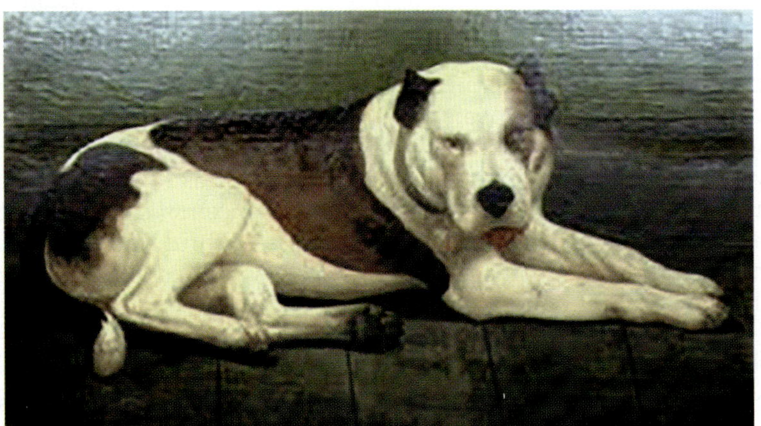

The 102nd mustered out on June 28, 1865. Out of the original 2,100 soldiers that joined up, 10 officers and 169 men were killed or died from their wounds; 23 officers and 518 men were wounded, 1 officer and 37 men died of disease, and 5 officers and 131 men were captured or went missing. This added up to 39 officers and 905 men. Jack did several important jobs in his regiment. If the men were marching and got really thirsty, Jack ran ahead to find water, and then he hurried back to tell them by barking loudly. If the men didn't have any rations to eat, Jack went out and caught chickens for them. After a battle, Jack searched the field for wounded soldiers from his regiment. At the Battle of Malvern Hill, Jack got wounded, but he recovered. Subsequently rebels captured him at Savage's Station, but somehow he escaped from prison. Jack was wounded again at the Battle of Fredricksburg, and he almost died, but the soldiers in his unit managed to nurse him back to health. Later, during the Chancellorsville Campaign, Jack was taken prisoner again, along with 94 men, and this time he was held as a POW for six months at Belle Isle. After that, he got exchanged, just like any other soldier.

When Jack returned to his regiment, he went with them through the Battle of the Wilderness, the Spotsylvania campaigns and the siege of Petersburg. His men were so grateful to him that they collected $75 to buy him a fancy silver collar as a tribute. They gave the collar to him in a special ceremony on December 23, 1864.

While the 102nd was on furlough at Frederick, Maryland, Jack disappeared. The men looked everywhere for him and offered a big reward for his return but he was never seen again. It's very possible that Jack was stolen or killed by somebody who wanted his silver collar or may be he had some kind of accident or just wandered off and died at some place. There's really no way we will ever know what happened to Jack.

LEO

Leo, a Poodle, had been for years the most attached and faithful companion of Acton. He had been sheared and trimmed up into the shape and appearance of a most ferocious Lion, but this was only in outward resemblance otherwise he had a kind and playful spirit. He possessed wonderful instinct and sagacity, and performed many amusing pranks and tricks such as fetching anything from his master's room which he desired him to bring. His forte, however, was in aquatic displays, particularly in diving or leaping overboard and then scrambling up again by a rope thrown over the side. Leo was the constant attendant on his master on all occasions of bathing. Acton was part of a piratical expedition to Porto Bello in Panama in 1819 headed up by the "Cacique of Poyais" aka the adventurer Sir Gregor M'Gregor. On 30th April, 1819, Acton had been on an out-picket during the night and after returning on 1st May, 1819, he went for bathing. While enjoying this luxury, after the fatigue of the night, the enemy came suddenly. Acton was defenceless, escape was impossible and the enemy bayoneted him in cold blood. His faithful Leo made a vigorous attack on the barbarous miscreants and was severely wounded, in the vain endeavour to defend his master.

MOUSTACHE

The heroic and hair raising tales of Mascot Dogs in war speak volumes on their bravery, devotion and faithfulness for their masters. This brave dog was the pet of French Grenadiers regiment and took active part in various campaigns during the Napoleon wars. At the Battle of Marengo fought on 14th June, 1800, between French Forces under Napoleon Bonaparte and Austrian Forces, near the city of Alessandria, in Piedmont, Italy, the dog detected an Austrian spy, and thus saved the soldiers from a surprise attack by the enemy. His crowning achievement was at the Battle of Austerlitz fought on 2nd December, 1805, between the French Army and Russo-Austrian Army (Third Coalition), in Moravia, when a young ensign bearing the regimental colours, mortally wounded and surrounded by the enemy, with a dying effort attempted to save the flag by wrapping round his body. Moustache went to rescue and could understand what for the soldier had given his life. He successfully unfolded the strand with his teeth and paws and carrying it in his mouth, brought it back, in triumph to his lines, despite his leg wounded while saving the flag of the regiment. Moustache was awarded a medal of gallantry and his name was placed on the regimental books as a full-fledged soldier drawing rations and pay. This dog was decorated by Le Marechal Jean Lanes (Marshal of the Empire) on the eve of battle of Austerlitz and was entitled to wear a tri-colour collar with a silver medal, engraved on one side "Moustache, a French dog, a brave fighter entitled to respect". He was presented to the Emperor Napoleon for whom he performed various tricks, including his most famous one, lifting his leg at the mention of the Emperor's enemies. He followed his battalion when it was ordered to the Peninsula, and at the siege of Badajoz a cannon ball hit Moustache. The bravest dog fell dead on the ground and his comrades buried him where he fell. A stone was put to his memory with one word of tribute: "Brave' Moustache."

MOUTON

Mouton was a Poodle who was picked up in Spain in 1808 by a French Regiment and he accompanied the Regiment to Germany the following year. As a Regimental dog, Mouton participated in battle of Aspern-Essling from May 21–22, 1809 and battle of Wagram on July 5–6, 1809 in Austria. After the battle, Mouton followed his Regiment back to Spain in 1810. While en route, Mouton had all four legs frozen and could not walk. He was carried by a sergeant of his regiment on his back. Later, Mouton set off with the regiment for Russia in the spring of 1812, but got lost in Saxony. Subsequently, he recognized an echelon of the Regiment by the uniform, and followed it all the way for participating in more battles.

MUCHUCH

After the battle of Talavera July 27–28, 1809 in south west of Madrid, General Thomas Graham, afterwards Lord Lynedoch, was told of a large Poodle dog, marked with brown patches and part of his one ear shot off in battle, lying on the grave of a Spanish officer. It is difficult to visualize the sequence of events leading to the death of his master and his efforts to save him in the battle field but the Poodle was still guarding his master's grave. On hearing the story, General Graham desired the dog to be brought to his quarters, but the servant returned without him, and said the dog would not allow him to come near. General Graham then ordered him to take as many soldiers as were necessary to secure and bring him away. The dog was brought with difficulty and stayed with General Graham for some time. Later, the Poodle was sent to Scotland to the Graham of Fintry, who was a friend of the General. There the dog stayed with the new master and very soon became friendly to the environment. In those days the guns from the Castle announced many victories, and when they were fired Muchuch was noticed in a state of great excitement. Once the house-door was opened, he used to run direct to the Castle and straight to the battery amongst the men. After a while he became most popular with troops and was regularly expected and welcomed on such occasions. The soldiers loved and appreciated his gestures. Mochuch lived the remainder life peacefully at Fintry.

It will be interesting to know about General Thomas Graham, a Scottish landowner, born on 19th October, 1748 and began his military career at the age of 50 years. His wife Mary's poor health led the couple to live mainly abroad in warmer climates. They went in the spring of 1792 to the south of France, but the expedient proved unavailing, and she died on board ship, off the coast near Hyères, on 26th June, 1792. As her body was returning to England for burial, her coffin was callously opened and searched by French Revolutionary Authorities causing Graham to develop a passionate franco phobia and he decided to take revenge. He volunteered for British Army's action in 1793 against the French at Toulon, one of the few places which held out against the French Revolutionary Government.

Napoleon Bonaparte was then a Lieutenant of artillery and rose to prominence through his part in the siege. The following year he raised 1st Battalion of the 90th Regiment of Foot (Perthshire Volunteers). Despite his obvious passion and talent, Graham was not initially given a permanent commission, but still served with the Regiment as its Colonel at Quiberon. In 1796, he became a liaison officer with the Austrian Army in Italy. Graham saw extensive service with the Austrian Army fighting against the French. His next campaigns came with Sir John Moore, firstly to Sweden in 1808 and then into Spain. After the battle of Corunna in Spain on 16th January 1809, his temporary status was made permanent and Colonel Graham was promoted to the rank of Major General. He was appointed, in the summer of 1809, to command a division in the fatal Walcheren expedition. A year later he was promoted as Lt General and took command of the British troops at Cadiz. He served with the British Army, notably in the Peninsular War where in 1811 he led the victory over the French at Barrosa. In 1813, he fought at Vittoria and San Sebastian before taking command of a British force sent to Holland in 1814. On 3rd May, 1814, he was raised to the peerage by the title of Baron Lynedoch, of Balgowan in the County of Perth. He was promoted to the full rank of General in 1821 and in 1829 was appointed Governor of Dumbarton Castle.

OLD HARVEY

Old Harvey, a Pit Bull Terrier, was the Mascot for the 104th Ohio Infantry. The dog had a great love of music. He provided companionship and humour for the troops. Harvey would show his great love for music by swaying from side to side while the soldiers sang campfire songs in the evening. He was wounded in two different battles but survived each time. Harvey's tag read "I am Lieutenant DN Stearns' Dog. Who's Dog Are You?"

The 104th had a portrait of Harvey commissioned so that he could still be part of their reunions after his death. Harvey is remembered by the Western Reserve Historical Society in Cleveland, where a portrait of the troop features a proud Harvey posing with his fellow soldiers.

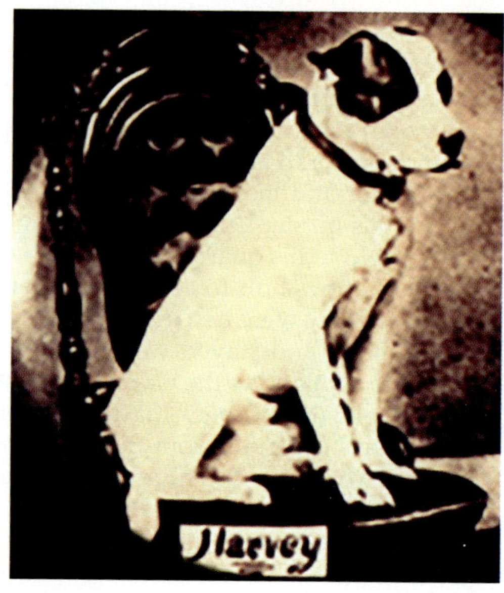

Old Harvey

SALLIE

During the American Civil War 1861 to 1865, the Eleventh Regiment of Pennsylvania Volunteers was organized in May, 1861, under the command of Colonel P Jarrett to put down the rebellion. One morning a civilian presented a four-week-old pup to 1st Lt William R Terry, the Captain of one company and she was soon named Sallie Ann Jarrett, after the names of the Commander and a young lady of the nearby town. Sallie, a Pit Bull Terrier, pug nosed and brindle in colour, friendly and loving became the official regimental mascot. Sallie won the affections of the regiment and very soon came to know the drum roll and participated in exercises. In April, 1862, the regiment proceeded south to engage the rebels, and remained active in the bloody struggles of the next three years. Sallie went everywhere with her men and inspired them with her remarkable endurance. She was never confused about who was in "her" regiment and who wasn't, recognizing her own even when they were out of uniform.

During the spring of 1863, one year after entering the active phase of the war, the regiment, while encamped across the Rappahannock River at Fredericksburg, VA, march passed along with other regiments at a review of the Union Army. The President of USA, Abraham Lincoln, sat in the centre of the reviewing stand. Sallie as usual at the head of her column marched along with her soldiers. The Commander-in-Chief raised his hand in a half-salute of recognition to some officers in the preceding regiment, and noticed Sallie. He doffed his stovepipe hat as a special tribute, possibly thinking of his own beloved dog, Fido. The little Sallie, seemed as proud as her men to be thus honoured by their Commander-in-Chief.

True to the traditions of man's best friend, Sallie never deserted her companions, even when the fields were crowded with fallen soldiers. She licked the hand of those victims who still moved and guarded those who didn't. At the battle of Gettysburg (1st July–3rd July, 1863), during the first day of battle, the regiment was forced to retreat back to town from Oak Ridge and lost track of Sallie in the commotion. She was located 3 days later at their original position guarding the lifeless bodies of her comrades. On May 8, 1864, Sallie was shot in the neck at Spotsylvania and had to be taken to the hospital, but the bullet (a Minie ball) could not be safely removed. A few days later, she returned to active duty. Her first performance "was to tear the seat out of the pants of a young conscript from another regiment" who ran and tried to retreat through the ranks of the Eleventh Regiment. Several months later, the cyst in her neck, developed into the size of an egg and ruptured, releasing the foreign object, the minie ball. The wound began to heal in time leaving a noticeable and honourable battle scar.

By the beginning of 1865, it became obvious that the South could not hold out much longer. On 5th February, 1865, in the morning hours, the troops marched with Sallie at the head, to a position near Petersburg (Battle of Hatcher's Run), Virginia, where the regiment encountered fierce opposition. Among the dead of the Eleventh were one Sergeant and one of the privates whereas two men were badly wounded. In the middle of this group lay the "Brindle Bull Terrier", shot through the head. Sallie had served faithfully from the beginning of the war which was to end barely two months later. However, for her and so many of her friends the war had an earlier end. While still under attack, the men buried her where she lay on the battlefield. In 1890, a monument was erected and dedicated to "Those in the Regiment". It recognizes all those who fought and died on the Gettysburg Battlefield from the 11th Pennsylvania Infantry. At the base of this great bronze and marble structure lays the resemblance of Sallie facing the west from where the rebel forces had approached. One ear is cocked as if listening for the rustle of leaves that would call her to act again.

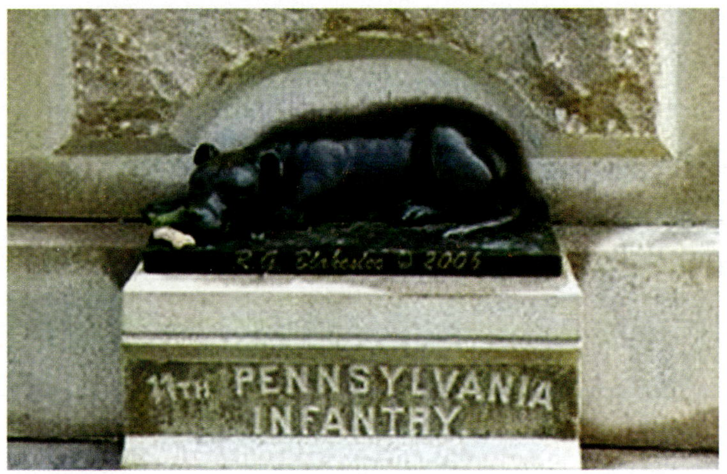

Sallie

SANCHO

A large white Poodle was rescued from the battlefield at Salamanca in France on 22nd July, 1812, and adopted by the Marquis of Worcester (Lord Worcester, Henry Somerset, 1792–1853). This faithful Poodle had been found lying on the grave of his master, a Lieutenant in the defeated French army. The dog was found exhausted and nearly starved to death. Sancho was forced away from becoming a sacrifice to its fidelity. A print was issued showing Lord Worcester with his Poodle, Sancho. The story of Sancho's devotion and faithfulness proved to be extremely popular and subsequently another print was issued showing the dog lying upon his master's grave.

5

War Dogs of World War I

"A dog is the only thing on earth that loves you more than he loves himself."

... Josh Billings

During World War I, the dog became a symbol of patriotism and a literal soldier serving alongside both the Allied and Central Powers in Europe. Ernest Baynes, a journalist, journeyed to the war zone in order to document the particular uses of dogs, among other animals. He reported that Mascots brought from home, while untrained, were familiar and helped men to cope up with life in the trenches. Messenger dogs served a dual purpose, to spare the lives of human runners and to speed delivery time. Other dogs served as Sentries or Scouts, accompanying night patrols and alerting their handlers to nearby combatants. Hefty Draught Dogs were used to transport ammunitions over long distances. Most famously, dogs assisted the Red Cross workers by locating and transporting wounded soldiers back to hospitals. Jack Russell Terriers, small dogs with a penchant for hunting rats patrolled the trenches to keep vermin away from soldiers and supplies. The YMCA used small Terriers to distribute free cigarettes to the troops known as "Cigarette Dogs." The war elevated the status of the useful and heroic dog to a nearly human level for the benefit of the nation's prospects in the trenches.

The Russian Army Command did not give due attention to the use of dogs before World War I. Russian Sanitary Dogs were trained to search for the wounded and guide rescuers to them. There were no more than 300 dogs in the Russian Army during World War I. In 1914, the Russian Imperial Army put its dog programme on display. The exhibition proved that dogs could carry heavy loads, work under gunfire, transport ammunition, etc. It is interesting to know that although the United States Army expressed interest in a war dog programme as early as 1896, when it translated and distributed a collection of essays on the treatment, training, and employment of war dogs in the German Army, yet during World War I, they did not have their own Military Working Dogs. American Troops had to depend on the French, Belgian and British troops for trained Sentry and Courier dogs. At one point, the US Army borrowed French-trained dogs for sentry duty, but the plan was eventually aborted because the dogs only responded to commands in French. However, Mascot Dogs of various formations and units participated in war and some American Troops brought dogs along with them in battle field unofficially. It was typical for soldiers to outfit their dogs with masks made for humans prior to the development of specialized animal masks. Many reporters used sentimental language and editorialized photographs of service animals with their human counterparts.

Of all the Allies during World War I, the French used more dogs and in the most ways. The French War Dog Service was established shortly after the beginning of World War I in 1914, and its success was largely due to the untiring efforts of Sgt Paul Megnin, who later became Chief of the Service. Even though the French Military had used sentry dogs as early as the 18th century, Sgt Megnin still had to overcome the prejudices of commanders who could not be easily convinced to use the dogs tactically in the war zone. The French War Dog Service organized two kennels near Paris and a third in Normandy for the training of dogs and a fourth was being contemplated at the time the Armistice was signed in 1918. As soon as the four-footed defenders had completed their training, the handlers were sent to the school at Satory for an eight-day course in dog handling. During this time they became thoroughly acquainted with the particular animals with which they were to work at the front. Besides using Auxiliary Sentry Dogs, the French also had what they called Enclosure Dogs and training of such dogs lasted from ten days to two weeks. These were simply efficient watch dogs who were set free at night inside an enclosed area, such as a factory yard. Tracker Dogs were trained for at least three months. Pack and Driving Dogs (these were large powerful breeds not qualified for other army work) were used for pulling machine guns, mortar and supply carts and as Pack Dogs. The French Messenger Dogs were divided into two classes, i.e. Estafettes, who were trained to run with a message from one point to another, and the Liaison Dogs, trained to return with an answer to the message.

The French employed Chiens De Brie, large sheep dogs, in sentry duties During severe winter in 1915, some 400 Sled Dogs mostly Huskies, were brought by France from Canada to operate in deep snow. Heavy winter snows in the Vosges Mountains

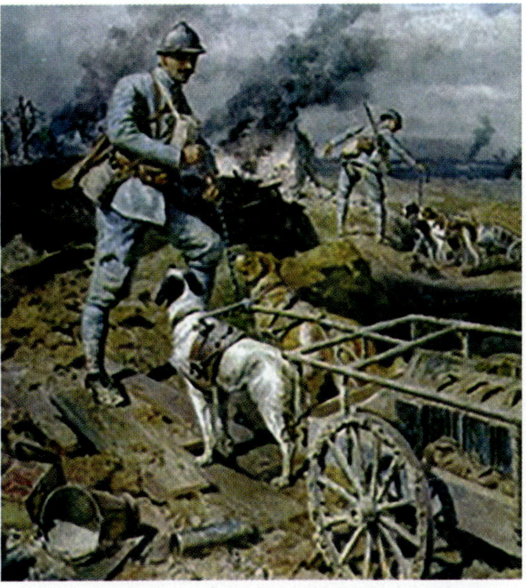

French dogs pulling ammunition carriage

were holding back French supply lines, mules and horses could not breach the impasse to move artillery and ammunition. More than 400 Sled Dogs were brought from Alaska to Quebec, where the dogs boarded a cargo ship bound for France. These dogs hauled ammunition, aided soldiers in the work of laying communication lines and helped transporting wounded soldiers to field hospitals. Even when the shells were singing, one could see half a mile long line of dog teams tearing down the mountain to the base depot and every blue devil whooping and yelling, while trying to pass the one ahead.

In 1916, the French Army issued a special citation to the memory of "Medor No. 6", a Messenger Dog that completed his mission to deliver a message despite being struck with bullets along the way. Similarly, Jacques, whom the soldiers spoke of "as they would with a fellow soldier" won special recognition by defending his machine gun company against assault and facilitating the capture of five German Soldiers. Sgt Helen Kaiser, an American-bred War Dog serving in the French Army, survived poison gas attacks and shrapnel wounds. Her regiment awarded her the "Croix de Guerre"(France's highest military honour) twice. Even President Wilson showed his appreciation for war dogs by inviting Nellie, the twice-injured Mascot Dog of the Belgian Army, to a garden party at the White House. During the war, French used 20,000 dogs. The casualties of dogs during the war exceeded 3500 whereas 1500 were declared missing. At the end of war, French Army had to dispose off more than 15,000 dogs.

In 1915, the Belgian Army used Carabineers, strong-muscled dogs called Bouvier des Flandres, to haul heavy cannons to the front. These Draught Dogs easily pulled, towed gun carriages. Italians used 3000 dogs during this war. In Alpine areas, climbing narrow paths where horses or mules could not venture. Germany had a long tradition of military dogs and had the war's best-trained canine force. In the 1870s, the German Military began coordinating with local dog clubs for training and breeding dogs for combat. They established the first Military Dog School in 1884. During the Herrero Campaign (1904–1907) in German South West Africa, (a former German colony (1884–1919) that is now the nation of Namibia), 60 war dogs were deployed by the armies and these dogs saved the troops from enemy ambushes in the dense terrain. When hostilities were declared in August, 1914 the German Army had 6,000 trained war dogs ready for action. In addition, the army was able to call on a reserve pool of trained dogs from the German Police Force. Messenger Dogs became an acknowledged part of the organization in the German Army. An infantry regiment was allocated a maximum of twelve dogs, while a battalion might have six. The allocations were made by the Messenger Dog Section (Meldehundstaffel) at the Army Headquarters. The breeds chiefly employed for message-carrying work were German Shepherds, Dobermans, Airedale Terriers and Rottweilers. The Germans, unlike the British, employed the dogs on the double-journey liaison principle, that is, two handlers per dog. At the end of World War I, some German dogs were taken over by the allies for use and breeding. Many more, however, were destroyed, following the German defeat as military restrictions and the overall economy could not sustain anywhere near previous peacetime numbers. However, Germany under Hilter ignored the Versailles Treaty and military numbers were slowly increased. With a restricted army of 100,000 men, Germany found the war dog to be a great force multiplier. They founded the Military Kennels at Frankfurt in 1934 and by 1939 had about 50,000 trained war dogs ready for use. As German

Forces advanced into both Belgium and France, they lost no time in taking control of all suitable dogs and sending them back to Germany to be trained. Once trained, the dogs were drafted to kennels. Each army platoon had one kennel from which dogs were issued to the front-line troops. At the peak of the war, Germany's dog force numbered more than 30,000 which included Messengers, Sanitatshunde (Red Cross dogs), Draught animals and Guards, etc.

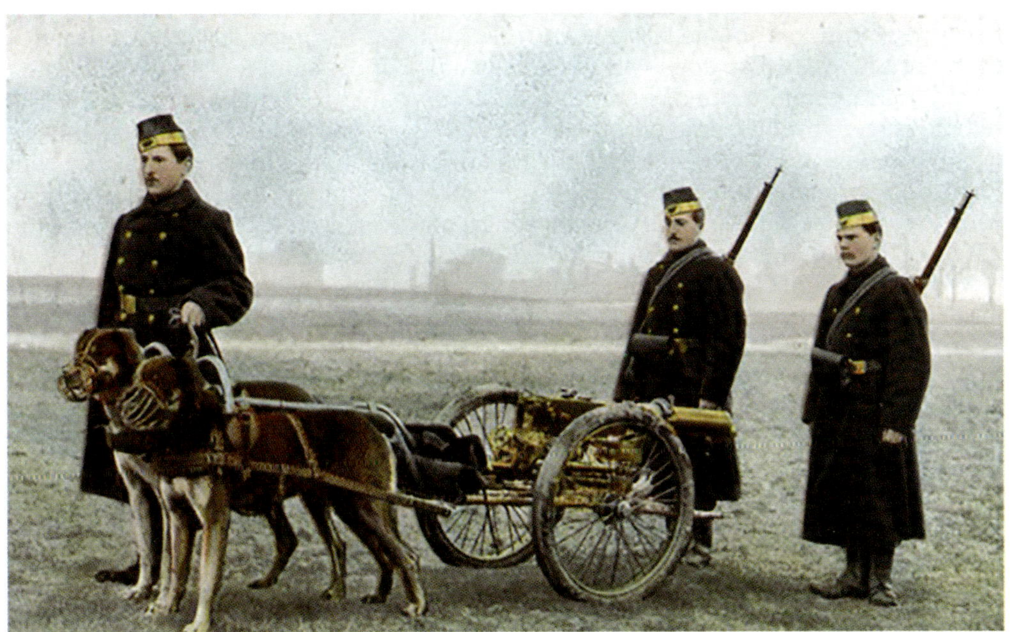

Dogs pulling the Belgian Machine Gun

In Britain, when war broke out in 1914, there were no Military Dogs attached to the British Army except one sole Airedale, who served with the 2nd Battalion Norfolk Regiment as a sentry and accompanied the battalion to France where it was eventually killed by a shell on the Aisne. The British War Dog programme was underway. Lt Col Edwin Hautenville Richardson, a dog enthusiast, after attending Sandhurst and serving in the Sherwood Foresters, he settled down at his farm with his wife Blanche, a fellow dog-lover. Richardson was convinced of the essential role, dogs could play in wartime and had built up a large kennel of dogs at his farm. They started experimental training of the Red Cross dogs on the farm at Carnoustie on the east coast of Scotland. In early August, 1914, Richardson offered his services to the British Red Cross Society and travelled with some trained dogs to Belgium, but when he arrived in Brussels, the Germans were entering the city and so left immediately and made his way back to Britain via Ostend. It soon became clear that the Red Cross dogs could not be used practically since they were being shot and killed without regard to the wearing of the Red Cross. Hence, Richardson began to train and supply dogs for sentry and patrol work. He concluded that Airedale Terriers displayed the ideal combination of qualities. Later, in the winter of 1916, an Officer from the Royal Artillery wrote to Richardson for training of Messenger

Dogs for his regiment to facilitate communication in battlefield, as the trained dogs would be able to keep up communication between his outpost and the battery during a heavy bombardment, when noise and communication difficulties rendered telephones practically useless and the risk to human runners was enormous. Richardson, after a number of experiments, successfully trained two Airedales to carry messages for two miles without a hitch and on New Year's Eve, the two dogs, named Wolf and Prince, departed to France to be used as message carriers. One of their first tasks was to carry a message four miles to Brigade Headquarters from the front line through a smoke barrage and this task was completed within an hour. It soon became clear that dogs were faster, steadier, more nimble across shell holes, muddy terrain, and more difficult to spot as compared to human messengers. The two dogs were trailblazer and both served with great success with the 56th Brigade RFA, 11th Div. at Wytschaete Ridge. Airedales were then widely trained and sent to the front for many different and highly important military jobs such as Messengers, Sentries and Red Cross Dogs. The sterling work performed by these dogs made Airedale Terrier, the most popular breed in Britain during and after the war.

With Wolf and Prince having proved the usefulness at the front, demand for more Messenger Dogs grew and Lt Col Richardson was asked by the War Office to establish his British War Dog School in 1917. The Official sanction of the use of dogs in war was given with the opening of the War Dog Training School (WDTS) in Shoeburyness, in order to train dogs principally to act as messengers and sentries close to the front line. Major Waley, was appointed supervisor of all dog operations in the field, once the dogs arrived in France. The main kennels were at Etaples under the command of the RE Signal Corps, who took over the operations in early 1917. Sectional kennels were set up not far behind the front line. Each Sectional kennel had on an average, one Sergeant-in-Charge, 16 handlers and 48 dogs and all of them from RE Signals Corps. The dogs then went to the active sectors at the ratio of 3 dogs to 1 handler, who then handed them over to selected individuals from the Infantry Battalions in the designated Brigade. The original handler was then based at the Brigade Headquarters to oversee the dogs operations.

At the British War Dog School (WDTS), in the beginning the dogs came from the Battersea Dogs Home in London for training. As demand grew, dogs were obtained from Bristol, Liverpool, Birmingham and Manchester Dogs Homes. More and more demand of trained dogs, outstripped the 'suppliers', and an official order was issued to all police forces in the UK to send all strays to the War Dog School. Even the general public was requested to send in any dogs they were unable to keep properly with the ration system in effect. The response was excellent and many family pets were soon doing their bit for king and country. Many of the letters accompanying the donated dogs were heart-rending. One little girl wrote, 'We have let Daddy go to fight the Kaiser, and now we are sending Jack to do his bit', or a lady whose letter read, "I have given my husband and my sons, and now that he too is required, I give my dog." Certain breeds were considered better suited to the task, particularly Sheep dogs, Collies, Lurchers, Irish Terriers, Welsh Terriers, Deerhounds and of course, Airedales. Fox Terriers were considered too fond of play, Retrievers were too compliant and unlikely to show an independence of thought while any dog with a gaily carried tail, which curled over its back or sideways, was considered rarely of any value. The WDTS at Shoeburyness continued to train and send out dogs not only to France and Belgium but also for use as Guards and Sentries on the

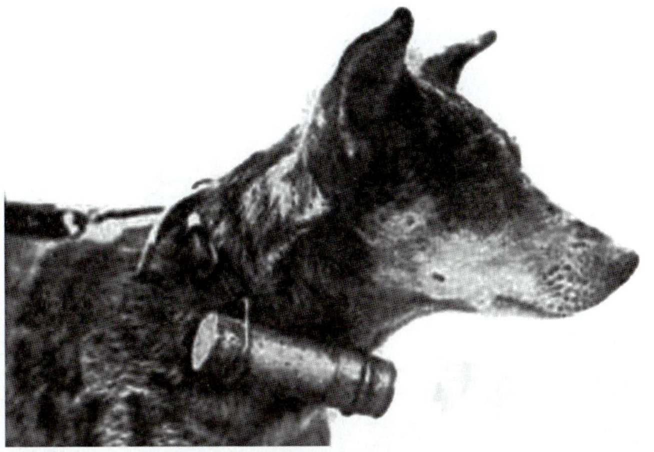

Messenger Dog with a canister

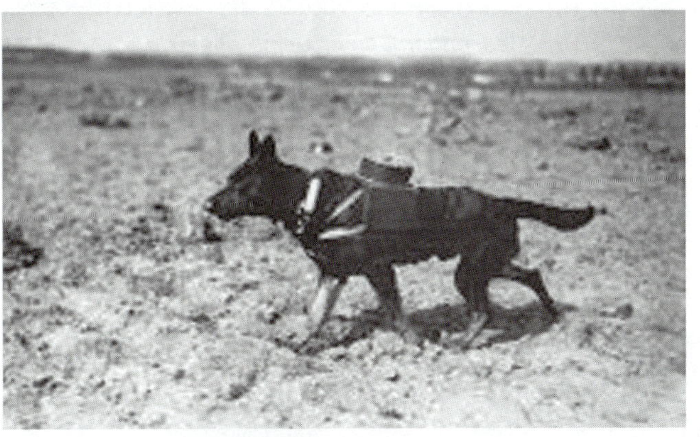

Messenger Dog in action

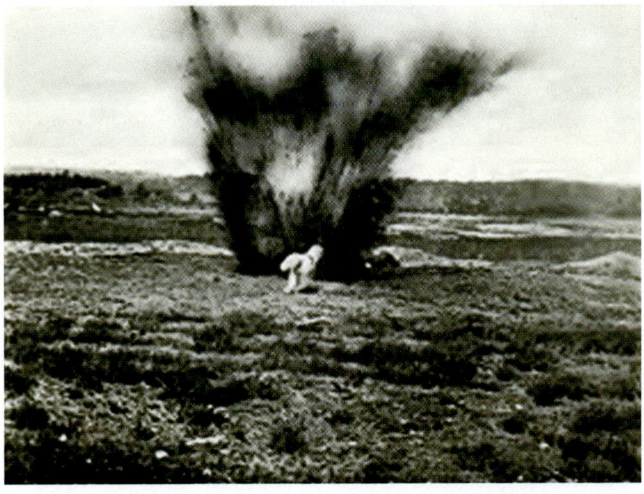

Messenger Dog running before an explosion

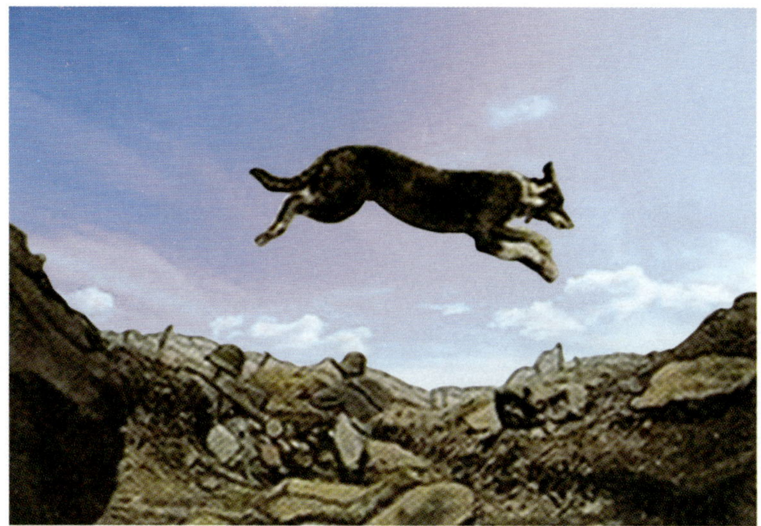

Messenger Dog crossing obstacle

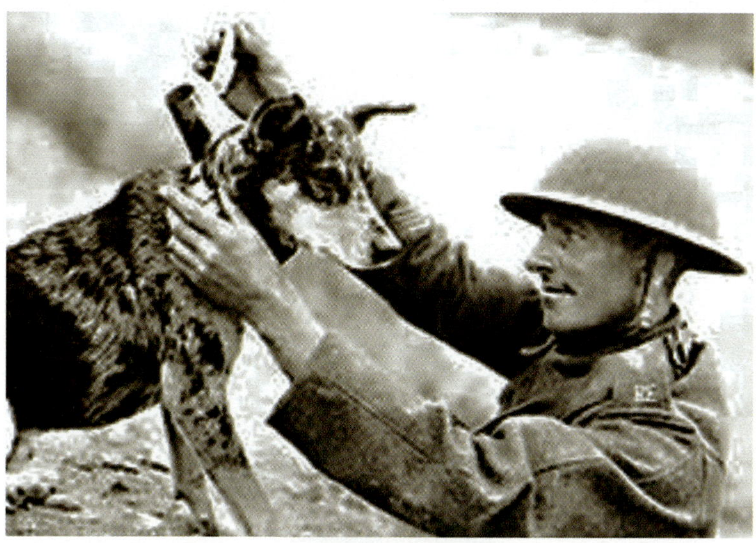

Retrieving message

home front, as well as in Salonika. The WDTS was later moved to Matley Ridge, Lyndhurst in 1918 and it was finally moved to Bulford on Salisbury Plains in May, 1999. The value of Messenger Dogs was demonstrated in war for traversing heavy, sticky mud which was a major obstacle to movement. Perhaps the ultimate accolade for the dog's role in the British Army came from Field-Marshal Haig who "acknowledged their essential role in his final dispatch of the war".

Every War Dog who contributed towards the combat efforts was a hero, however, it is not possible to describe each hero in this text, hence, some bravest of the brave considered to be the legendary dogs of World War I, have been chosen as representatives of a large number of famous War Dogs of World War I era.

AIREDALE JACK

Jack, an Airedale dog recruited by the British Army from the Battersea Dogs Home in London and trained at the War Dog Training School. He was sent to the trenches in France where he worked as a Messenger Dog. Every day, Jack went from area to area, through no man's land, often when battles were raging. During a particularly fierce battle his battalion came under heavy fire and was in severe danger of being overcome by the enemy. The Battalion needed immediate reinforcement and ammunition. It was also well-known that no human runner would survive the barrage of gunfire to get a message out. Lt. Hunter of the battalion slipped a message into the Jack's collar and said, "Goodbye Jack. Go back boy". Jack ran off, staying close to the ground, taking advantage of whatever cover there was and running through deep swamps. The Germans were advancing and Jack's Battalion held out little hope of survival. Everybody in Battalion was thinking that, will it be possible for the brave little animal to make it through the battlefield and deliver the urgent message asking for reinforcements. Previously, Jack had proved time and again that he was an efficient and brave 'soldier' but this seemed to be an almost impossible task even for him. The soldiers were beginning to resign themselves to certain death but their final hope was Jack. When Jack left the trenches with his message, the soldiers must have wished him well but without a great deal of optimism as he left under heavy fire. The battalion watched Jack stagger on and soon he began to get hit and a piece of shrapnel smashed his jaw. A missile ripped open his black and tan coat from shoulder to thigh but still he continued using shell holes and trenches for cover. Suddenly, his forepaw was hit and he fell. Jack dragged himself along the ground on three legs and despite a very seriously wounded leg, and a broken jaw, he arrived at his destination covered in blood and in an appalling condition. But the message was delivered. Despite all odds, Jack had made it through. The battalion was saved, thanks to his heroism, but his wounds were too serious for him to survive. Within minutes of delivering his vital message, Jack slipped away. He was posthumously awarded the Victoria Cross for his bravery.

MARQUIS

Marquis, a regimental dog of the 23rd Foot, was picked by the French Regiment outside St Etienne. This dog was carefully smuggled into the train as a play thing for the soldiers. Subsequently, he was trained to carry messages in battlefield and served as a Dispatch Dog with the French army. Marquis never cared a bit for the firing line, the shells, or the bullets and accomplished the given task with courage, speed and diligence. In November, 1914, Marquis was sent out on a fatal mission to deliver an important message through heavy fire when it was considered unsafe to send an human messenger, owing to the intensity of German fire. He moved with great speed crossing the hurdles but while jumping over a trench, he received a bullet wound and fell. Marquis managed to crawl back to his location with the message undelivered and letting it drop out of his mouth, stained with blood at his master's feet. Marquis was one of the earliest casualties of the war in 1914. The French Government acknowledged his sacrifice by announcing his death among the other human casualties of the day. His soldier comrades buried him and raised funds to erect a monument over his grave duly inscribed "Marquis-Killed on the field of Honour."

A poem dedicated to the brave dog Marquis, on the occasion of the centenary of the First World War 1914–1918, to remember the war animals who gave their lives for us, is reproduced below:

The regimental dog of the 23rd Foot killed on the field of honour
So the campaign is done at last
O! Little soldier dog
Thy brief, brave course is run out at last
Good little faithful dog
***
Just picked by the regiment
Outside St Etienne
You were carefully smuggled into the train
As a play thing for the men
***
You 'went for' a German in uniform
As the 'Tommies' taught you to do
But you carried messages round your neck
When they found how much you could do
***
So you played a game of life and death
And it was just a 'game' to you
But the messages hid in your curly fur
Their import you never knew
***
And you never cared for the firing line
The shells, or the bullets a bit
And it seemed that the luck was all on your side
And you really could never get hit
***
But they got you at last, little 'soldier dog'
Within two bounds of the trench
And when the soldiers saw you fall
I'll bet that was a wrench
***
For there was another messenger
Who went even faster than you
And he caught you up as you galloped along
But you got your message through
***
And just as they got that message off
And the last knot untied
Did you know the 'game' was done at last
And so, little dog, you died?
***
There are plenty of dogs who will bark at a 'Hun'
And lie down and die for a King
Yes, and jump up the moment we've counted to ten
But, by jove, you have done the real thing
***

So they've put your name on the honours roll
Amongst the casualty list
"Marquis" on the field of honour killed
And I can't see your name for a mist
***
O! theres many a man in England today
Who would envy the death you died
Though only a dog, you have died for your King
You have died for a nations pride
***
And you've earned for yourself a soldiers grave
Although you're only a dog
And you lie where your masters and playmates lie
A soldier's 'Soldier Dog'
***

NELLIE

Nellie, the celebrated war dog was a wire hair Fox Terrier and the pet of a British Officer. In October, 1914, she participated with her master in first battle of Ypres in western Belgium also called Battle of Flanders which continued till November, 1914. Nellie faithfully remained besides her master even while facing rain of shrapnel and high explosive shells. During the course of battle, while boldly facing the storm of firing and explosives, the British Officer fell and died. Nellie was wounded and wandered about "No Man's Land" until picked up by Major Osterreith of the Belgian first Regiment of Guides and she transferred her allegiance to her new master.

Nellie lived in trenches for many months with the Belgian Regiment. She was always ready to "go over the top" with her new friends. She was wounded twice by shrapnel but she never thought of deserting. When Major Osterreith came to Washington, USA, with the Belgian Mission, Nellie accompanied her master. Even President Wilson showed his appreciation for war dogs by inviting Nellie, the twice-injured Dog Mascot of the Belgian Army, to a garden party at the White House. Thousands of Americans saw her little twinkling eyes and her stubby wagging tail acknowledging their attention and kindness.

Nellie died in October, 1917 due to age and after effects of shrapnel wounds sustained in war. Her passing caused more grief among the Belgian mission staff with whom Nellie was very friendly. She will always be remembered by her comrades as a real hero who went into the battle without faltering and was faithful to her master and friends to the very last. Her obituary column was published in Lewiston Maine Evening Journal on Tuesday, 23rd October, 1917 under the heading "Nellie, Celebrated War Dog dies of wounds and age in US."

RAGS

Rags was a Cairn Terrier mix who served as the mascot of the 1st Infantry Division during World War I. He joined in 1917 in France, and held his title until his death in 1931. Rag was recruited by Private James Donovan in peculiar circumstances. James overstayed his leave in Montremere and was declared absent without leave (AWOL). One day as a coincidence, two military policemen noticed him and enquired his where about. Just in a confused state of mind that he will now be caught, he tripped over a passerby small stray dog and replied that he was part of a search party, sent out to find the Division's Mascot. Thus James was out of hot water and Rags had a name and a job. Though he was a small dog, Rags relayed messages from the front lines. His greatest moment of heroism came during the Meuse-Argonne Campaign in 1918, when he ran a vital message through falling bombs. Although Rags was seriously affected by gases and was partially blinded, he survived but his master, however, was not so lucky and died during the campaign. In 1920, Rags was adopted by the family of Major Raymond W Hardenberg and lived his remaining life peacefully. He is buried at Aspen Hill Memorial Park, an Animal Sanctuary in Maryland.

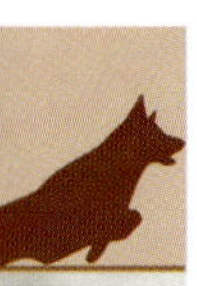

RIN TIN TIN

Celebrity dog RIN TIN TIN was considered as the most recognized name in the history of German Shepherd dog and likewise one of the oldest continuous bloodlines in this breed's history. On 15th September, 1918, when an American Infantry Regiment was checking a German war dog kennel in Lorraine, France, during World War I, they found the only survivor, a mother German Shepherd Dog and her litter. Corporal Lee Duncan of this unit picked one small pup of this litter and named after tiny (one inch tall) French puppets called Rin Tin Tin, that was given to American soldiers for good luck. After the war, Rin Tin Tin came to America with his master. In Feb, 1922, this dog while participating in a show organized at Shepherd Dog Club of America, amazed everyone with his ability to perform by jumping 11 feet and 9 inches. Subsequently, He became a matinee idol and acted in 26 films including the famous films such as "Jaws of Steel" and "Man from Hells River" produced by Warren brothers, the name of fledging studio on the verge of bankruptcy. Public loved Rin Tin Tin's performance in the films showing his heroic abilities. This dog was referred as mortgage lifter and credited with saving of the studio from financial ruin during the silent film era. He added to the folk lore and popularity of German Shepherd breed. This famous American dog is buried in a cemetery named as the "Cimetiere des Chiens" in the suburb of Asnieres by the side of River Seine in France. His tombstone is made up of fruity-black onyx with a gold leafed "star of the cinema" inscription.

SATAN

During one of the most horrifying battles of World War I, "German siege of Verdun", a French garrison was trapped, surrounded by enemy guns. The Siege of Verdun lasted for almost 10 months, and the death toll on both sides was heavy. By autumn of 1916, the German Army had surrounded the city taking possession of a ridge above the town and put them in position to prepare for a final attack.

Verdun was strategically vital to France, so it was important for the French Military stationed elsewhere to know the details of the battle regularly. At French Headquarters, Commanders were aware that the situation had taken a turn for the worse, and they wanted to get word to the soldiers and people of Verdun town that more military units were being sent. They were also hoping that somehow a message about the current situation might be sent back so that they could plan for what awaited them. During 1916, the year of the battle, seventeen French Soldiers had been killed carrying messages. Hence, a Messenger Dog named Satan, a black Grey Hound Collie

Mongre, was selected for the task. His handler was in Verdun so the Commanders felt that only Satan could get a message through. The first mile and a half of involved terrain had bushes and other forms of cover, Satan ran and crouched and again ran and crouched, watching his surroundings carefully. The last stretch for Satan, however, involved crossing open fields and making that part of the journey was dangerous.

Back in Verdun, French Soldiers were on the point of losing all hope as the garrison having run out of ammunition and food. Suddenly, soldiers on watch in Verdun happened to note that something seemed to be coming in their direction which was looking like a large-headed monster with wings. The watch command in Verdun alerted the Commandant, and as the military leader looked through his field glasses, the vision he was seeing was becoming clearer, a dog in a canine gas mask and something bulky attached to his back, flying at record speed. The dog was weaving in a zigzag pattern (as he had been taught) to make himself a more difficult target for a marksman. As it moved closer, the handler of Satan realised that it was his own messenger dog. He was wearing a gas mask and carrying two wicker baskets on either side of his back. Despite his best maneuver, as the dog was approaching towards garrison, he was hit and wounded by a German Sharpshooter. He staggered to his feet, reeling and dizzy and dropped on the ground and moments later, he paused to re-orient himself and continued on with slower pace. As he was nearing destination, Satan took another bullet in the leg but by now he was close enough and he could hear the men calling to him. He kept going, hobbling as fast as he could on three legs. All the soldiers at the French garrison were anxiously watching Satan's dare devil actions and utmost bıavery while negotiating various hurdles in the face of direct enemy fire in the battle field. Finally, Satan wounded with bullets reached near the French line and immediately soldiers stepped out to pick him up bringing him to safety. The message carried by the brave dog on his collar was retrieved, pleading the garrison to hold on and wait for the relief that has been sent. There were also two baskets on Satan's back, in each basket there was a pigeon.

The Commandant immediately wrote the details of the situation, specifying the exact locations of the German Troops. He wrote the same information twice, one note was rolled and placed into the quill carried by one pigeon and the other note was placed in the quill of the other pigeon. Both pigeons were released to take the message back to Headquarters and the French garrison watched with bated breath. The Germans, however, were expecting this and one pigeon was brought down almost immediately but the other escaped and flew away. One hour later, the French at Verdun got their answer. The pigeon had made it back to Headquarters. Long-range guns of the French Military took perfect aim at the German Battery encamped on the ridge above the town. Soon additional military reinforcements arrived and Verdun was saved. Subsequently, Satan recovered from his injuries and retired as a French hero. The heroism of Satan in delivering the message speak volume by itself.

SERGEANT HELEN KAISER

This brave dog was born in Potomac Park and was adopted by Private James White of 372nd Infantry Regiment. She moved in battle field with her owner and proved brave and dedicated while supporting the troops on the front lines. Sgt Helen Kaiser became the heroic war mascot of the First Separate Battalion, District National Guard, and was deployed with her owner James White of the 372nd Infantry Regiment of the 93rd Infantry

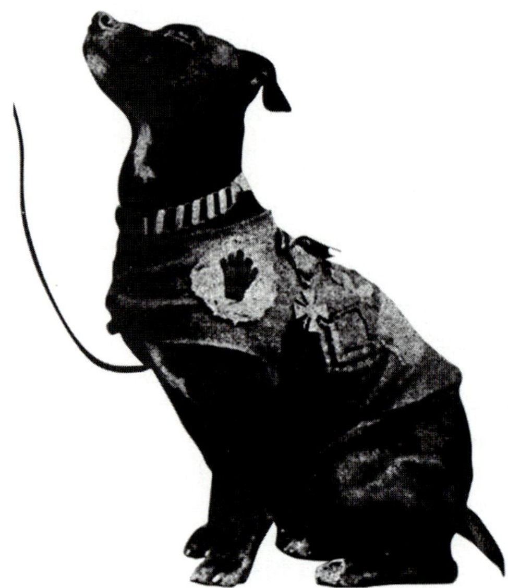

Division, an African-American division serving alongside the French Army in World War I. The Division comprised four Infantry Regiments, including the 372nd Coloured Infantry Regiment (staffed by 900 men from the 9th Separate Coloured Infantry Battalion of the Ohio National Guard and 9th Battalion units from Springfield). In 1918, the United States' Military Commanders refused to let black and white Americans fight side by side, but French leaders had no such objection. So when the 372nd Infantry Regiment arrived in France they were immediately assigned to the 157th Infantry Division of the French Army, the renowned "Red Hand Division", to help fight in the famous Meuse-Argonne Offensive and Battle of the Argonne Forest, fought from 26th September, 1918 till the Armistice on 11th November, 1918. In the combat, the 372nd suffered 616 casualties and 107 deaths but their advance was decisive in ending the war and the entire unit received the "Croix de Guerre" (France's highest military honour). The French Commanding General paid tribute, stating, "The 'Red Hand' sign of the Division, thanks to you, became a bloody hand, you have well-avenged our glorious dead."

During the war, Helen was wounded by shrapnel while in the Champagne Sector, fighting with the Red Hand Division. She was also exposed to blinding mustard gas but thankfully survived. Helen Kaiser was twice decorated with the "Croix de Guerre" by her Regiment for bravery in the trenches and promoted to the rank of Sergeant. She was the first American Dog to enter German territory. Helen survived the worst times in war and soon after the war was over, she returned to the USA with her owner James White. She lived a more peaceful existence thereafter in Washington, USA. On 10th March, 1919, Washington Times published a column on front page about Sergeant Helen Kaiser along with her photograph under the heading "DC War Hero, First American Dog to enter German Territory".

SERGEANT STUBBY

The most famous and bravest dog of World War I was a Pit Bull Terrier named Stubby who befriended American Soldiers at Yale University's football stadium.

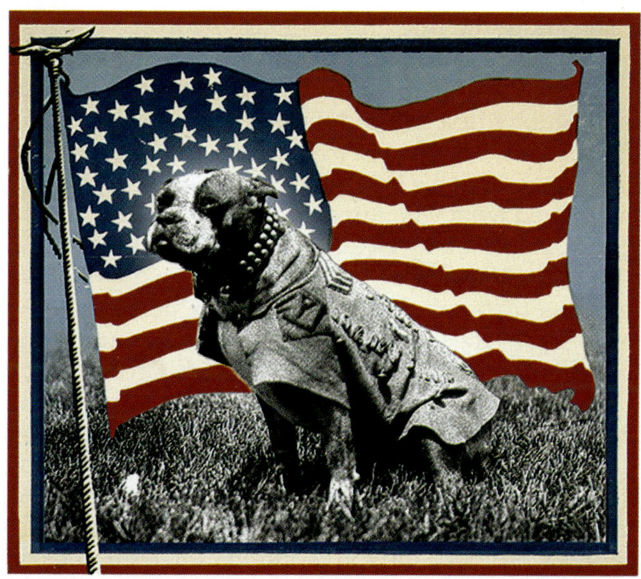

It was the site of Camp Yale, where the soldiers of the 102nd Infantry Regiment, part of the New England-based 26th "Yankee" Division, were doing basic training prior to their deployment. On a steamy summer morning, a non-descript dog wandered onto the massive field where the soldiers were doing exercises. He was not an impressive sight being short, barrel-shaped, with brown and white brindled stripes. The dog lingered around Camp Yale and J Robert Conroy, a 25 years old Private from New Britain, Connecticut, forged the closest bond with the mutt. The two were soon inseparable and he named the adopted dog as Stubby. Conroy had managed to keep the stray as a pet throughout his three-month training in Connecticut. In September, 1917, the 102nd Infantry Regiment was ready to ship out to France and Conroy was now facing problem as dogs were forbidden in the US Military. He felt that getting Stubby to Europe would be a more daunting challenge. The troops travelled by rail to Newport, a newly designated port of embarkation for soldiers heading to France. Here the 26th Division was slated to board one of the largest freighters navigating the Atlantic, the SS Minnesota. Conroy eluded the ship guards by concealing Stubby in his Army-issue greatcoat. He then hid him in the ship's coal bin but this arrangement did not last long as during the turbulent Atlantic crossing, Stubby was found out. However, the dog charmed his way into the good graces of the officers who discovered him by lifting his right paw in a salute. Out of hiding and free to roam the freighter, Stubby proved popular with the crew. By the time the troops disembarked in the port of Saint-Nazaire on France's Western Coast, Stubby was the 102nd Infantry's unofficial Mascot. Subsequently, Stubby became official Mascot of the 102nd Infantry Regiment and most famous American War Dog in World War I.

During February, 1918, the 102nd Infantry was bunkering along the lines of Chemin des Dames, the French-held "ladies path" on the Western Front, nervously anticipating the Germans' launch of a spring offensive. On St Patrick's Day, bells and klaxons, the signal of a poison gas attack rang out along the hillside in the Marne where Stubby and Conroy were stationed. For a full 24 hours, German gas shells rained down but somehow the dog and his master survived. It was at Chemin des Dames that Stubby reportedly saved the 102nd from a gas attack. One morning, while most of the troops were sleeping, the division was assaulted by an early morning gas launch. Stubby first smelled the gas then ran up and down the trenches barking and biting soldiers, working to rouse them from slumber and getting them to safety. On April 5, Stubby got his first military rank and became a Private first class. 26th Division soon moved from Chemin des Dames to nearby towns of Saint-Mihiel and Seicheprey. The 102nd Infantry Headquarters were set up near a dangerous spot 1 1/2 miles north of Mandres-aux-Quatre-Tours known as "Dead Man's Curve" because the hazardous turn required oncoming vehicles to slow down and the location made easy prey for the German Artillery. Stubby and company were placed in support positions to wait for a German breakthrough. On April 20, near Seicheprey, the Germany Infantry led one of its first attacks against American Troops. Almost 3,000 German Stosstruppen (Shock Troops) fired on, and overwhelmed a small contingent of 600 American Soldiers from the 26th Division. Fighting was so intense that Maj George Rau, Commander of the 102nd, ordered his cooks, truck drivers, and even the marching band into the fray. The Germans claimed victory, leaving 81 allied troops killed, 424 wounded, and 130 captured. Seicheprey sustained the heaviest losses in the Saint-Mihiel Sector. Stubby got his first war wound at Seicheprey, when a German shell fragment lodged in his left foreleg.

By June, however, Stubby had recovered and was back in action. When the 102nd reached Chateau Thierry in July, the dog had evidently learned to distinguish the uniform of Americans from that of German Soldiers. Stubby became the dog hero of 17 battles including 4 offensives. He took part in the brutal offensives of Saint-Mihiel, Aisne-Marne, the Champagne-Marne and the Meuse-Argonne. In the battle of Argonne, Stubby sniffed out a lost German Soldier hiding in nearby bushes. The dog gave chase and holding on to the seat of his pants, kept the stunned German pinned till the soldiers arrived to complete the capture. To the victor go the spoils, the Iron Cross medal that had been pinned to the German's uniform thereafter adorned Stubby's army coat. Stubby became the most decorated dog in war, wining several medals and even the "Honorary Rank of Sergeant". The French also awarded him a Victory medal and French women knitted him a blanket on which his well earned medals were pinned. When the war ended on November 11, 1918, Stubby was in Meuse-Argonne. The process of demobilization was protracted, and troops stayed on for several months after Armistice. While waiting out for the trip home from France, Stubby had the honour of meeting the American President, Woodrow Wilson, on Christmas Day 1918 in Mandres en Bassigny, and the two reportedly shook "hands." Four months later, on April 29, 1919, Stubby and Conroy were demobilized at Camp Devens, Massachusetts.

After the war, Stubby came home with his master Corporal J Robert Conroy to a hero's welcome. On July 6, 1921, a ceremony took place at the State, War, and Navy Building on Pennsylvania Avenue in Washington. The occasion was honouring the Veterans of the 102nd Infantry of the American Expeditionary Forces' 26th "Yankee" Division, who had seen action in France during the Great War. The hall was packed with members of the 102nd Infantry of all ranks including Generals but one soldier in particular commanded the spotlight and this soldier was "Sergeant Stubby", a short brindle Bull Terrier mutt, who was now officially a decorated hero of World War I. The ceremony was presided over by Gen John J Pershing, Commander of the American forces in Europe during the war. Pershing made a short speech, noting the soldier's "heroism of highest calibre" and "bravery under fire." The General solemnly lifted an engraved solid gold medal from its case and pinned it to the Stubby's uniform. The award was not the formal US Military Commendation, but was commissioned by the Humane Education Society, the forerunner of current Humane Society. It symbolically confirmed Stubby, who had also earned one wound stripe and three service stripes, as the greatest war dog in the nation's history. He was the first dog ever given rank in the US Army. His glory was even hailed in France, which also presented him with a medal. After the war, Stubby was ubiquitous. He attended the 1920 Republican National Convention, which culminated in the nomination of Warren G Harding as President of the USA. Harding officially received Stubby at the White House in 1921. In 1924, the dog passed review for Harding's successor, John Calvin Coolidge, three times. When his master Conroy went to study law at Georgetown, Stubby became the university's official mascot, a predecessor to the Hoya Bulldog of the present day. After that Conroy worked as a bureaucrat, first for the Bureau of Investigation (predecessor to the FBI) at the Justice Department, then with Military intelligence and finally on Capitol Hill as secretary for a Connecticut congressman. Stubby continued to stay with him and became lifetime member of American legion. The hero dog was seen leading victory parades and also became the lifetime member of the Red Cross and YMCA. In December, 1922, The New York Times reported that "Usually closed doors were flung open for Stubby for the first time, the exclusive Hotel Majestic on Central Park had broken its own rules and allowed the dog to stay over night."

Stubby died in his sleep in Conroy's arms in 1926. Today, he may be the last decorated World War I Veteran who you can still see in the flesh. His taxidermied remains are on view at the Smithsonian National Museum of America History in

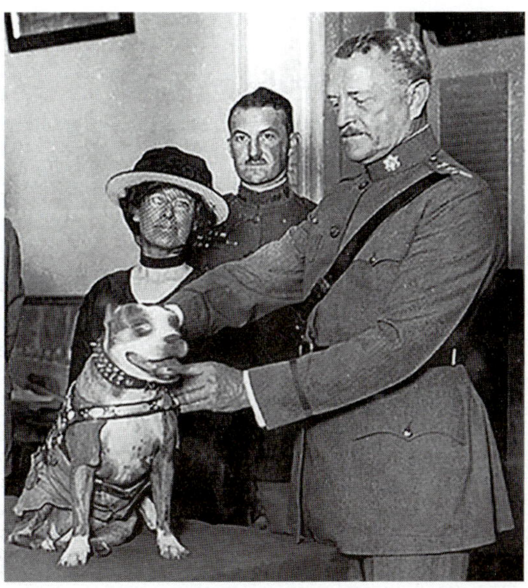

Gen John J Pershing, commander of the American Forces in Europe during the war, pinning a gold medal on Stubby

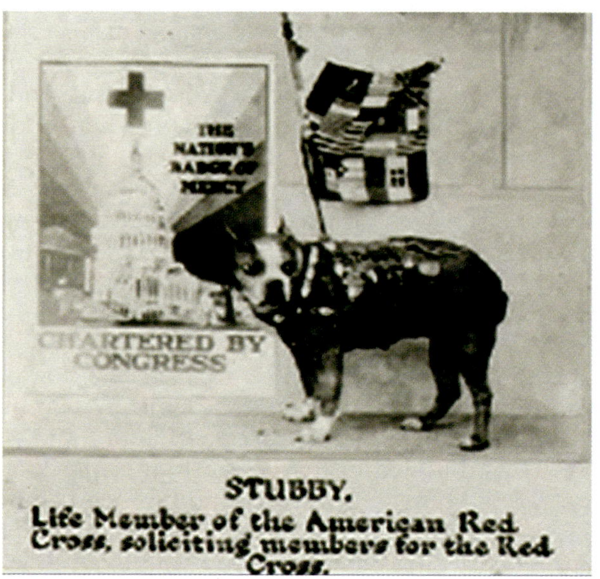

STUBBY.
Life Member of the American Red Cross, soliciting members for the Red Cross.

Washington, in the division of armed forces history. Stubby's ears are pointed up, and he wears a gruff expression. He looks like a ramrod Sergeant, tough, unsmiling, no nonsense, with a coat covered in medals. There is also a fascinating artifact, a leather-bound scrapbook, kept by his master Conroy. The book is crammed with documents, fan letters, poems, drawings and an invitation to the White House from President Wilson. There are also newspaper clippings of the press coverage of Stubby. The Pit Bull-centric website, StubbyDog.org, is named after him, and "Stubby Award for Canine Heroism" was instituted in his honour.

THE FAITHFUL SPANIEL

It is the story of a Zouave Soldier and his Spaniel dog during the time of World War I, in a battlefield location near Aubervilliers, France. This soldier was accompanied by his dog while on his mission. A German shell shattered his foot and severely wounded him in several body parts. He was almost buried under the earth, feeling suffocated and almost lost his consciousness. Probably, he would have died due to suffocation but for the timely action by his Spaniel, the faithful dog made herculean efforts by using his nose and paws to remove earth and exhumed his master. The dog while licking the wounds of his master, so as to avoid setting in of gangrene, began to howl loudly. This noise attracted the attention of French Ambulance to the spot. The wounded soldier was immediately taken to Field Hospital. After initial treatment this Zouave Soldier along with his dog was evacuated by train going to Paris for further treatment. On being taken out of train at Aubervilliers, the Surgeon Major on duty gave instruction to shift him to nearby American Hospital. The Zouave Soldier requested that his companion dog be permitted as he saved my life Monsieur (Major) and let him go with me. The Spaniel was licking the hand of the wounded soldier as he spoke. The Officer showed his inability and said it is impossible, I would like to comply your request but the hospital is not made for dogs. The Zouvave became very anxious and noticing his state, the manageress of the canteen at Aubervilliers relieved his anxiety by giving an undertaking that she will look after his dog during his hospitalization. While bidding farewell to his Spaniel with heavy heart, the wounded soldier narrated the story as to how this faithful Spaniel saved his life. When the ambulance took Zouvave to hospital, everybody present there was feeling sorry that the poor dog has been left behind. The Spaniel refused to take his daily feed provided by the canteen manageress for three days. Finally, she took the dog to hospital and met the director. She told the story of this faithful companion saving the life of his master, the wounded Zouvave Soldier, now admitted in the hospital. The Director of the hospital was impressed and permitted the Spaniel to stay with the soldier. On seeing his dog the Zouvave had a joyous meeting with his companion which brought tears into the eyes of those who saw it. This heart touching story was published in New York Times on 21st February, 1915 under the heading "Dogs of War in European Conflict".

RED CROSS AMBULANCE DOGS IN WORLD WAR I

It is in Egypt that dogs were used for the first time to find the wounded in battle. At that time it was thought that to lick the wounds was beneficial to their healing. Later on, Germany started the health dog training because during the war of 1870, there were significant loss of life (The Prussians counted 40,741 killed and 4,009 missing, the French 136,450 killed and 11,914 missing). The breeds used were Dalmatians, Wolves, Pomeranian, Scottish Collies and Airedale Terrier. It was a great annoyance to Germans to use dogs from most other countries, so they created a Shepherd Breed combining the qualities stem from Thuringia, Franconia and Wurttemberg. Captain Von Stephanitz was the real creator of the German Shepherd and he encouraged the use of these dogs in the army for the search of wounded in 1880. During the same period, trials in this regard were going on in Belgium and Professor Reul of Veterinary School Cureghem and two journalists, Van der Snick and Sodenkampf, set up demonstrations "Op Search Dogs" near Ostend, Belgium in 1885. The effectiveness of these dogs led to the establishment of "The Society of Sanitary dogs" in that country.

In 1890, health dogs were integrated into the German Battalion of Chasseurs of the Guard followed by almost all Regiments. The training kennel was located at Oberdollendorf and it was very frequently visited by other interested parties and served as a model to several countries. Captain Von Stephanitz, in his book published in 1921 on the German Shepherd, states that 4,000 health dogs had been used during the war and they had saved the lives of many soldiers. "Society health dog" was formed in 1893 and by 1914 it had about 2,000 dogs trained to search wounded soldiers. In 1916, it was reported that 1,600 health dogs saved 31,000 wounded.

Kaiser Wilhelm II, The last Emperor and King of Prussia, ruling German Empire and the Kingdom of Prussia from 15th June to 9th November, 1918, knew the value of Red Cross dogs (Sanitatshunde). While visiting a hospital behind German lines on the eastern front, he saw a soldier on one cot and a dog beside him on the next. He was told the story:

Lieutenant Von Wieland led a team of men in an attack on the Russian trenches but soon he got wounded. Seeing the task hopeless on account of the Russian fire, he sent back the men who had set out with him. He continued to lay in trench, in the blood, muck and filth of the battlefield. The Russian fire was so murderous that no one dared to bring him in. Suddenly, a dark form bounced from the German trenches, rushed to Lieutenant Von Wieland's side, grasped his coat between his teeth and dragged him foot by foot, to safety. Once but only for a moment, did he loosen his hold, and that was when a bullet creased him from shoulder to flank. The blood gushed from the wound, but the dog took a fresh hold and finished his job at the edge of the trench where willing hands lifted the lieutenant down to safety. They had to lift the dog down, too, because just then a bullet broke both his forelegs. The emperor was impressed and gave each an iron cross, handing one medal to the man and tying the other to the dog's collar.

In Switzerland, cynologist and animal painter, J Bungartz, established in 1893, the "Association for Health Dogs", and in 1903, Captain A Berdez, from Berne, published the first book on the subject "Guide for the training and use of Health Dog". In the following year, it led to the creation of "The Swiss Association for Health Dogs and Dogs of War" in Zurich. On 14th August, 1904 first review for war dogs and police dogs was undertaken and not only presented especially Airedales and Collies but the German Shepherd were also chosen for its nose and abilities. The fame of these courses transcended borders and several countries requested trained dogs, to the extent that the Federal Council put a ban on export of dogs on 7th August, 1914. The first course for Military Dogs was conducted in Bern, under the direction of Captain Studer. This was the group "Solothurn Sheepdog" who organized the first public health tests dog. Colonel Henri Guisan managed to generalize the dog of the army in 1928 and created a centre in Bex (Valais) in 1934.

The concept of training sanitary dogs or Sanitashunde as German call them, was debated at length in Germany. It was originally intended to amalgamate messenger and ambulance dog training, but it was soon realized that a combination of such different tasks was not suitable. A man from Dusseldorf, the animal painter Herr Bungartz, was the first to call attention to the necessity of making a radical distinction between these two types of Army Service dogs. In 1893, he founded the "Deutscher Verein fur Sanitatshunde" (the German Society for ambulance dogs). Initially, Medical Department of the Ministry of War had shown little interest in the use of ambulance dogs, but a demonstration was held in July, 1914 on the range at Zossen under conditions as nearly corresponding to those of war as possible. In this trial, which was continued throughout the night, dogs of the Ambulance Dog Society and of the Berlin Police Department had been allowed to compete, besides the dogs of the SV (the German Shepherd Society). The demonstration was successful and sanitary dogs were introduced gradually as the war unfolded. The Ministry of War established the Dog Replacement Depot at Fangschleuse near Berlin.

In France, the French Army was using Belgian Sheep Dogs to seek out injured soldiers who were unable to walk or crawl to an open space where they could be discovered. A private initiative led in 1906 to the creation of a "Society for the Study" for taming health dogs. In 1908, the company became the National Society of Dog Health, held by volunteers. Its purpose was to prepare the dogs to search for the wounded on the battlefield. The Societe Nationale des Chiens Sanitaires (National Society of Dog Health) had eight training and breeding kennels. Further, the dogs were trained not to bark when they found a disabled soldier. They were also taught to disregard dead soldiers. Each dog had a box containing first aid remedies and appliances tied to its neck. Upon locating a helpless soldier the dog would go close to him so that the box could be opened. The animal tore a piece of the uniform from the soldier and then returned to the kennel to which he was attached. When a dog returned with evidence of a wounded soldier, the follow-up action as envisaged at that time was described as follows:

The trained dogs return to the kennel, bark and turn back in the direction from which they came to indicate that they have found an injured soldier. The medical team attached to the kennels follow the dogs to the injured men. Many times soldiers are found at the bottom of deep ravines, and other sequestered places where only dogs with a keen sense of smell could locate them. Sometimes, it takes a whole day to get the soldier he has found, because of the hazardous work of carrying him to a road. They named such specialized dogs in search for the wounded as "Medic Dogs" and to prevent the enemy from shooting them, these dogs wore chabraque with Geneva cross. The dog having a harness or "chabraque" wearing a cross could be easily identified by soldiers as a lifeguard, and in principle do not shoot the dogs. From the beginning of the military conflict, 250 Sanitary dogs were pressed into service and they saved many lives. One of such dogs was "Gizmo", a Beauceron who located 148 injured.

This organization obtained the sponsorship of the concerned Ministries and on 14th March, 1911, the War Department created first Military Kennel "Dogs Dressage Health" led by Captain Tolet under the health service of the War Department. In December, 1915, the creation of "Service Dogs of War" was finally approved (dog health liaison, patrol, etc.) and attached to the Infantry. It was due to the effectiveness of Health Dogs that France opted for Dogs of War. The French Army mobilized a total of 15,000 dogs during the 1914–18 war and at the end of war about 5,300 were missing or killed. On 21st November, 1918, a ministerial circular demobilized war dogs.

In England, an article appeared in the British Medical Journal in 1910 indicating that the training being developed by Lt Col Edwin H Richardson was being kept secret, as regarding the best cross-breeds to be used for training of Red Cross Dogs. The article describes the equipment of a British Red Cross Dog as: "the dog is equipped with a waterproof canvas saddle, with a pocket at each side. In these pockets are placed eight triangular bandages, while slung round the dog's neck is a small cask of brandy or rum, and a bell for use after dark. A biscuit for himself is a wise provision."

Richardson made sustained efforts to interest the British War Office in Red Cross Dogs. Finally, the War Office requested him to attend the camp at Stobs for the autumn maneuvres. He was attached to the 42nd Black Watch and General Sir Charles Tucker, Commanding in Scotland, put the dogs through very severe tests, and as a result recommended their adoption. As the war began, Richardson settled on training Red Cross Dogs. However, when the French Army hurriedly sent some of their Red Cross Dogs with their keepers to the front in the earliest feverish days, the first thing happened was that, although both men and dogs wore the Red Cross, the enemy brutally shot them down whenever they attempted to carry out their humanitarian work. It was also found that, when the opposing forces settled down into trench warfare, the opportunities on the Western front were closed. As such, this idea was deemed unsuccessful as early as the battle of Antwerp and the French infact banned the use of Red Cross Dogs within a few weeks of the war beginning. Lt Col Richardson then started training Sentry and Patrol dogs.

In the United States, The Surgeon General of the US Army, WC Gorgas, testified before the Congressional Committee for Military Affairs that Germany had 6,000

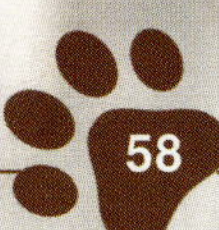

Red Cross Dogs. Gorgas gave this number as a means of trying to get the War Department to devote more attention to expand the American programme, arguing that a few dogs of the US had at Fort Vermont at the time were a drop in the bucket to what the US should have had.

TRAINING OF RED CROSS DOGS

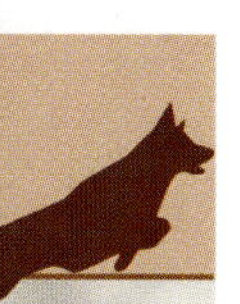

Red Cross Dogs were called by various names such as Ambulance Dogs, Medic Dogs, Sanitary Dogs, Mercy Dogs, Search and Rescue Dogs, etc. and to learn the importance of a wounded man, was the principal business in their lives. As such, they were first trained to distinguish between the uniform of their country and that of the enemy. Secondly, they must be able to communicate the news of the wounded to their master and must not bark, because the enemy always shoots.

Ideally, the training of a Red Cross dog involves only one handler, but the dog's loyalties also go to members of his unit, while he will come in touch with all its members more or less daily. As such, efforts should be made that no one fondle or coax him or try to distract his attention from whatever work he may have in hand. The dog should not be interfered with, even if not in training at that time, or on duty. Such dog must recognize his trainer/handler and next to him, a few members of the squad, as his masters. However, after completion of training, if needed, he may be taught to obey anyone belonging to that unit and to transfer his fidelity to any soldier in the familiar uniform. A well-trained dog will soon get the proper esprit de corps and will know and obey every member of the unit to which he is attached.

The training of war dogs in general was imparted into obedience lessons and field lessons. The obedience lessons were Heel, Down, and Retrieve. However, for a Red Cross dog, "Down" was supposedly be the greatest obedience exercise that a trainer has to ground into the very being of the dog.

Those days, field lessons for war dogs in general included the following commands:

1. S-sss, S-sss. This was a command and caution to increase the dog's attention, given in a whisper, and may be given with the hand signal for Down in order to preclude barking.
2. Advance. A command to send the dog forward into the immediate area to detect hidden or advancing enemies and avoid a surprise attack. This command was taught in stages until the dog can reconnoiter without a handler.
3. Report. This was taught so that the dog can deliver a report from an advance post. This command was also taught in several stages.
4. Report-Advance. This command was used after a dog has been sent from a unit at the front to bring back help and the commander of the base determines to let the dog leads the support column to the forward unit. The dog may also receive the command, Slow, that it would not lead the support column too quickly into the same danger, the advance unit has encountered.
5. Guard. This command was used when required to assist in guarding prisoners. Guard-Attack was used to recapture an escaped prisoner.

The ibid fourth command, "Report-Advance", was particularly relevant to Red Cross dog training.

There are various ways in which the dog could communicate with his master about his discovery. One method is, if no wounded has been discovered, he trot back and lie down whereas if he has found a wounded man, he urges his master to follow. Although the easiest way for a dog to announce that it had found a wounded soldier was to bark but it was realized that the enemy could shoot in the direction of the sound. The greatest silence, therefore, is just as imperative as the avoidance of any light, and thus the return of the dog to make his report is the only possible method. However, the problem was as to how to do it. As such, dogs were first taught to bring back objects, such as a soldier's cap. This worked well in the beginning of the war but subsequently this technique poised its own set of problems. Not finding a cap or helmet, the dog would pull a piece of uniform, a bandage, or even hair to accomplish the job at hand. This increased in frequency as the war went on and forced the allies to rework their training methods. The new training regimen had the dog lie down if no wounded were found or beckon the handler to return to the site if indeed a soldier was still alive. The Germans also faced the same problem at the beginning of the war but went in a different direction with much better results. They devised a short stick or leather tug that is suspended from the collar of a trained dog called a Bringsel. Upon finding a wounded man, the dog would return with the stick in its mouth. Conversely, if the stick hung loose, no wounded or perhaps only the dead were to be found. Thus, a leather 'sausage' was hung from the dog's collar by a leather strap. The dog (sometimes the wounded soldier) put this object, 'bringsel' (the object to be brought) into his mouth and returned to the dog leader, nicknamed the "Wow-Wow-Lieutenant." The leader then leashed the dog who then took him back to the wounded man. It will be interesting to know that the Bringsel method was devised by a German psychoanalyst named Pfungst from Berlin, who had no experience with dogs at all.

These Mercy Dogs were trained to provide wounded men with two essential service. Firstly, they carried medical supplies and small canteens of water or spirit, so that wounded soldiers, if conscious, could avail themselves of these supplies. Secondly, the mission of Red Cross Dogs was mainly to search and rescue soldiers, who were not able to move. If the wounded man was behind his own battle line, the Mercy Dog had simply to call for his handler. If they had to work in no man's land, the dogs were trained to return to their handler carrying the helmet or a piece of his uniform in order to inform the medical unit that someone who needed urgent help had to be rescued.

RED CROSS DOGS IN WORLD WAR I

These dogs, were useful for open warfare since in trench warfare or in defensive actions, there is little opportunity for the Red Cross Dogs to function. The real chance comes when the troops are advancing in the open and one such opportunity for open warfare was after the first two weeks on the Eastern, the South Eastern and the Southern fronts, i.e. in Russia, Romania, Balkans, Italy, and even in Asia Minor. The Red Cross dogs that were used with great success were the Sanitary Dogs (Sanitatshunde), as the Germans called them, when the Russians were retreating on the Eastern front. They carried medical supplies and small canteens of water or spirits that were typically attached across the dog's chest or with a saddlebag arrangement. The wounded man, if conscious, could avail himself of these supplies. These dogs fully justified the confidence placed in them, whenever they arrived in time and in sufficient numbers. It is not yet known, and probably never will be, as to how many thousands of wounded soldiers owe to them, their restoration to health. These dogs were deployed particularly at night when the battles were not raging and it was impossible to try to find the wounded with lights, which would expose soldiers to the enemy. The dog must run to and fro, and in an area of something like 220 × 54 yards, smelling out the tracks of the wounded, and announce them to their leaders. The dogs were also trained to distinguish the particular smell of the wounded and not to point out corpses.

Staff correspondent of "The Times", who visited forward areas in December, 1914 wrote an article under the heading 'Dogs of war save many German lives'; 'Sanitatshunde' finds who would otherwise die on the battlefield. It was published in "The York Times" on 21st January, 1915. The contents of the article are reproduced here:

Berlin, December 31—The Kaiser's canine conscripts, the "Sanitatshunde," or Ambulance Dogs, have proved such a success in the west, where they have been employed for several months, that by special order of the Minister of War, the number of dogs attached to each ambulance company is to be increased to eight, and at the urgent request of Field Marshal Von Hindenburg, 250 additional dogs have been sent to the east. How they worked is vividly described by the Commander of a Dog Division (sanitatshundfuhrer) in the following report:

"At 7 in the evening, we started for the battlefield, where we were already eagerly awaited by our grieviously wounded comrades. We learned that the enemy had been driven back two or three miles. It was a pitch dark night with heavy fog and at the command "Hunt the wounded", the dogs dashed ahead into the woods. We followed them as rapidly as possible so that they wouldn't have to bark too long and draw enemy's fire on us as we were now close to his trenches. It is not long before we heard barking and head in the direction of the bark, the dog came running back to meet us and guide us ahead until we came upon the poor devil who lay on ground groaning, his eyes fixed on the dog. For God's sake give me something to drink, he cried out to us. I gave the poor fellow some coffee from my flask then put him on a stretcher and had him carried back, while we again pressed on, we heard more barking ahead. And so it went all night long till we had thoroughly searched the battlefield. Fourteen wounded who were found in dark woods by our dogs could never have been found by our ambulance men and would have been left to their fate. You cannot picture the horror of it. At the day break, we went back to camp with our four-footed brothers in arms and all heads dropped in their tracks for a much needed sleep."

Similarly, from the Military Hospital at Bonn, a member of Engineer Corps wrote the following testimonial to the Ambulance Dog:

"I was wounded in the ankle and with several other comrades including a First Lieutenant, all wounded, hid in a cellar of a small village. We were locked in either by inhabitants or by other French, who tried to drown us out by running water into the cellar. For three days and nights we stood up to our breasts in water without food and had given up all hope of being saved, when we heard a dog sniffing around a small opening in the wall and then to our great joy, saw the dog's head. The Officer grabbed off his helmet cover and stuck it in the dog's collar, and the dog ran off again, but in about four hours, ambulance men came and liberated us. I am convinced that we would have died a miserable death in that cellar, if the dog hadn't found us".

The following is quoted from the diary of a captured German Red Cross worker:

"We left for the battlefield at two O'clock in the morning. We could only work on the lead, as we were less than 400 metres from the French lines. 'Treu,' my dog, in a short time found five wounded, three severely wounded and two slightly wounded, which even with the sharpest eyesight you could not have found as they were so well-hidden. They had been out on the battlefield for a day and a half."

The German soldiers rescued by of Red Cross Dogs, showed their gratitude by establishing a hospital for sick and wounded animals at Jena.

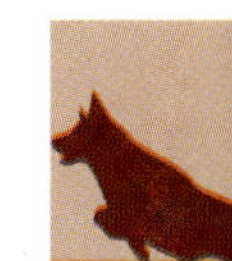

Similarly. French Red Cross Dogs also did a yeoman service. At the beginning of the war, the innate sense of retrieval bred into many dogs led to the way they were trained, meaning the return of a cap or helmet indicating that a wounded soldier was located.

There is also textual evidence in respect of few French Red Cross Dogs as narrated below:

Captain

This French Red Cross Dog located thirty wounded men in a single day. Every time the dog located a soldier, he returned back with the soldier's cap or helmet to report that he has found the wounded.

Pluto

Pluto was a French Red Cross Dog trained to search and rescue the wounded soldiers in the battlefield. On the fateful day, while on duty, his keen sense of smell took him towards the edge of the parapet which gave him a view of the precise location of the injured soldier. Soon he came straight to the body but as he was smelling the wounded soldier, several bullets were fired from the enemy's trench. Pluto, the superb rescuer showed indifference to the enemy firing. He raised the soldier a bit and after tossing and turning, grabbed his shoulder and started dragging him to safety. Pluto and the soldier were nearing to reach own lines when a bullet hit the dog's leg and he fell on his knee with a shattered leg. The journey was not finished, it was still a few metres, Pluto again started his efforts and at last, he dragged the injured to the parapet. But then a bullet hit him right in the head, Pluto rolled and the four paws were in the air. Troops caught him in turn, after obtaining the soldier but the dog fell heavily to the bottom of the trench. He stood there, motionless, already stiff, clenched jaws, a trickle of blood on this beautiful all white furrow between the eyes. The brave Pluto was dead, but the French wounded soldier was saved.

Prusco

Prusco, a Red Cross Dog of French Army, looked like a white wolf. He was credited with saving more than hundred men. The dog, would drag men into protective craters and trenches before alerting his master. Prusco is believed to have once allowed three soldiers in sequence to hold onto his collar while he dragged them to a depression where they could be safe from enemy fire in one battle. Several dispatches from different regiments mentioned the heroic efforts of this dog.

Testimony of a stretcher bearer on the capabilities of dogs that accompanied stretcher is summarized below:

"The Battle of the Meurthe lasts a whole week. We can, despite prohibitions, make three or four rounds. It was dangerous in the woods near St Benoit and we found each time two or three wounded in extremely dense forests. In a single afternoon, in the area of Suippes, we could find more than thirty wounded in the woods while the stretcher unaccompanied dogs, return empty-handed..."

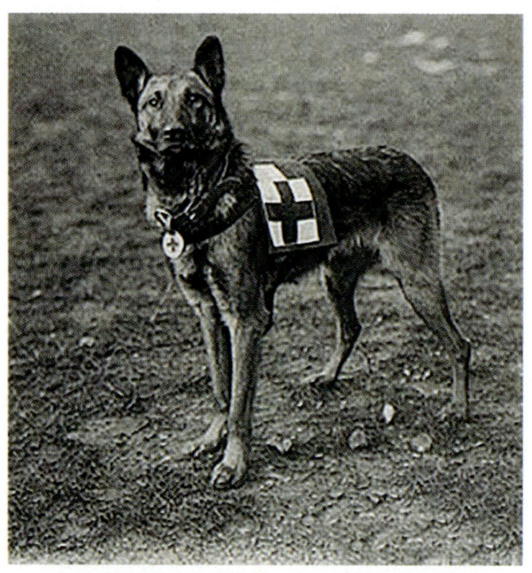

A French Red Cross Dog ready to move

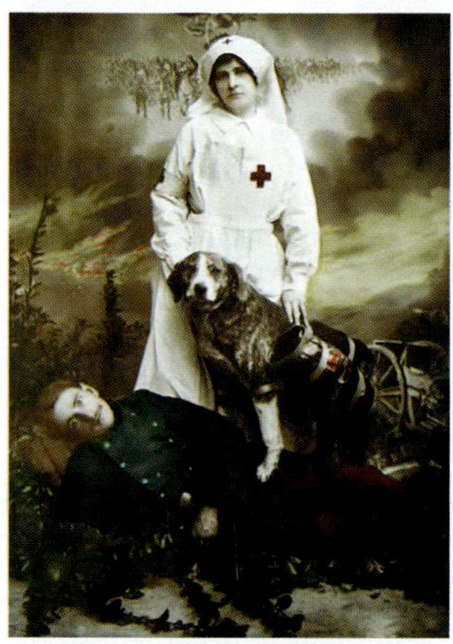

French Red Cross Dog with nurse and injured soldier

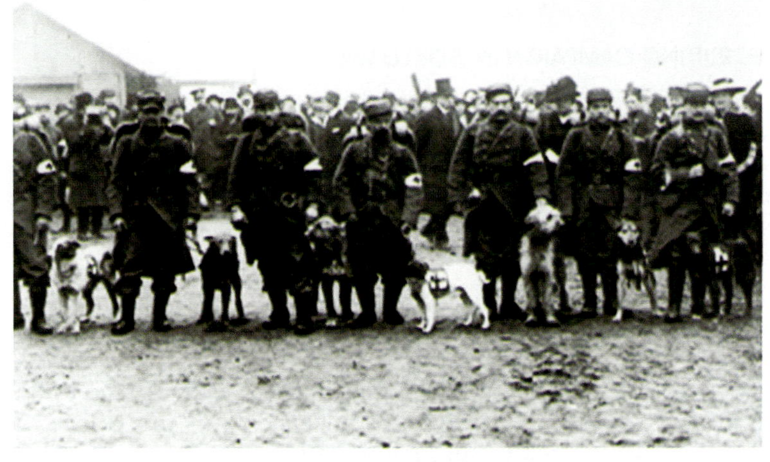

French Red Cross Dogs

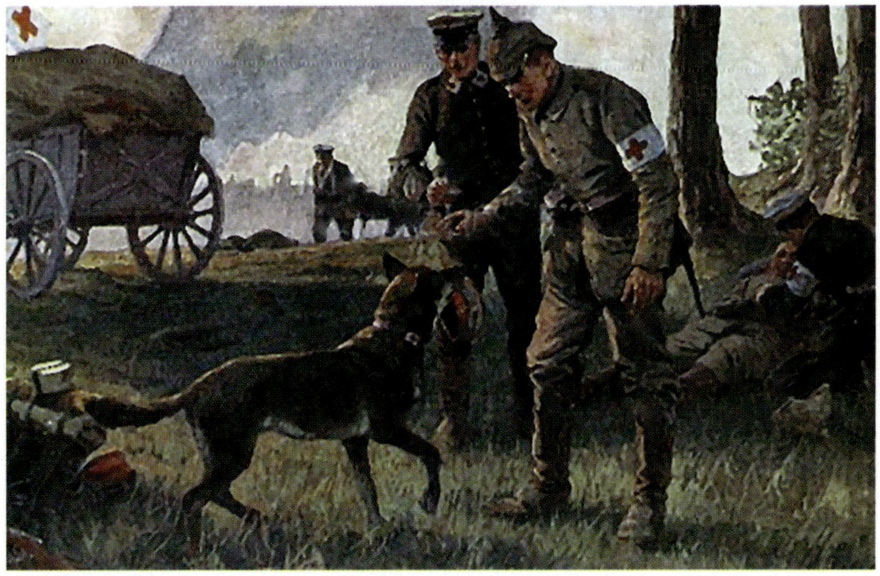

German Red Cross ambulance dog with medical team and injured soldier

To accomplish their mission, the Red Cross dogs had to deal with deadly gases, slit trenches and artillery. Thousands of soldiers owed their lives to these Mercy Dogs during the Great War; and it is, therefore, not astonishing that a special cemetery was dedicated to these animals in New York, the Hartsdale Canine Cemetery. The monument of a German Shepherd, dedicated to all dogs, as we can read, "For the valiant services rendered in World War, 1914–1918."**Currently, only**

Switzerland has Health Dogs that participate in competitions on a programme that approximates real conditions with obedience exercises and search of persons or objects.

DOGS IN RECRUITING CAMPAIGN IN WORLD WAR I

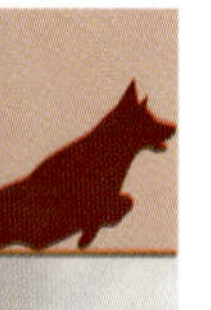

Military and Red Cross campaigns featured dogs prominently in their advertizing. Newspapers reported relentlessly on the work of dogs at home and overseas. Publishers welcomed narratives that featured a dog as the central character. No matter a dog's national affiliation, the print media inundated the public with the doings of dogs overseas and the war dog as a class was mentioned honourably and lovingly by all the men of every nation in the struggle.

The United States' Military also employed dogs in its recruiting campaigns. The one US Army recruiting poster depicts a dog with the insignia of the Red Cross draped across its flank. The dog stands a top a pile of rubble, panting, while the city in the background burns. The artist has set this canine's expression into what might be a smile, the animal presumably pleased with the rescue work it has accomplished. The caption below this image challenges its human audience: "**EVEN A DOG ENLISTS, WHY NOT YOU?**" By communicating to the viewer that even an animal without will can "volunteer" for war. This propaganda piece attempts to convince potential soldiers that as men they ought to do more for their nation than the beasts did. The Marine Corps also used dogs in its propaganda. One widely produced recruiting poster welcomes the viewer into a canine chase sequence. A burly Bulldog, playing the role of an American Marine, pursues a German Dachshund, which flees with head turned in trepidation and tail set firmly between its legs. The breeds convey clearly which nation each dog symbolizes. The artist had also inserted another clue, while the Bulldog wears a simple helmet over its square skull, the Dachshund sports a crested headpiece emblazoned with an eagle wings outstretched, a recognizable emblem that denoted a Prussian Regiment. The poster declares that German soldiers had already nicknamed the American Marines "Teufel Hunden," meaning "Devil Dogs." It matters little that the origins of this moniker are mythical. The military's use of the dogs as tools for raising money and recruiting men stands as evidence of how the American people reshaped the role of their dogs to serve the war effort, in this case imagining them as Soldiers themselves, nearly human.

Americans seemed eager to volunteer their own dogs for war service. Red Cross Magazine chronicled how American citizens on the home front supported the war effort through their pets, an indicator of how dogs and civilian mobilization were intertwined. In the November, 1917, issue of the Red Cross Magazine, Walter A Dyer, a journalist, editor and prolific writer of canine-centric fiction, had written about the contribution of Red Cross Dogs to the war effort, adding that more were needed to help with hospital work. Immediately, the public responded to his call by donating dogs generously. By January, 1918, the Red Cross National Headquarters had to turn dogs away and issued a statement begging "No More Dogs, Please."

In Japan, the most famous wartime dog was the cartoon character Norakuro (1931–41), a Mongrel Orphan, who rose from Private to Colonel in a dog army whose feats, blunders and victories captured the popular imagination. Depicting the emperor's army as a pack of dogs was always risky and it is not surprising that the Norakura series was terminated after irking military authorities when he decided to retire from the army and engage in some profiteering in Manchuria.

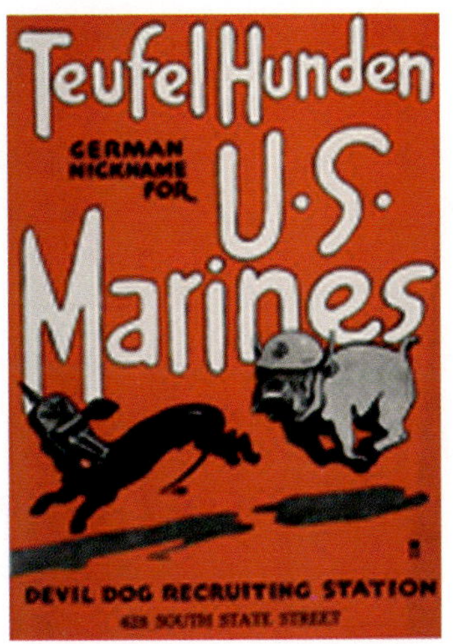
Teufel Hunden
GERMAN NICKNAME FOR
U.S.
Marines
DEVIL DOG RECRUITING STATION

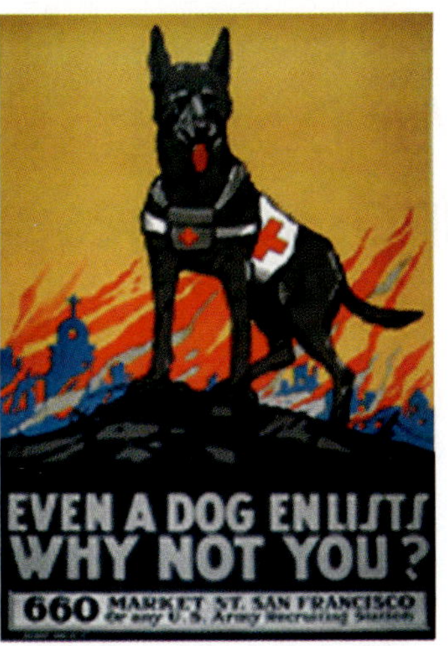
EVEN A DOG ENLISTS
WHY NOT YOU?
660 MARKET ST. SAN FRANCISCO

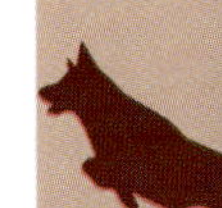

6

War Dogs in Sino-Japanese War

"I have found that when you are deeply troubled, there are things you get from the silent devoted companionship of a dog that you can get from no other source."

... Doris Day

After the end of First Sino-Japanese War which was fought between Qing, dynasty China and Meiji Japan from 1st April, 1894 to 17th April, 1895, Korea became a part of Japan. However, the Treaty of Shimonosekii (1895) declared Korea independent and provided for the cession of Taiwan, the Pescadores, and the Liaodong Peninsula by China to Japan. China also had to pay a large indemnity. Within a week of the treaty signing, the diplomatic intervention of Russia, France, and Germany forced Japan to return the Liaodong Peninsula to China. Under a subsidiary commercial treaty (1896), China yielded to Japanese nationals the right to open factories and engage in manufacturing in the trade ports. This right was automatically extended to the Western maritime powers under the most favoured nation clause.

Japan took her troops along a railroad from Manchuria to Korean ports-of-trade. This railroad was used to transport raw materials and other finished goods to Korean docks to be shipped to Japan. Japanese Troops controlled this railway and wanted more free resources from Manchuria. Therefore, the Japanese started to attack Chinese Troops and succeeded in gaining control of Manchuria. Japan aimed at taking all roads, railroads, and cities, in order to gain total control. Despite the fact that Japanese forces were controlling the Eastern coastal region, guerrilla fighting continued in the conquered areas. The Chinese Nationalist government had been forced to retreat to a transitory capital at Chongqing. However, Japanese did not have the capability or intention of directly controlling all of China. So they set up friendly "puppet" governments which would favour their interests. These governments were not very popular especially after Japan refused to negotiate with China's Communist Party. China, on the other hand, was not ready for war. Moreover, she had a few mechanised divisions, lacked significant military industrial strength, and had no armour support. China largely depended on the League-of-Nations to come to her aid and offer countermeasures to Japan's assault. Furthermore, the Koumintang, or the Chinese Nationalist Party, was caught up in an internal fight against the Communists. Due to all these disadvantages, the Chinese were forced to come up with a strategy which aimed at preserving their army strength but the occupied areas would continue to exert pockets of resistance in order to disturb Japanese Forces and make their control of China as difficult as possible. The origin of the Second Sino-Japanese War (1937 to 1941) can be linked to such developments after 1896. Further, when Japanese bombed the Pearl Harbor in 1941, the United States and China declared war against Japan. This merged the second Sino-Japanese War into World War II. Although Chinese had insufficient resources, they managed to fight back especially after receiving economic help from the Soviet Union and the USA.

The Japanese Military on the Asian Continent relied heavily on animal-based logistics, i.e. horses for transportation, pigeons for long-range communications, dogs for short-range communications and sentry duties. One subject that greatly interested Japanese Army leadership was the Germans' extensive use of Military Working Dogs and Carrier Pigeons. Accordingly, in 1913, The Army Infantry School at Tendai in Chiba, began research into Military Dogs, on the orders of its Commandant. All the German Shepherds at the school descended from 11 German Colonial Police Dogs confiscated in Qingdao, China which was occupied by the Japanese during their limited engagement in World War I. Until the arrival of the Japanese, Qingdao had been a de facto German colony. Captain Itakura became the chief of the War Dog Training Centre in February, 1930 at Army Infantry School in Chiba. A year later, Itakura was transferred to Mukden where, Lt Col Sadao Yoshida, already has founded the Mukden Garrison's War Dogs Section. Captain Itakura, a well-known researcher of Military Dogs, arrived in Manchuria from the Japanese home islands in March, 1931 along with three German Shepherds (Kongo, Nachi and Meri). He lived in an area of Mukden known as Inaba, where he looked after his unit's dogs. Of all the Hounds he housed, his favourites were the Meri, Nachi and Kongo. Itakura trained them to deliver messages and patrol with their handlers at night.

During the intervening period, there had been many clashes between the Chinese and Japanese Forces. Japan used Military Working Dogs in support of its troops.

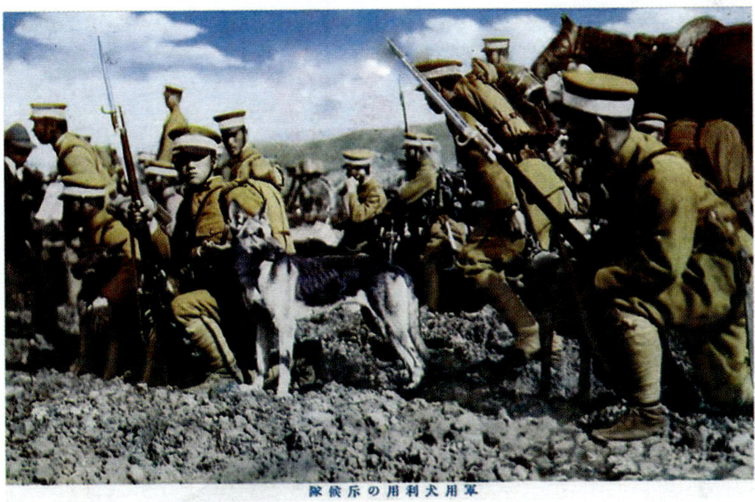

Postcard of Military Dogs in a large-scale Japanese Army exercise in 1932

There were approximately 10,000 dogs in service with the Imperial Army as Messengers, Sentries, Trackers and Sled Teams. As Japan marched across Manchuria and later China, the military recognized the need to ensure a steady supply of animals. It asked the citizens of the empire to donate their pets to the military for use in Manchuria, which officials described as a "Working Dog's Heaven."

The story of three heroic dogs of Sino-Japanese clashes at Manchuria in September, 1931 is narrated here:

MERI, NACHI AND KONGO

On September 18, 1931, an explosion destroyed a section of railway track near the city of Mukden (now Shenyang). The Japanese, who owned the railway, blamed Chinese nationalists for the incident and used the opportunity to retaliate and invade Manchuria, northeastern part of China, where Japan established its puppet state of Manchukuo six months later. However, others speculated that the bomb may have been planted by mid-level officers in the Japanese Army to provide a pretext for the subsequent military actions.

As the artillery thundered on Peitaying Barracks during the night, Meri, Nachi and Kongo put their skills to work, from 11 pm to 4 am. The handlers dispatched the dogs to and from Battalion Headquarters carrying messages from 1st Company out in the field. Meri was with his handler Private. Ueno and he joined the assault on the barracks. As Ueno's squad closed on one of the buildings, a hand grenade exploded and Chinese Soldiers leaped up, forcing the Japanese into close-quarters combat. A Shrapnel gashed Ueno's leg and while in severe pain, he desperately tried to hold onto Meri, but the dog slipped away and dashed inside the barracks. Ueno attempted to run after him but Meri vanished into the smoke and dust. Elsewhere, Kongo and Nachi had also been cut off from their handlers and were also missing. The Chinese retreated in the morning and Peitaying Barracks were again in Japanese hands. However, the three dogs were nowhere to be found, even when Itakura went out whistling for them to come back. Three days later, the bodies of Nachi and Kongo were found covered in wounds and lying in blood-stained snow nearby the mauled bodies of Chinese Soldiers. Both dogs still had the bitten-off scraps of enemy uniforms clenched between their teeth. The dead bodies of both Heroic Dogs were buried honourably under the supervision of Capt Itakura.

Clashes between Japanese and Chinese troops further escalated in the aftermath of the Mukden Incident. Anti-Japanese Volunteer Army troops invaded Jinzhou on 27th November, 1931. The Kwantung Army dispatched its own troops from the Mukden Independent garrison in armoured trains to fend off the Chinese advance. Captain Itakura also left Mukden at 0540 hours on an armoured train heading west towards Shanhaiguan. At 0930 hours, the Japanese train suddenly came under fire. As shells burst around them, the chief of the train's guard element, 1st Lt Shimoshiba, ordered the train's mountain guns to return fire. The attacking train's front carriage came into view and it was the eight-carriage Chinese Zhongshan. Captain Itakura delivered a situation report to the Battalion Commander and received further orders. He arranged ammunition supply to the forward train car and as he opened the carriage door to continue down the tracks, an artillery shell exploded, spraying him with shrapnels. Itakura fell on the floor as the shrapnel had penetrated the left side of his abdomen deep into his gut and shredding everything insides. He was bleeding out when the Battalion Commander Kojima lifted Itakura onto his shoulder and rushed him back inside the train. The fighting raged until the Chinese train beat a retreat at 1,500 hours, leaving one of its carriages completely destroyed. In recapturing Raoyanghe, several of Japanese Non-Commissioned Officers were wounded or killed. Captain Itakura was the only Commissioned Officer killed in the attack. He was posthumously promoted to the rank of Major for his actions that day.

On 5th July, 1932, during the first award presentations for animals of the Imperial Army, Kongo and Nachi, each received the highest honour, "An Honorific Collar," which is now kept in the museum on the grounds of the controversial Yasukuni Shrine.

The Mukden Independent Garrison Headquarters also requested public recognition of the dogs' efforts and the citation reads:

"On the night of 18th September, 1931 the 2nd Battalion was dispatched for the offensive on Peitaying near Liutiaoman. Kongo and Nachi, war dogs attached to 1st Company participated in the battle. On the battlefield they were responsible for carrying orders between the Company and Battalion Headquarters through darkness and under enemy fire and performed with distinction.

In addition, at the height of the battle 1st Company broke through under machine gun fire, the dogs broke into the ranks of the enemy volunteers, killing and wounding with their bites, causing much loss and menace, aiding the company's battle efforts before being honourably killed in action. For their meritorious deeds we put them forward for Highest Honours".

On 9th July, 1933, the dogs were commemorated by dedicating a Monument to the Loyal Dogs at Enmei Temple in Zushi. Itakura's widow, Army Minister Sadao Araki and former minister of war and soon-to-be Commander of the Kwantung, General Jiro Minami attended the ceremony along with other political and military dignitaries. More than 2,000 schoolchildren who had raised the funds to erect the statue sang in the dogs' honour called "Nachi and Kongo's War Feat."

7

War Dogs of World War II

"Dogs do speak, but only to those who know how to listen."

... Orhan Pamuk,

By the beginning of World War II, the Germans upped the ante, training more than 200,000 dogs for a variety of duties. The German Army made extensive use of the War Dogs in a variety of roles, such as guarding airfields, railway heads and logistical areas against sabotage and commando-style attacks. They were also employed behind the lines to track down partisan groups and in the front lines as Scout Dogs. It also cannot be ignored that the War Dogs were also used in some distasteful role, such as guarding concentration camps as a terror weapon. One Guard Dog could in effect secure an area that might have required 50 soldiers, thus freeing up manpower to fight on the front. Such was the brutal use of some of these dogs, and left a negative opinion of the War Dogs that took several years to overcome. During the Winter War, in the frozen desolate hinterland of the north, the German Sixth SS Mountain Division (Nord) was the only German Military unit to have dogs as part of its official establishment. The dog section comprised three different groups of dogs, i.e. Scout, Messenger and Sled known as Ziehhunden. There were 30 men assigned to the dog section known as "Hunderfuhrer" or dog drivers. Their task included haulage of supplies to the front lines and evacuation of the wounded. There is no official estimate of their success, but one soldier's diary stated in 1943 that he and his dog evacuated more than 340 wounded troops from the front alone. Sled Dogs were often operated alone or typically in a three-dog tandem harness between wooden shafts pulling a pulkka, or akja, a Finnish Boat-like wooden Sled.

The attack upon Pearl Harbor ensured the sudden entry of the United States into World War II which greatly stimulated interest in the use of dogs for sentry duty. At the time of attack on Pearl Harbor, Sled Dogs were the only working dogs employed in the army. About fifty of these animals were assigned to military stations in Alaska, where they were used when snow and ice precluded other transport. In 1941, dogs were used by the Air Corps Ferrying Command to rescue airmen forced down in snowbound and desolate parts of Newfoundland, Greenland and Iceland. As World War II started in Europe, and the US Army began to prepare for its role, it was initially estimated that 200 dogs might be needed whereas in actuality, about 10,000 dogs were trained for the Army, Navy, Marine Corps and Coast Guard by

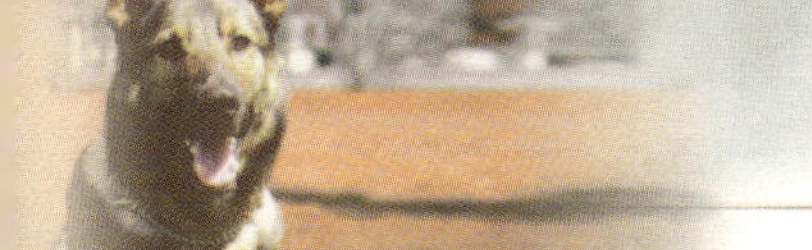

the time the war ended in 1945. The first effort to procure and train dogs for the US Military was based on volunteers. A civilian organization, Dogs for Defense, Inc. was formed in January, 1942, to work with qualified civilian trainers, who offered their services without pay. In the summer of 1942, a new training programme was developed, and responsibility for procuring, handling and training dogs was placed with the Quartermaster Remount Branch. With the rapid expansion of industrial plants and army installations during the war, the threat of potential damage that might be done by saboteurs or enemy agents saw an increase in the use of Guard Dogs. By early 1942 German submarines began to operate in large numbers near the Atlantic and Gulf coasts and the landing of saboteurs was a possibility. In all, the Coast Guard fielded 2,000 dogs and so successful were they that in 1944 the Coast Guard dog trainers were sent to China to train similar beach patrol units there. In May, 1942, the US Army established the K9 Corps and 595 dogs were trained for scouting duties. The War Dog Platoon, although trained by the Quartermaster Corps (QMC), was a Combat unit. Each squad contained eight dog handlers who trained and handled four Scout and four Messenger Dogs. After training at a Quartermaster War Dog Reception and Training Centre, a War Dog Platoon was attached to an Army Corps or Division, as determined by the theatre Commander. The Scout and messenger Dog Teams, were further attached to lower units as needed for work with reconnaissance, combat and security patrols, and as needed for communication purposes. The Commanding Officer of the War Dog Unit advised the Commanders of using units on the proper use of the handlers and dogs. Fifteen War Dog Platoons served overseas in World War II. Seven saw service in Europe and eight in the Pacific. Sentry Dogs were most commonly needed and over 9,000 of the dogs trained were used to patrol beaches, security of military installations and military protected sensitive civilian locations. About 800 dogs participated directly in war effort and were employed as Scouts, Messengers, Sentries and Mine Search Dogs in both the European and Pacific theatres of War. Scout Dogs were used to sniff out snipers and other dangers whereas Messenger Dogs were used to courier materials between soldiers in both combat and non-combat situations. Army War Dogs were used not only in the Pacific but also in the Europe, China, Burma and India. The 38th War Dog Platoon was attached to the 85th Division in Villa Di Sassonero, Italy, and conducted many operations under mountainous conditions. The 42nd War Dog Platoon was heavily engaged during the Battle of the Bulge and later transferred to guard supply dumps in Belgium due to the presence of saboteurs. The US War Dog Platoons were active throughout the Pacific, in New Guinea they were used as Patrol and Scout Dogs in dense jungle. Such dogs were so feared by the Japanese that they became a prime target for Japanese snipers. Army War Dogs of Company G 106th Regiment 27th Division on Okinawa were often used on patrols at night. Dogs were used to guard lines of communication support and supply bases as well as operating ahead of Infantry Patrols.

On 1st November, 1943, the 1st US Marine War Dog Platoon was attached to 2nd Marine Raider Regiment to mark the first appearance of the Devil Dogs, as the Raiders were to call them, during the Bougainville operation. This platoon was composed of 24 dogs (21 Doberman Pinschers, 1 Belgian Shepherd and 2 German Shepherds). To facilitate training and control in the field, for every 5–6 dogs there was a Marine responsible for their well-being. The squad organization consisted of thirteen men, as in the rifle squads at that time. The Raiders generally used only the

Scout and Messenger Dogs whereas Sentry Dogs were used extensively by the Coast Guard. The Casualty Dogs were trained to find wounded military personnel in debris and heavy cover. The dogs were also used to lay communication wire from a spool or spindle attached to their back or side. The Pack Dogs were useful in northern and mountainous areas to transport small amounts of ammunition and medical supplies. Sled Dogs were also used to some extent by the ski troops. The Messenger Dogs carried messeges in the small first aid pouch that was attached to the dog's collar. Each Messenger Dog was married up with two handlers, i.e. one at the dispatching location and other at receiving location. All dogs were issued a leather leash, a choke chain and a leather muzzle. While lowering dogs from ship rail to landing craft, a marine fatigue jacket was put backward on the dog, inserting his front legs through the rolled up sleeves, buttoning the collar backwards around his neck by the first three buttons and then tying the remainder of the jacket in a knot and securing it. This resulted in a comfortable and secure vest or sling which the dog accepted stoically during the lowering into the Higgins Boats where his other handler waited. Most of them were Doberman Pinchers, black, lean and tall. Dogs were assigned to the handlers on a one-to-one basis and were not to be petted or fooled around with by anyone else. These dogs were of immense help, for example, Jack, a three-year-old Belgian Shepherd acted bravely while getting through with a message to send stretcher bearers immediately, a vital message since all telephone lines had been cut. Jack made the run in spite of being shot in the back. Another dog named Rex, a two-year-old Doberman Scout Dog forewarned his group of marines of the presence of Japanese during the night. They were ready and waiting when the attack came at dawn and successfully repelled it. Similarly, a four-year-old Doberman named Otto, while working ahead of a reconnaissance patrol warned the marines of a Japanese machine gun position located 100 yards away. This gave the marines time to disperse and take cover before the machine gun opened fire. Dogs made very significant contribution to the war effort by foiling night infiltration attacks and discovered enemy patrols and troop movements in the jungles of Pacific. In 1943, the US Army sent one hundred dog teams to China, Burma and Indian theatre. Some dog teams were also sent to support "Merrill's Marauders", officially named the 5307th Composite Unit (Provisional). It was the United States Army's long range penetration special operations jungle warfare unit, which fought in the South-East Asian theatre of World War II. The unit became famous for its deep-penetration missions behind Japanese lines, often engaging Japanese forces superior in number.

In Russia, the Red Army leadership took several steps to develop military dog breeding and training to boost their war efforts. On 23rd August, 1924, the Revolutionary Military Council of the Red Army issued an order to establish the Central Experimental Military and Sporting Dog Kennel in Moscow (Kuskovo) to conduct experiments on the use of dogs for military purposes. The Combat Training Directorate of the Red Army was asked to set up the kennel/school under the Higher Small Arms Firing and Tactical School in Moscow, immediately and the school was to commence by 1st November, 1924. Further, District kennels to be set up in Red Army units in order to train dogs for scouting, communication, sentry, delivering first aid and assisting defence depot guards. On completion of theoretical and practical dog training, the Combat Training Directorate of the Red Army and the Command of Districts and Armies were asked to set up special commissions in order to assess the dogs' level of training and the advisability of further training.

Colonel Nikita Evtushenko, whose military occupation was communications, became the first head of the Military and Sporting Dog School, though he was not familiar with his new occupation but even before this appointment he had been involved in dog training as the first head of the Central Section for Working Dog Training under the Hunters Union, and later under the OSOAVIAKHIM (Union of Societies of Assistance to Defence and Aviation-Chemical Construction of the USSR). Colonel Evtushenko's initiative and administrative skills ensured establishment and development of military dog training.

The Army was supplied with 68,000 dogs from different regions of the country through dog training clubs and individuals. Those dog fanciers who gave their dogs to the school gained the right to get a puppy from the School's kennel at no cost after the war and as promised, the kennel gave 1,200 puppies of working and hunting dogs to clubs and individuals after the war. The Soviet Army had no dedicated dog trainers, therefore, they recruited hunters, circus and police dog trainers for the purpose. Several leading animal scientists were also involved, in order to organize a wide-scale training programme. German Shepherd Dogs were preferred for their physical abilities and ease of training, but other breeds were used as well. The idea of using dogs as mobile mines was developed in the 1930s, together with the dog-fitting mine design. In 1935, Anti-Tank Dog Units were officially included in the Soviet Army. The Soviets tested Anti-Tank (AT) Dogs during the military conflict with Japan in 1939, destroying several Japanese light tanks.

During 1934, experimental work on the possibility of air dropping dogs behind enemy lines and using them for target demolition was undertaken. This job for dogs was called Airborne Dog Service (during World War II, it was called diversionary service). Training covered three aspects: rail demolition, railway and highway bridge demolition and oil tank demolition. In order to train the staff and dogs, a parachute tower and a 100 metres railway was constructed at the unit training site. The test for Airborne Dogs were held at the Monino Airfield in Moscow region in June and October, 1934. Training of Airborne Dogs did not cause any difficulties due to available experience with Anti-Tank Dog training. With the Airborne Dog Service, the focus was on training personnel who would be able to define a tactically correct target and choose the right moment to release a dog. Such operations were to be preceded by proper reconnaissance of designated objectives.

During the Great Patriotic War (1941–1945), the Central School did not carry out any special airborne or diversionary dog training for combat operations. However, it was Sub-Colonel Alexander Mazover's personal initiative to use a dog from his Mine Detection Dog Unit No. 37 to demolish a railway on the Belorussian front in 1943. On 19th August, not far from Polotsk, Private Filatov released a dog called Dina. The dog covered the distance between the hideout to the railway, dropped a special separable pack on the railway track and quickly returned to its handler. Fifteen to eighteen seconds later, an explosion destroyed the railway bed and wrecked a troop train since the dog had been re-released towards the approaching train.

The Soviet Forces during the war had 168 units and subunits ranging from separate Platoon and Companies to special Regiments which include 2 special Regiments, 21 Battalions, 45 Detachments and 100 Platoons. In addition, special services were provided, 13 Anti-Tank Dog Detachments, 18 Mine-Detection Dog Detachments, 36 Sled Dog Detachments, 4 Messenger Dog Detachments, 2 Special Regiments and

69 Separate Sled Teams. In order to staff all the units, a total of 43,000 personnel which included, 3,000 Officers, 8,000 Sergeants and 32,000 handlers were trained.

The use of Anti-Tank Mine Dogs also known as AT Dogs, was a new tactic adopted by the Russian Army in an attempt to hold the advancing Germans in check. Dogs strapped with explosives also known as dog mines, dog bombs were sent out to disable and destroy enemy tanks. The explosive was detonated by tilt of a lever when the dog ran beneath the tank and also blow themselves in the process. The German Panzers were quick and powerful vehicles of war, and dynamic weapons were needed to stop them. Each Hound was taught to dive under the tank so that a wooden lever protruding from their packs would be triggered, setting off the explosives and blowing the tank crew and dog to smithereens. In August, 1941, Soviets Military had ten army units of AT Dogs. Each AT Dog unit also had a Rifle Platoon with snipers for killing the missed dogs with explosives. The Soviet AT Dogs were used to the familiar diesel-engine smell of the static Soviet tanks and not on the petrol scent of their German counterparts. As such, many a times, they refused to dive under tanks that were not static but moving. Further, these dogs were frightened off by the unknown noise of gunfire. The persistent dogs that ran beside tanks waiting for them to stop were shot, while those that retreated back to the trenches often jumped in and detonated the charge, killing and injuring Soviet soldiers. Out of the first group of 30 dogs, only four managed to detonate their bombs near German Tanks, while six exploded upon returning to the Soviet dugouts whereas three were shot and taken away by the Germans. Partly through their capture, the German Army soon learned of the Soviet tactics and took measures to shoot any dog encountered on sight. However, during the battle of Moscow in autumn 1941, the 28th Unit of AT Dogs destroyed 42 German tanks and two armoured cars during the Battle of Stalingrad Airport and won the appreciation of one and all. In battle of Kursk, fifteen of seventeen dogs managed to reach the German tanks. The dangerous drawbacks of using these Anti-Tank Mine Dogs outweighed their advantages, and this practice rapidly declined after 1942. Although, AT Dog units were disbanded in 1943, yet considering that AT Dogs were employed in the biggest battles of Moscow, Stalingrad and Kursk and destroyed a sufficient number of tanks, the survivors were considered worthy of the honour of taking part in the victory parade in the Red Square.

Messenger Dogs delivered 200,000 messages whereas Communication Dogs and specially equipped Sled Teams pulled 7,883 kilometres of telephone cable. The Red Cross Dogs searched many wounded on the battlefield and the Ambulance Teams evacuated 4,500 casualties. Sled Teams evacuated 500,000 Soldiers and Officers and their arms from the battlefields, and transported 3,682 tons of different loads.

The French used considerable number of the War Dogs at the beginning of World War II but due to France's quick defeat they did not get a chance to prove themselves in operational service. Many French War Dogs were taken over by the occupation troops and used as Guard Dogs, against their old masters.

Japan has a long history of employing dogs in wars and during World War II, dogs were used by them in sentry roles. It is also believed that attempts were made to train Suicide Dogs who would run towards enemy emplacements prior to exploding with a timed fuse but no such evidence is on record and can not be given much credence.

In Britain, after World War I, the government had reduced defence spending and one of the first services to go was the dogs. The main argument was that technology

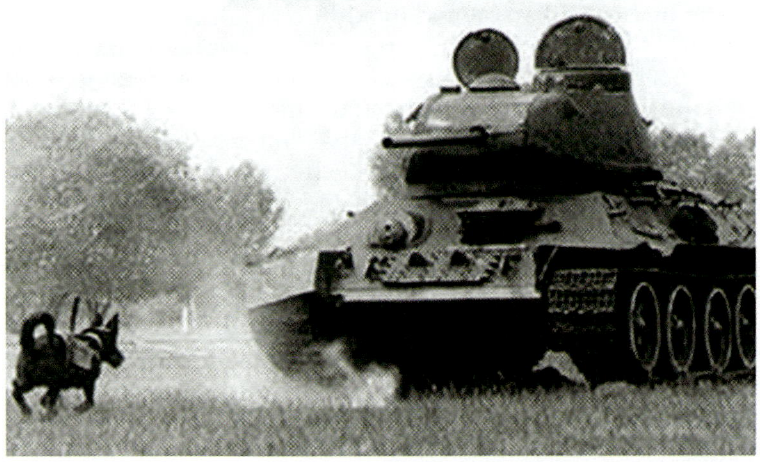

Anti-Tank Mine Dog strapped with explosives, approaching the tank

would make War Dogs obsolete. This same argument is still used today, but in the 21st century, MWDs are on the increase as never in the previous hundred years. As a result, in the British Invasion Force's plan of World War II, only Guard Dogs of the Royal Military Police (RMP), a small number of Parachute Regiment Patrol Dogs and Mine Detection Dogs (MDDs) of the Royal Engineers (REs) were included. MDDs were found to be far superior to metal detectors operated by men because a Mine Detection Dog Unit could detect wooden, plastic and glass mines laid by the Germans. In 1939, on the outbreak of World War II, forces saw the need for the Royal Army Veterinary Corps (RAVC) to expand rapidly from 190 to nearly 4,500 personnel before hostilities ended in 1945. While most personnel were to serve with equines during World War II. It was fortunate that the RAVC had developed wartime skills in the training and deployment of dogs, since the post-war involvement in equines was to decline rapidly. The British Army started the "War Dog Training School" in Hertfordshire in 1941 and the British War Office made radio appeals for dog-owners to secure canine donations, as a result, many excellent dogs were "volunteered" for the war effort. This led to the first batch of animals at the training school. In 1942, the RAVC became responsible for the procurement of dogs for all service agencies. German Shepherd were widely used, proving superior in intelligence, stamina, loyalty and courage. RAVC personnel ran the Army Dog Training School, which was located at the Grey Hound Racing Association kennels at Potters Bar near London. In 1945, this School moved to Belgium as an RAVC unit. Subsequently, it moved to Sennelager in Germany. This unit provided technical support for all animals on the continent. The RAVC also required a permanent depot and moved to the old Remount Depot at Melton Mowbray, east Leicestershire, in 1946, where it remains to this day as the Defence Animal Centre, that trains animals (mainly dogs) for all three Armed Forces as well as for British Defence Organizations. It also prepares dogs for the UK Immigration Service, HM Prison Service, HM Revenue and Customs, other UK government agencies and Overseas agencies.

In January, 1944, the school undertook Parachute Dogs Training. "One of the dogs selected from the training school in Hertfordshire was 'Bing' a two-year-old Alsatian-Collie cross and was the smallest of his litter and due to wartime rationing he was given up by his civilian owner. In addition to Bing, two other dogs selected for training were Monty and Ranee, both German Shepherds. These three were to be among Britain's first ever Para-Dogs during the war, with Ranee being the only female parachuting dog in the war. The 13th (Lancashire) Parachute Battalion of the British Army enlisted these dogs into their ranks. The so-called "Para-Dogs" (short for "parachuting dogs") were specifically trained to perform tasks such as parachuting, locating mines, keeping watch and warning about enemies. They also served as a mascot for the troops.

A large number of Mascots and other War Dogs trained and utilized for specific tasks were deployed by the Armies of various countries and the allied forces used approximately 250,000 dogs in their war efforts. Heroism of some of these war dogs was recorded in texts whereas others were only fondly remembered by the surviving buddies of these heroes. Keeping in view the very wide spectrum of heroic actions only a few representatives of the legendary War Dogs of World War II period are described here:

BING

Bing was an Alsatian-Collie cross, born in 1942 and named as Brian by his owner Betty Fetch and her family from Loughborough, Leicestershire. The family donated Brian to army during World War II, as they could no longer afford to keep him due to war-rationing. Bing joined army in 1944 and began his basic training at Army War Dog Training School, near Potters Bar Heartfordshire. After qualifying as Patrol Dog, he was posted to the Sniper Reconnaissance Platoon,13th Parachute Battalion of 6th Airborne Division and got training in parachuting. He trained hard to become a tough paratrooper for his deployment with the British Army. After a few practice runs, he was back in Blighty. He was deployed with the elite 6th Airborne Division over Normandy on 6th June, 1944 with his handler and trainer Ken Bailey. While participating in "Operation Overlord (D-Day)", heavy anti-aircraft fire raked his plane and history records that he needed an encouraging boot to propel him landwards. Unit personnel would see Bing falling to earth with his forepaws up and rear legs down, just as trained—ears flapping in the wind.

Bing landed on a tree and was shot at by German troops and got wounded in his neck and eyes but after first aid, he joined Ken Bailey in the line. Bing was one of the first dogs to be dropped behind enemy lines with British Paratroopers and put his paws on Normandy soil on the D-Day. Once on ground, he was ready for action and when something didn't look quite right, he would freeze and point towards the danger with his nose. During rest breaks, he kept watch over sleeping British Troops and while on the move he pioneered the advance through potential danger zones. Bing went on patrol with the Red Berets of the 13th Battalion and his fearless excursions through perilous terrain and behind enemy lines were credited with saving many lives and hundreds of soldiers from ambush. He was wounded by mortar fire and was evacuated for treatment and recuperation to Veterinary Kennels at Chillbolton, Downs near Stockport.

Once fully recovered and fit for duty, he was taken to Ark Hill in Salisbury and assigned a new handler Corporal Jack Walton with whom Bing participated in "Operation Varsity", the Pivotal Rhine Crossing and advanced into Germany on 24th March, 1945. Troops landed in enemy strong points and the Germans began firing. Now the task was to clear the machine gun post and head towards the Baltic.

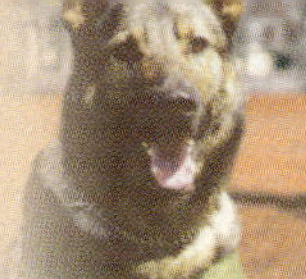

After achieving the goal, the Platoon embarked on marching, 20-mile-a-day towards the Baltic. The duo of Bing and Jack proved very useful, especially while passing through danger zones where they used to be ahead of the column for locating mines, explosives, booby traps and enemy personnel. He would sniff excitedly over Mine/Booby traps for a few seconds and then sit down looking back at the handler with a quaint mixture of smugness and expectancy. On a night march the dog sensed something and indicated to the handler. The Platoon shouted 'hands up' and German Soldiers came out and surrendered. During the march there were moments of humour too. One hot day everyone was suffering from thirst and Bing struck lucky in a roadside barn. He squeezed under a barn door and reached up to a drip tray which was under a barrel of white wine. He drank the lot and was obviously sloshed, wobbling all over the place. After the end of war, Bing was taken back to Britain and returned to his owner, Batty Fetch and her parents and he resumed civilian life as 'Brian'.

On 26th April, 1947, he was awarded the prestigious **"PDSA Dickin Medal".** His citation reads: "This Patrol Dog was attached with 13th Parachute Battalion, the 6th Airborne Division. He landed in Normandy with them and having done the requisite number of jumps became a qualified paratrooper. His selfless acts of bravery throughout Operation Overlord (D-Day) and Operation Varsity (Rhine Crossing) saved many men's lives."

Bing died of natural causes on 26th October, 1955 and the former Para Dog was buried in a cemetery of honour for animals northeast of London. Today, one can also find a true-to-life replica of this four-legged hero in the Parachute Regiment and Airborne Forces Museum in Duxford. He is naturally shown wearing his parachute and next to his medal of honour, which bears the words "For Gallantry" and "We Also Serve."

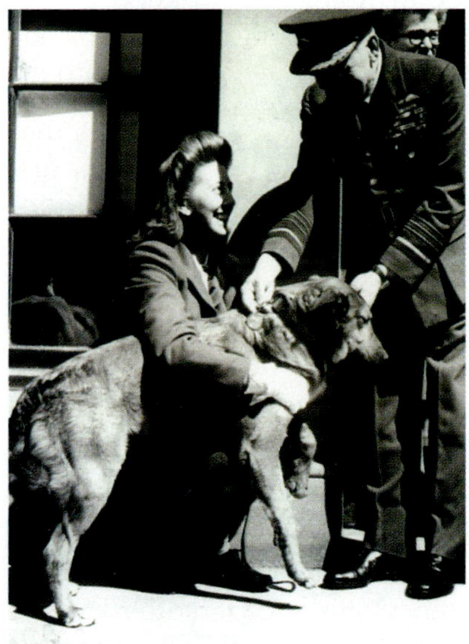
Bing receiving Dickin Medal

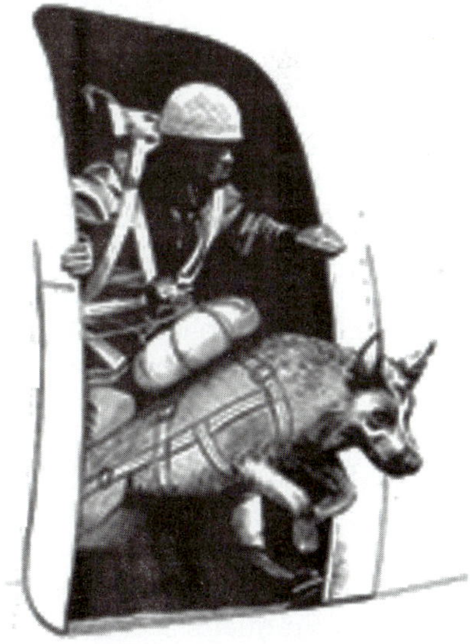
Bing and Jack Parachuting

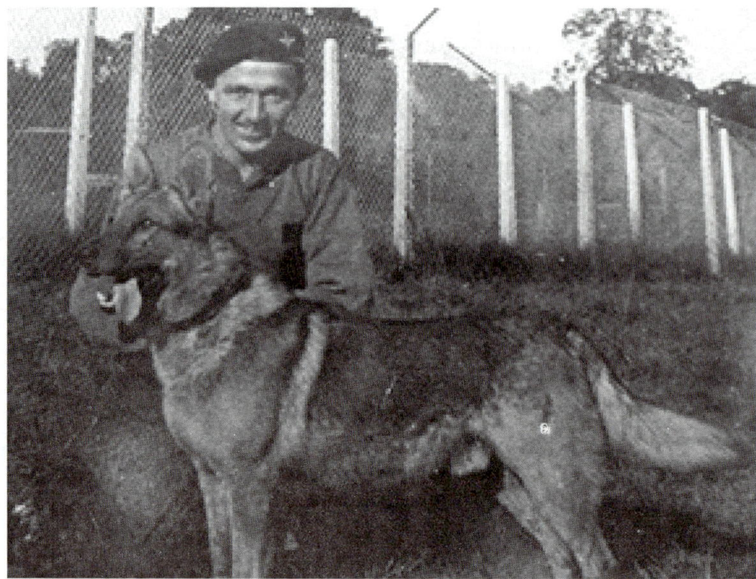

Bing with handler Jack Walton

A Children's book has now been written on Bing, titled "The Amazing Adventures of Bing, The Parachute Dog" by Gil Boyd BEM, a former paratrooper who served in 2nd Battalion, The Parachute Regiment.

BLONDI

A German Shepherd was given as a gift to Adolf Hitler by Martin Bormann in 1941 and was named as Blondi. In May, 1942, Hitler bought another young German Shepherd "from a minor official in the postoffice in Ingolstadt to keep Blondi company". He called her Bella. However, Hitler was very fond of Blondi and this dog stayed with him even after Hitler Moved into Fuhrerbunker located underneath the garden of Reich Chancellery on 16th January, 1945. Hitler always kept Blondi by his side and allowing her to sleep in his bedroom in the bunker. This affection was not shared by Eva Braun, Hitler's mistress (and later his wife), who preferred her two Scottish Terriers named Negus and Stasi (or Katuschka). Blondi had a litter of five puppies on 4th April, 1945 and Hitler named one of the puppies as Wulf, his favourite nick name and the meaning of his own first name, Adolf (Noble wolf). Blondi played a role in Nazi propaganda, portraying Hitler as an animal lover. Dogs like Blondi were coveted as "Germanischer Urhund", being close to the wolf, and grew very fashionable.

During the course of events on 29th April, 1945, Hitler learned about the death of his ally Benito Mussolini who had been executed by Italian partisans. This, along with the fact that the Soviet Army was closing in on his location, led Hitler to strengthen his resolve not to allow himself or his wife to be captured. That afternoon, Hitler expressed doubts about the cyanide capsules he had received through Heinrich Himmler's SS. To verify the capsules' potency, Hitler ordered Dr Werner Haase to test them on his dog Blondi, and the dog died as a result. Hitler became completely inconsolable.

According to a report based on eye witness accounts, Hitler's dog handler, Feldwebel Fritz Tomow took Blondi's pups and shot them in the garden of the bunker complex on 30th April, after Hitler and Eva Braun committed suicide. He also killed Eva Braun's two dogs. Tornow was later captured by the allies. Hitler's nurse, Erna Flegel, said in 2005 that Blondi's death had affected the people in the bunker more than Eva Braun's. After the battle in Berlin ended, the remains of Hitler, Eva Braun, and two dogs (thought to be Blondi and her offspring Wulf) were discovered in a shell crater by a unit of SMERSH, the Soviet counterintelligence agency. The dog (thought to be Blondi) was exhumed and photographed by the Soviets.

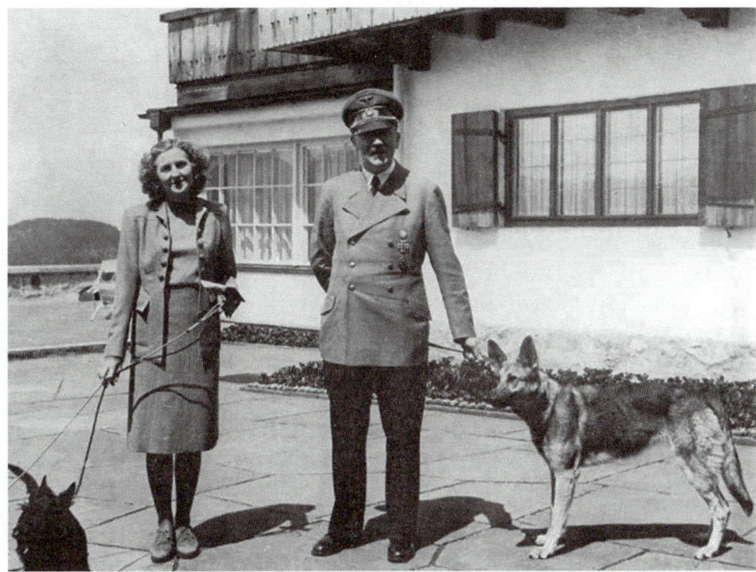

Adolf Hitler and Eva Braun with favourite German Shepherd Dog Blondi

BOB

Bob, a Mongrel was Mascot of an Infantry Unit, 6th Battalion Queens Own Royal West Kent Regiment in Africa in 1944. One day Bob was travelling with his unit when he froze suddenly and refused to move. A noise was then heard which revealed the presence of the enemy. Because of Bob's actions, none of the men of his unit were killed or captured. Bob was the first dog to be awarded the **"PDSA Dickin Medal"** (the UK's highest honour for animals that have displayed conspicuous gallantry or devotion to duty while serving with any branch of the Armed Forces or Civil Defence Units) on 24th March, 1944. Bob's citation reads:

"For constant devotion to duty with special mention of patrol work at Green Hill, North Africa, while serving with the 6th Battalion Queens Own Royal West Kent Regiment".

CAESAR

On the Bougainville Campaign, probably the most famous of the dogs was Caesar, a German Shepherd. During the time that "M" Company, 3rd Raider Battalion was holding a road block on the Piva Trail, Caesar made nine runs between the road block and the Battalion Command Post when lines were out and radios would not carry in the heavy jungle. Caesar was wounded on the third day when, during the early morning, he attacked a Japanese who was in the act of shoving a hand grenade into the foxhole of his handler, PFC Rufus Mayo, and thus saved his life. Caesar being a big beautiful male was the obvious favourite of the troops. He had a regular Marine record book and carried the rank of PFC. On the 3rd day ashore, word got around that Caesar had done such an outstanding job that he was given a spot promotion to Seargent (SGT) and troops saw Caesar come trotting down the muddy Piva Trail ignoring everybody as he was trained to do. He also invited taunts from the ranks—"Ear Banger," "Brown Nose," "Ass kisser" and so forth but these did not have any effect on Caesar.

CHIPS

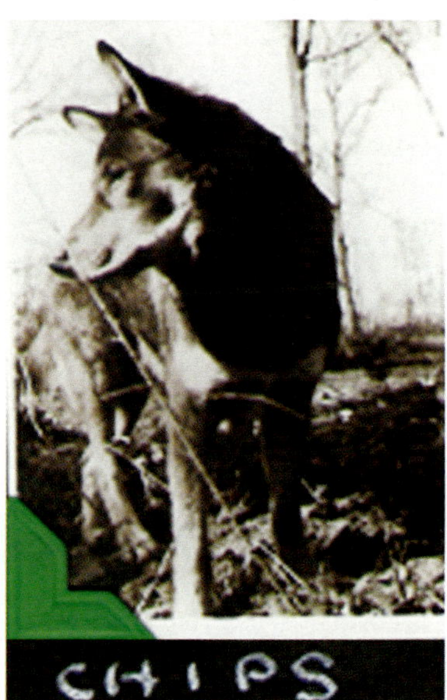

Chips was a German Shepherd-Collie-Siberian Husky mix, owned by Edward J Wren of Pleasantville, New York. Chips was well-loved by his family and was very protective of the Wren's two daughters, Gail, 8, and her younger sister Nancy. In his role as "protector" he was also known to be aggressive and had also bitten a local garbage man. During the war, private citizens were requested to donate their pet dogs for war efforts and Wren family also decided to donate their pet for military duty and Chips be trained by the military so that his aggression could be used for the sake of the country. He was sent to the War Dog Training Centre in Front Royal, Virginia, in 1942, and was trained to be a Sentry Dog. Private John P Rowell was Chips' handler and both made a good team while serving with General Patton's Seventh Army and the US Army 3rd Infantry Division. On one occasion, Chips alerted to an impending ambush. Then, with a phone cable attached to his collar, Chips ran back to base, dodging gunfire so that the endangered Platoon could establish a communications line and ask for the backup, they so desperately needed. The duo accompanied the Division in Africa, Italy and other parts of Europe. Chips proved to be a valued team member as soldiers on sentry duty were sometimes killed by the enemy at night when the attacking forces had the advantage of darkness. Once dogs like Chips began to be deployed on sentry duty, no soldier on guard duty with a dog was ever killed as the dogs alerted their masters about the approach of strangers. Chips and Rowell encountered their first battle when their ship landed at French Morocco. As the soldiers came up the beach, they were under attack, so Rowell quickly dug a shallow foxhole for himself and another for Chips. When it quieted down, Rowell started to deepen his foxhole to make it more safe, and Chips got the point and started digging deeper as well. Chips and Rowell served as sentry at Casablanca, Morocco, for the historic conference between the President Franklin Roosevelt and British Prime Minister Winston Churchill and their Military Commanders in January, 1943.

Chips' heroism became legendary during fighting in Sicily in July, 1943. One early morning, at about 04.20 am while Rowell and Chips were on duty, they noticed a grass covered hut and Rowell hoped they might rest there for some time. As the duo was approaching the hut, they were suddenly fired upon by a machine gun. Chips pulled away from Rowell, and moments later he was in the pillbox (a dug-in guard post, usually with holes from which soldiers could shoot). He seized one man and made four others to surrender by forcing them out of the pillbox. One of the soldiers shot him with his revolver that grazed Chips' scalp. The complete crew of Italians was captured and loss of many lives averted. Chips sustained a scalp wound and some powder burns but he was safe and required only first aid. Chips returned to duty that night with his master and he noticed a group of soldiers advancing towards their location, taking the advantage of darkness. He immediately alerted his master and the troops. This allowed his handler and Squad to organize themselves and as a result the group of ten Italians was captured. The Army awarded Chips with the **"Purple Heart and Silver Star"** (later revoked because at that time honouring an animal was "contrary to army policy"). However, the company took matters into their own hands, and they unofficially gave him a Battle Star and Ribbons of all the Eight Campaigns. Chips was also known for an embarrassing situation. After the Battle of Salerno in which Chips and Rowell had taken part, General Dwight D Eisenhower came to congratulate the unit, and he bent to pet Chips but Chips was trained to be touched by his handler only and so Chips responded as he was trained. Despite this gaff, Chips was well-respected. Chips along with his master participated in campaigns in Italy and then moved on with his unit to southern France. He served in the French Rhineland, and Central Europe campaigns. By early 1945, Chips was getting weary and his family had requested his return after service, so in the fall of 1945, he was taken back to Front Royal where he was retrained so that he could go back to his family. Chips was honourably discharged in December, 1945 and he returned to the Wren family as the most decorated War Dog of World War II. Chips travelled home to Pleasantville, riding in the baggage car of a train. He was accompanied by six reporters and photographers who wanted to cover the story. Mr and Mrs Wren and son Johnny, who was only a baby when Chips left, met Chips at the train, and the girls ran home to see their dog as soon as school was over. Chips lived only four months before his kidneys gave out, but as one of the first Military War Dogs, he blazed a trail. Disney made a TV movie based on his life, titled "Chips, the War Dog" in 1990.

DICK

A scout dog donated by Edward Zan of New York City, was cited for working with a Marine Corps patrol in the Pacific Area. On 4th February 1944, T/4 Boude with his Scout Dog, Dick, went out with a Marine Reconnaissance Patrol of about fifteen men from K Company. The mission of the patrol was to locate and reconnoiter a trail through a portion of the island adjacent to Cape Gloucester. The terrain to be covered consisted of heavy jungle, forest and swamps. Rain fell throughout the period. On the third day, T/4 Boude and Dick were working as usual at the point of the patrol. Dick alerted, pointing to the right front. The handler, Boude, stopped and signalled the patrol leader, who came up and received the report. He and Boude went forward about forty yards and saw a Japanese bivouac of five huts. No Japanese were in sight. Boude and Dick searched to determine which of the huts were occupied. Dick alerted to one hut only. The patrol surrounded this hut, closed in, and found four Japanese who were subsequently killed in the follow-up action. There were no Marine casualties. The patrol proceeded on its mission, and some more Japanese stragglers were encountered. In each instance the dog alerted in time and the Japanese were captured or killed.

HORRIE

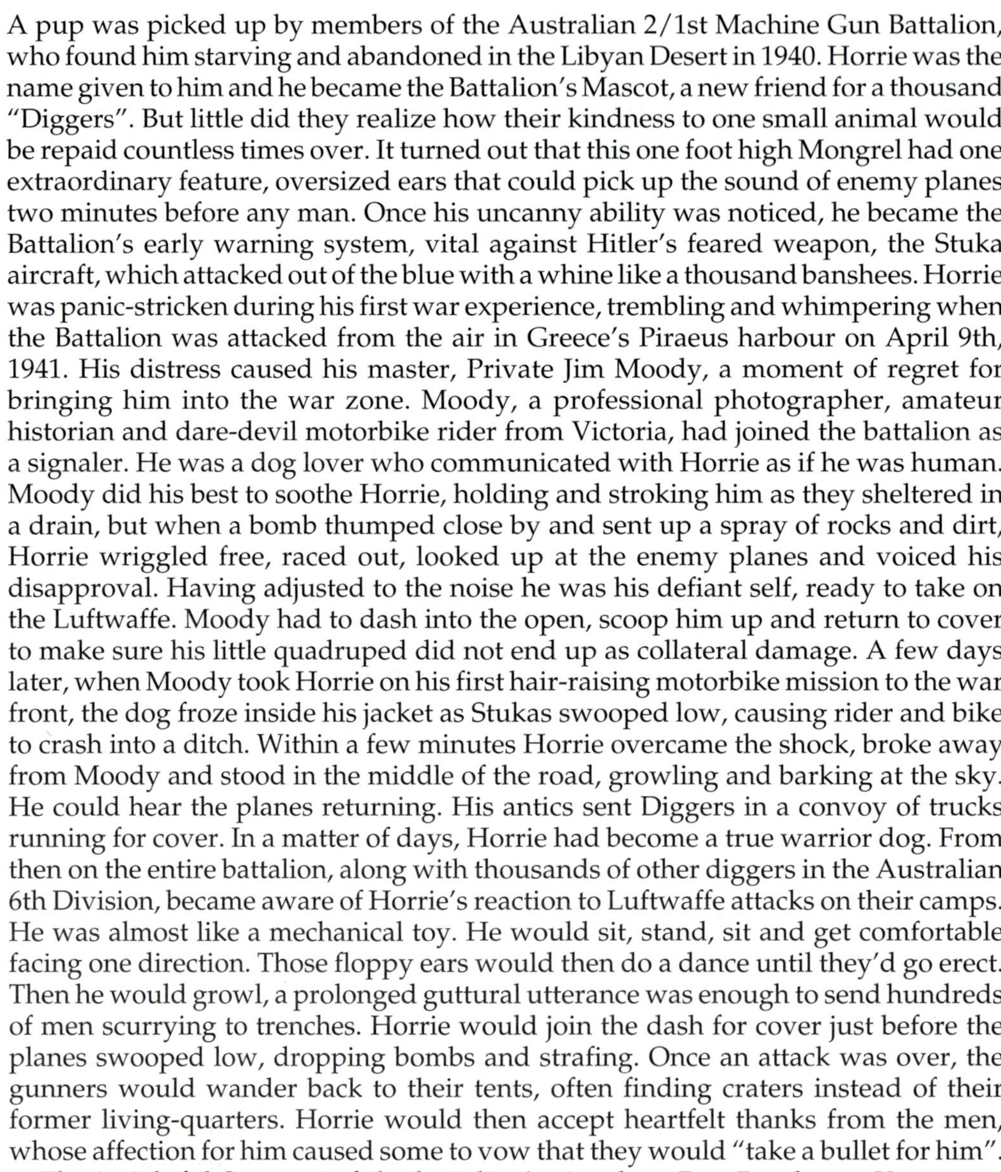

A pup was picked up by members of the Australian 2/1st Machine Gun Battalion, who found him starving and abandoned in the Libyan Desert in 1940. Horrie was the name given to him and he became the Battalion's Mascot, a new friend for a thousand "Diggers". But little did they realize how their kindness to one small animal would be repaid countless times over. It turned out that this one foot high Mongrel had one extraordinary feature, oversized ears that could pick up the sound of enemy planes two minutes before any man. Once his uncanny ability was noticed, he became the Battalion's early warning system, vital against Hitler's feared weapon, the Stuka aircraft, which attacked out of the blue with a whine like a thousand banshees. Horrie was panic-stricken during his first war experience, trembling and whimpering when the Battalion was attacked from the air in Greece's Piraeus harbour on April 9th, 1941. His distress caused his master, Private Jim Moody, a moment of regret for bringing him into the war zone. Moody, a professional photographer, amateur historian and dare-devil motorbike rider from Victoria, had joined the battalion as a signaler. He was a dog lover who communicated with Horrie as if he was human. Moody did his best to soothe Horrie, holding and stroking him as they sheltered in a drain, but when a bomb thumped close by and sent up a spray of rocks and dirt, Horrie wriggled free, raced out, looked up at the enemy planes and voiced his disapproval. Having adjusted to the noise he was his defiant self, ready to take on the Luftwaffe. Moody had to dash into the open, scoop him up and return to cover to make sure his little quadruped did not end up as collateral damage. A few days later, when Moody took Horrie on his first hair-raising motorbike mission to the war front, the dog froze inside his jacket as Stukas swooped low, causing rider and bike to crash into a ditch. Within a few minutes Horrie overcame the shock, broke away from Moody and stood in the middle of the road, growling and barking at the sky. He could hear the planes returning. His antics sent Diggers in a convoy of trucks running for cover. In a matter of days, Horrie had become a true warrior dog. From then on the entire battalion, along with thousands of other diggers in the Australian 6th Division, became aware of Horrie's reaction to Luftwaffe attacks on their camps. He was almost like a mechanical toy. He would sit, stand, sit and get comfortable facing one direction. Those floppy ears would then do a dance until they'd go erect. Then he would growl, a prolonged guttural utterance was enough to send hundreds of men scurrying to trenches. Horrie would join the dash for cover just before the planes swooped low, dropping bombs and strafing. Once an attack was over, the gunners would wander back to their tents, often finding craters instead of their former living-quarters. Horrie would then accept heartfelt thanks from the men, whose affection for him caused some to vow that they would "take a bullet for him".

The insightful Sergeant of the battalion's signalers, Roy Brooker, a Veteran of World War I, believed that the love for Horrie went beyond the gunners' gratitude for saving their lives. He personally had been in two big wars and recollected that once he told Moody and the others in the group of signalers that Horrie is a worthy recipient of all the gunners' love and sympathy. Moody, Brooker and the rest of the Rebels took responsibility for Horrie during the war, smuggling him in their packs through Libya, Egypt, Greece, Crete, Palestine and Syria and finally, in the most dangerous venture of all for them and the dog, back to Australia. The Captain of the Troop Ship, USS West Point, followed Quarantine directives and decreed that all "pets" on board had to be handed over. They were to be destroyed before reaching Fremantle, the first port of call for the 6,000 men of Australia's 6th Division, being brought home urgently by Prime Minister John Curtin, to meet the menace of marauding Japanese forces. When they refused to produce Horrie, the Captain, who had a reputation as a "Maritime Caesar", thundered that the ship would not dock at all if the dog was not handed in. He slowed the ship to a stop in sight of the Australian coast, much to the chagrin of all on board. Other animals, including a cat, were given up but not Horrie, who was hidden in the Rebels' cabin. In the stand-off, a delegation led by a defiant Moody made it clear to the Captain that he could not touch Horrie. The Captain in turn said he would have Horrie "thrown in the ship's furnace". "The men of my Battalion are wild enough to dish out similar treatment to you," Moody told him. The Captain only had to look into the faces of these hardened soldiers, who relished the prospect of fighting the Japanese in New Guinea, to know that this was no bluff. On top of that, he was reminded by an Australian liaison officer on board of what it might do to the Captain's commission and reputation if there was a mutiny on his ship. The USS West Point started up again and sailed into port. Horrie was smuggled into Australia and left with Moody's father in Melbourne's St Kilda.

Three years later, in 1945, Moody returned with the Rebels to Australia after fighting the Japanese. He was approached to bring the dog out of hiding to raise funds for the Sydney Red Cross. Horrie was already well-known as a "War Hero" and was about to feature in a book by Australian author Ion Idriess. Yet Moody was not convinced by the overtures from the publisher and Idriess. Horrie had not been quarantined on entering Australia and he feared the Department of Health, which was obsessed with slaughtering any pets brought home by returning diggers. Moody only agreed when Brooker managed to talk the Melbourne branch of the RSL into making Horrie an honorary member in recognition of the lives he had saved.

Horrie was taken to Sydney so he could be exhibited by the Red Cross, and was photographed wearing his special coat (which had been made for him during a cold winter in Syria), his colour patch, gunner's disc, identity tags and now Returned and Services League (RSL) badge. Moody and Brooker were in another photo with him. The accompanying newspaper articles were the beginning of what seemed to be a superb public relations exercise. Each piece mentioned his "amazing" war career. There was careful mention of a wound when a bomb splinter lodged in his leg, but that he was in rude good health, was a signal to any Quarantine official who might be thinking of pinning a disease on him. The second day after his "coming out", Idriess visited the Sydney home in which Moody and Horrie were staying and was photographed with the dog for the newspapers. Moody fielded hundreds of calls from journalists, battalion members and other soldiers and well-wishers. It led to a nationwide surge in interest in Horrie. On 24th February, 1945, press articles on Horrie reached the desk of Ron W Wardle, the Director of the Division of Veterinary Hygiene in Canberra's Health Department. He reckoned that he could sniff a crime and told his colleagues that Horrie's appearance was "nothing more than a money-making stunt for the publication of a book". He vowed to put a stop to it and quarantine official pounced. Moody was ordered to bring Horrie into its Abbotsford station within a week. It was still wartime and such a directive had to be adhered to or the rebels would face jail terms. Handing the dog over did not necessarily mean that Horrie would be put down. After all, this dog was disease-free and had been checked by a Veterinarian in Tel Aviv before being smuggled to Australia. Moody was told that Horrie would be given a medical examination and if he proved healthy, there was every chance he would be released. But Moody was suspicious. The speed with which quarantine official moved to impound the dog, worried him. Would the Health Department make an example of Horrie to demonstrate its diligence in tracking down animals with potential diseases such as the much-feared rabies? This led to a dilemma. If Moody handed over the dog the odds were that he would be put down. If he didn't comply, he would be jailed and Horrie would be hunted down and probably euthanized. Moody had to act. He did deliver Horrie to Abbotsford. Wardle was informed that the animal was in very good condition, a Sydney Veterinarian's report, which Moody had obtained, backed this up. There was no sign of any disease. John King, the Director at the Abbotsford station, rang the Veterinarians to verify the report's authenticity, but Wardle didn't care. He had made up his mind that the dog was to be executed. "Horrie must be made an example of," Wardle told King. "Can't have any soldiers smuggling pets into our country, Rabies kills, as you well know". As Moody feared, the animal was destroyed. But was it Horrie the War Dog? The public, newspapers, the military and government, Idriess and the publisher believed it was. The media went into overdrive, with newspapers running a campaign akin to a witch-hunt to assign blame for this "crime" against a certified saviour of diggers. The zealous Wardle became the main target as protest over his action reached the desk of Prime Minister Curtin. The questions were asked in the House of Representatives concerning the "Horrie tragedy". Parliamentarians responded to anger from their constituents and continued to pressure the government. There was a public rally at Sydney's Town Hall. Even while the war in the Pacific continued to rage, letters-to-the-editor correspondence was dominated by the issue. Wardle received scores of death threats. Typical was one from a person calling himself "Y.S", an old soldier of Sydney's Chatswood. He ended his letter with: "I hope and pray that when your day comes I will have the pleasure to put you to sleep in the same way that little mate Horrie died." More worrying was an unsigned message: "I was trained to kill in the Great War and I am still a very accurate shot. Your killing of this creature of God deserves a similar fate and I know how to do it." Moody and Brooker organized their Battalion to carry out a funeral for the dog, although there was no body in the coffin. Quarantine refused to hand it over, saying it had been incinerated. The press covered the funeral and a special service for Horrie was carried out on Anzac Day and a wreath in his honour was laid at the Cenotaph in Martin Place, Sydney.

GANDER

A Canadian Newfoundland Dog named "Pal" with his large build and goofy, friendly demeanour was loved by the local children. They would play with him and have him tow their sleds. One day while playing, one child got a scratch from the paw of the dog. His owner feared that the authorities would take action against their beloved dog so they donated Pal to a local Rifle Regiment. The soldiers were very happy to have a dog of high potential, renamed him Gander and made him their Official Mascot.

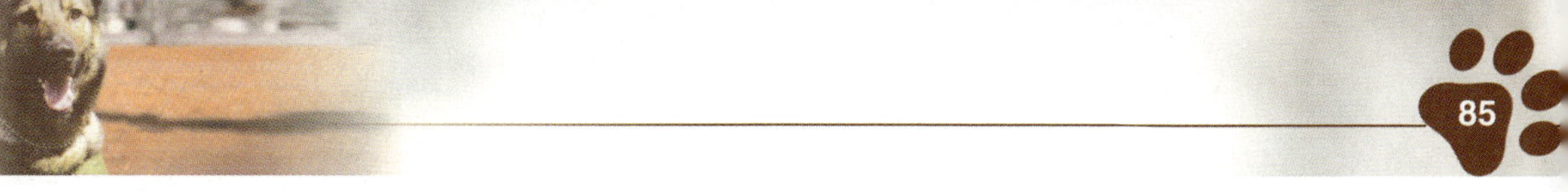

Subsequently, he was promoted to the rank of Sergeant. Gander adapted to military life well and the unit was sent overseas to assist in the Battle of Hong Kong in 1941. The Japanese attacked the unit under the cover of night, thinking of less resistance, in December 1941. Gander noticed the impending sneak attack and started barking furiously as well as attacking the Japanese Soldiers and did not allow them to move forward. After this heroic act, Gander noticed a second Japanese unit advancing on a group of injured Royal Rifles and again he roared down on the soldiers and ensured that the enemy fled. Gander then sat down to guard the injured soldiers. In the meanwhile Japanese opened fire and threw a grenade at the group of injured soldiers. Gander took a calm look at the grenade, picked it up and charged the terrified Japanese troops. The grenade exploded and Gander went out in an blaze of glory. For the unbelievable bravery, "PDSA Dickin Medal" was awarded to Gander posthumously on 25th October, 2000. Although, Dickin Medal was awarded last in 1949 but in 2000 it was revived to honour the brave dog Gander posthumously, for saving the lives of Canadian Infantrymen during the Battle of Lye Mun on Hong Kong Island in December, 1941. Gander also became the only non-human soldier whose name is included in the Hong Kong Memorial Wall in Ottawa.

The official citation of Gander reads:

"For saving the lives of Canadian Infantrymen during the Battle of Lye Mun on Hong Kong Island in December, 1941. On three documented occasions, Gander, the Newfoundland Mascot of the Royal Rifles of Canada, engaged the enemy as his Regiment joined the Winnipeg Grenadiers, members of Battalion Headquarters "C" Force and other Commonwealth troops in their courageous defence of the island. Twice, Gander's attack halted the enemy's advance and protected groups of wounded soldiers. In a final act of bravery, the War Dog was killed in action gathering a grenade. Without Gander's intervention, many more lives would have been lost in the assault."

GUNNER

Gunner, a small black and white Kelpie is one of the unsung heroes of World War II. Gunner was found in injured state on 19th February, 1942. On this day, first and the largest single air attack was mounted by Japanese on Darwin's harbour in northern Australia. During the bombing of Darwin also known as Battle of Darwin, 242 Japanese Aircrafts attacked ships in Darwin's harbour and the two airfields of this town. It was an attempt to prevent the allies from using these as bases to contest the invasions of Timor and Java. The ibid dog was found with a broken leg, he was named Gunner so that he could be treated legitimately and Leading Aircraftman Percy Leslie Westcott was made Gunner's master. The dog became known for his uncanny hearing and incredible ability to warn of approaching airplanes long before humans could hear them. It was believed that he could warn of Japanese Aircraft before they showed up on radar. He was so reliable that air-raid sirens were sounded when Gunner gave the warning and he successfully worked as "Canine Air-Raid Early Warning System".

JUDY

Judy was a pure-bred liver and white Pointer. She was born in a dog kennel in Shanghai, China, in 1936. She had escaped as a puppy and had been kept in a back alley by a shopkeeper until she was six months old. Following an altercation with some sailors from a Japanese Navy gunboat, she was found by a worker of the kennel and taken back. She was originally called Shudi, which was anglicized to become Judy. In the autumn of 1936, the crew of the Insect class gunboat HMS Gnat voted to get a Ship's Mascot. This was partly due to the competitive nature of the gunboats, with HMS Bee, Cicada and Cricket already having Mascots of their own. The Captain and the Chief Bosun's mate, Lt Cmdr J Waldergrave and Chief Petty Officer Charles Jefferey, purchased Judy from the kennel and presented her to the crew. It was hoped to train her as a Gun Dog, but the men began to treat her like a pet instead and Judy became their Mascot.

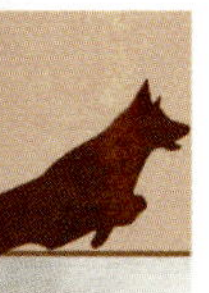

In June, 1939, several Locust Class Gunboats arrived on the Yangtze to take over operations from the existing Insect class vessels. Part of the crew of the Gnat was transferred to HMS Grasshopper, including Judy. Following the British declaration of war on Germany in September that year, several of the river gunboats including Grasshoper, were redeployed to the British Base at Singapore. Judy was initially sea sick, but the crew ensured that she was properly taken care off and exercised regularly. By the time the ship arrived at station, she had recovered and was absolutely fit. She proved her unimaginable ability to hear incoming aircraft and providing the crew with an early warning. She was on board of the ship during the Battle of Singapore, which saw Grasshopper evacuating the Dutch East Indies. It was sank enroute, and Judy was nearly killed having been trapped by a falling row of lockers. She was rescued when a crewman returned to the stricken vessel looking for supplies. When the ship sank, its crew made its way to an island that appeared to have no water. On the deserted island with the surviving crew, Judy managed to find a fresh water source saving them all. They made their way to Singkep in the Dutch East Indies and afterwards to Sumatra aiming to link up with the evacuating British Forces. After trekking across 200 miles of jungle for five weeks, during which Judy survived an attack from a crocodile, the crew arrived a day after the final vessel had left and became prisoner of war of the Japanese. She was eventually smuggled into the Medan Camp, where she met Leading Aircraftsman Frank Williams, who decided to adopt her for rest of her life. Williams convinced the Camp Commandant to register her as an Official prisoner of war, with the number '81A Gloergoer, Medan'. She was the only dog to be registered as a prisoner of war during the Second World War. In June, 1944, the men were transferred to Singapore aboard the SS Van Warwyck. Dogs were not allowed on board, but Frank Williams managed to teach Judy to lie still and silent inside a rice sack. When he boarded the ship, Judy climbed into a sack and Williams slung it over his shoulder to take on board. The conditions on board the ship were cramped with more than 700 prisoners. For three hours the men were forced to stand on deck in the searing heat, and for the entire time Judy remained still and silent in the bag on Wiliams's back. On 26th June, 1944, the ship was torpedoed and Williams pushed Judy out of a porthole in an attempt to save her life, even though there was a 15 feet (4.6 m) drop to the sea. He also made his own escape from the ship, not knowing if Judy had survived. Over five hundred of the passengers did not survive.

Frank Williams survived and was sent to a new camp without news of Judy's survival. However, stories were told of a dog helping drowning men to reach pieces of debris on which to hold, and others recalled how the dog would bring them flotsam to keep them afloat. The dog would also allow men to hold onto her back while swimming them to safety. She had been found in the water by other survivors of the sinking ship and once again hidden from the Japanese. Upon arrival at a dock, she was found by Les Searle who smuggled her once again into the next camp where she was reunited with Frank Williams who had almost given up hope of finding her. When she arrived in his new camp, Williams couldn't believe his eyes, as he entered the camp, a scraggy dog hit him square between the shoulders and knocked him over. He was very glad and so was Judy. After four weeks at the new camp, they were moved back to Sumatra by paddle streamer. After the end of the war, Judy's life was put in danger once again. She was about to be put to death by the Japanese Guards following a lice outbreak amongst the prisoners. However, Williams hid the dog until the allied forces arrived. Searle, Williams and others smuggled Judy back to the UK aboard a troopship and she spent the next six months in quarantine after arriving in Hackbridge. Williams and Judy were reunited on 29th April, 1946 and headed immediately to London. There Williams was given the "White Cross of St Giles" and Judy was awarded the "**PDSA Dickin Medal**", the animals' Victoria Cross, in May, 1946. Judy was enrolled by Major Viscount Tarbat MC, Chairman of the Returned British POW Association, as the association's only canine member. Her citation reads:

"For magnificent courage and endurance in Japanese prison camps, which helped to maintain morale among her fellow prisoners and also for saving many lives through her intelligence and watchfulness".

She was interviewed by the BBC for their coverage of the London Victory Celebrations of 1946 on 8th June and her barks were broadcast to the nation on the radio as part of the programme "In Town Tonight". Frank and Judy spent the year after the war visiting the relatives of POWs who had not survived. Frank remarked that Judy always seemed to give a comforting presence. On 10th May, 1948, the pair left to work on a government-funded groundnut food scheme in East Africa. There were some difficulties in getting permission for Judy to travel and it was feared that she and Williams would split up. This issue was promoted in the Evening Standard and after the involvement of William Lever, 2nd Viscount Leverhulme, permission was given for Judy to travel with Williams. After two years there, Judy

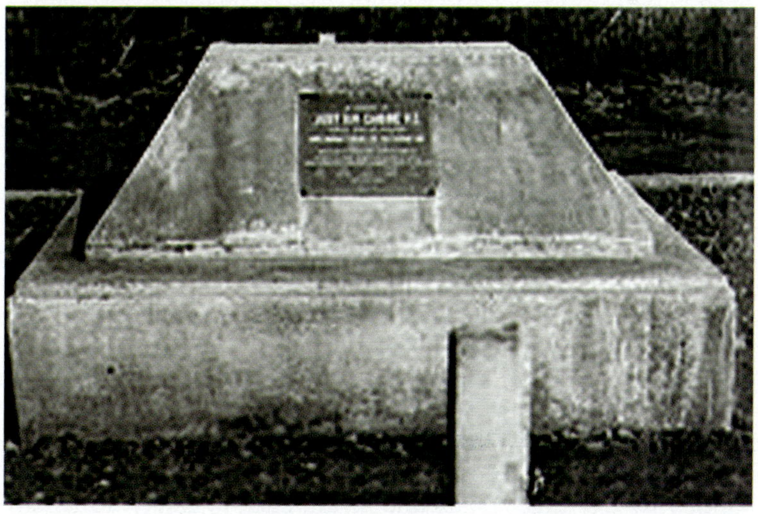

Judy's grave in Tanzania, Africa

was discovered to have a tumour and was put to sleep in 1950 at the age of 13 in Tanzania. William spent two months building a granite and marble memorial in her memory, which included a plaque that told of her life story.

On 27th February, 1972, Judy was remembered in church services across Gosport and Portsmouth, and in 1992 her story was featured in the British Children's TV show "Blue Peter".

In 2006, her Collar and Medal went on public display for the first time in the Imperial War Museum, London, as part of "The Animals' War" exhibition. It was presented to the IWM by Alan Williams, Frank's son.

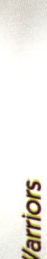

RIFLEMAN KHAN

War Dog No. 147, Rifleman Khan, a German Shepherd, was lent to the war office in the summer of 1942 by the Railton family from Tolworth, Surrey, London. He had simply been their family pet. He was named after the men from undivided India who served under the British. The dog was trained at the War Dog Training School and was considered a "star pupil" by Officers and trainers. He was soon an expert in finding explosives and on completion of training, Khan was assigned to the 6th Battalion of the Cameronians (Scottish Rifles) and Lance Corporal James Muldoon became his handler. Khan saw action in Normandy and across various centres of fighting in Western Europe. He proved his mettle time and again. However, his moment of glory came at the Battle of Walcheren Causeway in Belgium. It was of vital importance that the ports of the English, French, and Belgian Channels be cleared of German presence. Walcheren Island and the causeway that connected it to the mainland were guarded by the German 15th Division. The enemy had to be cleared before the allies could advance to Antwerp. From then on it would be a march to the aggressor's den—Germany itself!

In November, 1944, the battalion was part of the allied force and was sent to attack the Island of Walcheren in the Netherlands, as part of the Battle of the Scheldt. The island was of strategic importance and needed to be taken for the invasion of Germany. But clearing the well-entrenched and fortified German garrison from Walcheren was not easy. The responsibility fell on the 2nd Canadian Corps, which was to be supported by the 6th and 7th Cameronians. Five weeks of intense fighting led to more than 3,500 deaths on the side of the allies and the Germans were still there. On 2nd November, 1944 a fresh attack was launched by the 6th under the cover of darkness. Khan and Muldoon were in an assault craft approaching the island by sea when a spotlight came upon them and the boat came under heavy fire. Muldoon and Khan were on board a landing craft that was subjected to severe artillery fire by the enemy. Before long a shell destroyed the craft and sent the men flying into the cold black waters of the Sloe Channel. The men were even easier targets as they floundered to drown because of their heavy backpacks. Muldoon was not a swimmer. Rifleman Khan made to the muddy shore because he was not carrying any additional weight. On reaching the shore, he searched for his master. Upon hearing Muldoon's cries for help, Khan ran down 200 yards back through treacherous waters and waded up to his handler who was fighting a losing battle to keep his head above the water. He seized his handler by his tunic collars and swam back to safety. Rifleman Khan was awarded the **"PDSA Dickin Medal"** for bravery for this act on 27th March, 1945.

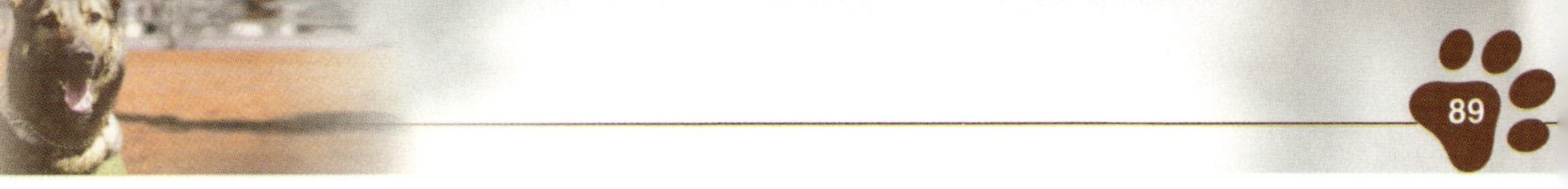

His citation read: "For rescuing L/Cpl. Muldoon from drowning under heavy shell fire at the assault of Walcheren, November, 1944, while serving with the 6th Cameronians (SR)."

After the Second World War, Khan returned to his former owner, Harry Railton in Surrey. On 25th July, 1947, Khan and Muldoon took part in a parade in the National Dog Tournament, in which 16 War Dogs who had received the Dickin Medal paraded. Railton was impressed by the bond that seemed to exist between Khan and Muldoon, and he handed the dog permanently over into the care of Muldoon.

ROB

War Dog No. 471/332, Rob, a Collie, was a working dog on a farm in Shropshire until 1942, when his owners, Basil and Heather Bayne, enlisted him as a War Dog. The dog was assigned to the Special Air Service at the Base in Wivenhoe Park, Essex. He was used as a Messenger and Guard Dog. When the troops based there departed for Arnhem in the Netherlands, he was not allowed on the ship and so was forced to stay behind. He took part in landings during North African Campaign with an Infantry unit and later served with a Special Air Unit in Italy as Patrol and Guard Dog on small detachments lying up in enemy territory. Rob made over 20 parachute jumps during World War II with the British Special Air Unit in Italy and even patrolled with the infantry in the North African Campaign. His presence alone was credited with keeping the men safe from discovery or capture when behind enemy lines.

Rob was awarded "**PDSA Dickin Medal**" on 22nd January, 1945 which he received in London on 3rd February, 1945. The citation reads:

"For service including 20 parachute jumps while serving with Infantry in North Africa and SAS Regiment in Italy."

Rob also won other medals for bravery, including an RSPCA Silver Medal. Following his military service, he returned to his owner in Tetchill, Shropshire. He died in 1952 and was buried on the family farm, marked with a stone memorial which reads: "To the dear memory of Rob, War Dog No. 471/322, twice VC, Britain's first parachute dog, who served three and a half years in North Africa and Italy with the Second Special Air Service Regiment. Died 18th January, 1952, aged 12½ years. Erected by Basil and Heather Bayne in memory of a faithful friend and playmate 1939–1952."

SERGEANT SOOCHOW

A small mixed breed Bull Terrier of unknown parentage who is believed to have been whelped in the Soochow District of Shanghai, China, in 1937. As a pup, he was found hanging around a Marine guard post in the autumn of 1938 and was befriended by a Marine Corps Private of "B" Company, 1st Battalion, 4th Marine Regiment, who was manning a sentry-box on Wu Chin Bridge. The friendship became a bond and wherever the young Marine went, the pup accompanied him. The pup won over the marine and he began to smuggle him into the barracks even though it was against regulations. The Mongrel puppy Soochow was named after the area where he was found (the Wu Chin Bridge was over Soochow Creek, called Suzhou Creek).

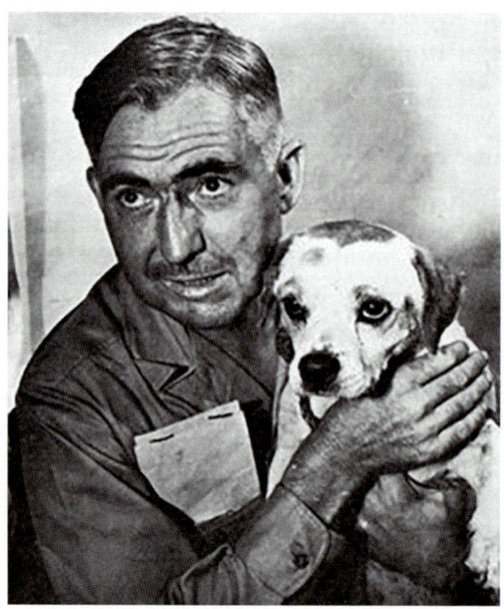

Soochow was small, but tough and was officially designated with the title of 4th Marine Regiment Mascot. Subsequently, he was actually enlisted into the Marine Corps and assigned to the 4th Marines with uniforms made for him by a local Chinese tailor. He even had a service record book and was awarded service decorations.

There are many stories of Soochow's Marine service in China. It is said that he would go to town with his Marines and imbibe in spirits with them and after getting sauced, his Marines would put him in a rickshaw for the trip back to the base and if the rickshaw driver tried to put him out before he got back to base, he would have to deal with Soochow's wrath and would have to take the little dog all the way to the barracks. Soochow also was caught urinating on the Regimental Flagpole and was sentenced to the cut on rations of champagne and cake. It was quite usual to see Soochow participating in parade reviews in full uniform and staying in step with the other Marines.

During late 1930s, the Imperial Forces of Japan were occupying a large portion of China, who had been fighting for many years. As the Japanese Military Forces began to increase in size in the Shanghai area, it became apparent that the contingent of "China Marines" stationed there would not be able to hold out should hostilities erupt. In November, 1941, orders were issued for the 4th Marines to leave China and sail to the Philippines and reinforce units there. Soochow was not allowed to go with his Marines and had to remain in China to fend for himself, even though he had been duly enlisted and was officially a member of the Regiment. One of the Marines, Bob Snyder, smuggled him aboard the US Ship Henderson and Soochow made it to Cavite Navy Yard, Philippines. A week after they arrived, the Japanese forces attacked Pearl Harbor, Hawaii, and the Philippine Islands.

During the Battle of Corregidor, Soochow was seen dodging bombs and taking cover in foxholes with his Marines. Everything the Marine defenders went through, Soochow went through as well. During the siege of Corregidor, he fought alongside his buddies by snarling and snapping at the Japanese. When Corregidor surrendered in May, 1942 and the allied troops imprisoned, so too, was the 4th Marines mascot.

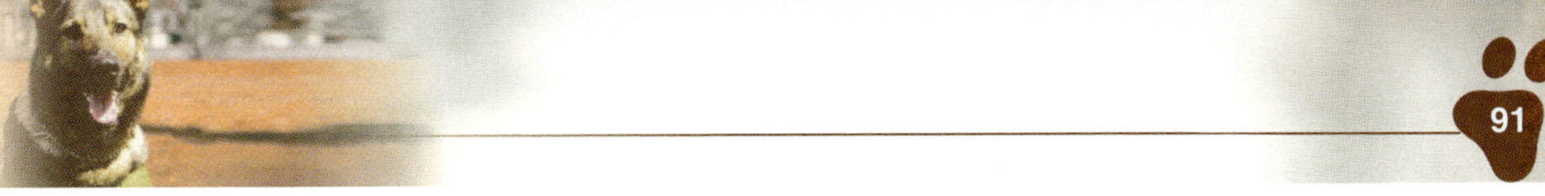

For three years Soochow was a prisoner of war (POW), continuing to stay with his Marines. It was reported that he hated the Japanese and would snarl at them continuously if they got too close but for reasons unknown, was never killed by them. His Marines kept him fed and Soochow still patrolled the area as he had done at Regimental headquarters in China. It wasn't long though until rations became scarce and the precious little the prisoners got to eat was coveted by all and only a few shared their food with the little dog. He lost weight but the tough little Marine endured and while his Marines died all around him, Soochow survived. When the prison camp was liberated in 1945, he was the first American prisoner repatriated in emaciated condition and covered with sores. He was flown to California with other POW (against regulations) and cared for until he recovered. In 1951, a book was published titled "SOOCHOW THE MARINE", written by Reginald Owen and Paul Lees (Lees was a former member of the 4th Marines) and the little dogs story went worldwide. Sergeant Soochow earned (but all were not awarded) the following badges/decorations for his service as a Marine Corps Mascot before, during and after World War II:

Combat Action Ribbon, Army Presidential Unit Citation Ribbon with Oak Leaf Cluster, China Service Medal, American Defense Service Medal with Base Clasp, Marine Corps Good Conduct Medal, Prisoner of War Medal, Asiatic-Pacific Theater of Operations Campaign Medal with bronze battle/campaign star, World War II Victory Medal, Philippine Defense Medal with Bronze Campaign Star and Philippine Presidential Unit Citation Ribbon.

Soochow was promoted to Mascot of the Marine Corps Recruit Depot (MCRD), San Diego, California. He had a Marine Corps Sergeant assigned, not only to take care of him, but to keep him out of trouble too. A full parade was conducted in his honour for his 9th birthday in 1946 and was promoted to the rank of Sergeant of Marines. While Soochow's health had greatly improved since his rescue from the POW camp, his time was running out and Soochow died in 1948. His death was greatly mourned by his Marines, especially those with whom he had shared a tablespoon of rice as a guest of the Emperor of Japan. A memorial presently stands behind the Recruit Dining Hall at MCRD honouring Soochow and other Marine Corps Mascots and war Dogs.

SMOKY

The smallest and the famous Military Dog Smoky was a Yorkshire Terrier. An extremely small breed of dog that was originally developed in Yorkshire England to catch rats in clothing mills. In 1944, Smoky was found in an abandoned foxhole in the jungles of New Guinea by an American Soldier who brought her back to camp and sold her to Corporal William A Wynne for $6.44. For the next 2 years Smoky lived with soldiers. Because she was not an official military dog, she did not get dog food or medical care. She shared Wynne's meals and slept beside him in his tent. Later she served in the South Pacific with the 5th Air Force and participated in 12 air/sea rescue and photo reconnaissance missions, secured in the soldiers backpack. Smoky survived 150 air-raids and saved Wynne on several occasions by warning him of incoming shells. In 1944, Yank Down Under magazine named Smoky the "Champion Mascot in the South West Pacific Area." Her largest contribution to the allied forces was with her incredible hearing and sense for danger. On multiple occasions, Smoky warned soldiers of incoming fire and saved their lives.

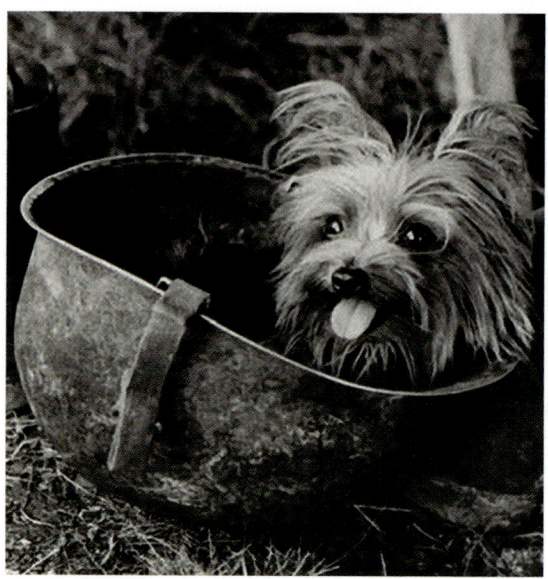

In 1944, Smoky made national headlines when she helped engineers build an airbase at Lingayen Gulf, Luzon. During the construction, a Signal Corps team needed to run a telegraph wire through a 70-foot-long (21 m) pipe that was 8 inches (200 mm) in diameter. Wynne attached the line to Smoky and she got the job done. Like many Yorkies, Smoky also loved to learn tricks and perform. She did so with the Special Services, entertaining soldiers in hospitals. At the end of World War II, Smoky was smuggled back into the United States hidden in a modified oxygen mask carrying case. After her return, Smoky became a National Celebrity and performed her skills for crowds, which included walking on a tightrope while blindfolded. She made television and public appearances in Veteran's Hospital until her death on 21st February, 1957 at the age of approximately 14 years. Smoky's exploits are chronicled in detail in the book titled "Yorkie Doodle Dandy", written by her adoptive owner William A Wynne.

TICH

Tich, a small black Terrier Cross (Egyptian Mongrel) who became the Mascot of the 1st Battalion King's Royal Rifle Corps during the Western Desert Campaign and onto Italy. Nicknamed "the Desert Rat", Tich rode into battle on the hood of her master's jeep. Serving for four years and seeing action in El Alamein in 1941 and Algiers in 1943, Tich unflinchingly went into battle by her master's side, Rifleman and Medic Thomas Walker. She never left her post and was a source of hope and joy to all those in the Battalion "For loyalty, courage and devotion to duty under hazardous conditions of war 1941 to 1945, while serving with the 1st King's Rifle Corps in North Africa and Italy," She was awarded "PDSA Dickin Medal" on 1st July, 1949.

WILLIE

General George S Patton, Jr had a personal liking for dogs and his favourite was a Bull Terrier. During World War II, on 4th March, 1944 at the height of Patton's fame, he purchased a white Bull Terrier named Willie, short for "William the Conqueror." For the rest of Patton's life, Willie and General Patton went everywhere together. Willie had his own set of "dog tags," and had quite a reputation with the "lady" dogs. General Patton doted on the dog and even hosted a birthday party for him. Not everyone was charmed by Patton and Willie. When Sgt Bill Maudlin, Stars and Stripes cartoonist, met Gen Patton in March, 1945, he described Willie this way:

"Beside him, lying in a big chair, was Willie, the Bull Terrier. If ever dog was suited to master this one was. Willie had his beloved boss's expression and lacked only the ribbons and stars. I stood in that door staring into the four meanest eyes I'd ever see".

On 9th December, 1945, Gen Patton suffered injuries as a result of an automobile accident. He died 12 days later, on 21st December, 1945 and buried in a grave at the US Military Cemetery in Hamm, Luxembourg, among the soldiers who died in the Battle of Bulge. Willie, Patton's constant companion during the war was sent to the United States, and lived out the rest of his life with the General's wife and daughters. A twelve-foot-high bronze statue of Patton and Willie has been erected at the General Patton Memorial Museum off Interstate 10 in Chiriaco Summit, CA, not far from the former site of the Desert Training Centre. It was there that Patton, as the first Commander in 1942, began developing the armoured tactics for Operation Torch in North Africa and later campaigns of World War II.

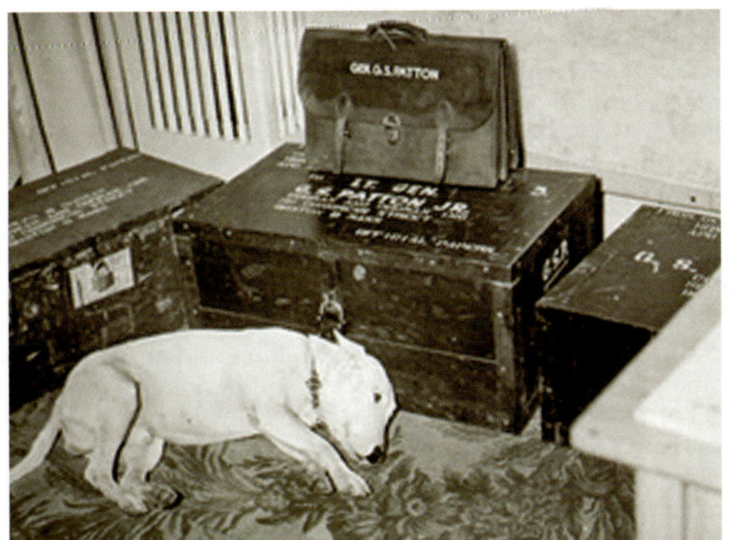

Photo taken right after Gen Patton's death, as Willie waits with personal belongings to be shipped to the United States

8

War Dogs in Korean and Vietnam Wars

"All his life he tried to be a good person. Many times, however, he failed. For after all, he was only human. He wasn't a dog."

... Charles M Schulz

KOREAN WAR

On 25th June, 1950, the Korean War began when approximately 75,000 soldiers from the North Korean People's Army poured across the 38th Parallel, the boundary between the Soviet-backed Democratic People's Republic of Korea to the north and the pro-Western Republic of Korea to the south. This invasion was the first military action of the Cold War. The US Army was in Korea on occupation duty after World War II and remained in the south after a Communist government was established in North Korea. By July, American Troops had entered the war on South Korea's behalf. As far as Americans were concerned, it was a war against the forces of international communism itself. After some early back-and-forth across the 38th Parallel, the fighting stalled and casualties mounted with nothing to show for them. Meanwhile, American Officials worked anxiously to fashion some sort of Armistice with the North Koreans. The alternative, they feared, would be a wider war with Russia and China—or even, as some warned, World War III. Finally, in July, 1953, the Korean War came to an end. In all, some 5 million soldiers and civilians lost their lives during the war. The Korean Peninsula is still divided today.

At the onset of War, the United States Air Force quickly established 12 Air Bases throughout the Korean Peninsula with major bases located at Kimp'O, Suwon, Osan and Kunsan. Each of the bases was assigned Air Police Squadrons, with Sentry Dog Sections of six to eight dogs attached for air base security and it was the beginning of defining a combat role for the USAF Air Police. By the time the Korean War ended, more than 500 dogs had been used by the combined United Nations ground forces.

In 1950, at the outbreak of hostilities more than 100 Army Dogs were stationed in Seoul on sentry duty to reduce theft around warehouses and storage areas. Some of these dogs were recruited for combat duty.

A new Army War Dog Receiving & Holding Station was activated at Cameron Station, Alexandria, Virginia on 11th July, 1951. The war dogs were conditioned before being shipped to the Army Dog Training Centre, Fort Carson, Colorado.

When the Korean War began, the 26th Infantry Scout Dog Platoon was in training at Fort Riley, Kansas. They were immediately sent to Korea for combat patrols. These dogs quickly established their value on patrol and Commanders demanded more dogs than the 26th could provide.

The outstanding results from the 26th Infantry Scout Dog Platoon led to plans for such Platoons for each Division in Korea, but only five Platoons were trained and shipped before the war ended. The 26th Scout Dog Platoon served with honour and distinction in Korea from 12th June, 1951 to 26th June, 1953. Platoon members were awarded a total of three Silver Stars, six Bronze Stars for Valour, and thirty-five Bronze Stars for Meritorious Service. The War Dog Receiving and Holding Station at Cameron Station was placed in a standby status on 4th May, 1954, after peace negotiations. At the end of the war, Scout Dogs not assigned to Infantry Divisions were retrained for sentry work to patrol the Demilitarized Zone (DMZ) that was established between North and South Korea. During the War, it was recognized by the military authorities that unbroken record of faithful and gallant performance of Scout Dogs in support of patrols have saved countless casualties through early warning to the friendly patrol of threats to its security.

Air Force also used Sentry Dogs which were trained for 3 weeks at the Sentry Dog Training Centre at Showa Air Station on the main Island of Honshu, Japan. The K9 Sentry Dog handlers, all volunteers from attached Air Police Units were sent to the school where they were matched to a dog and trained together for additional weeks in sentry dog tactics, before they were returned to their duty station in Korea as a K9 Team. The Sentry Dogs were used mostly at night, like the army, for patrolling the air base perimeters, guarding fuel storage sites, bomb dumps and supply areas.

During this conflict, the United States provided majority of the dogs used in the war, whereas Great Britain provided a few Mine and Tracker Dogs in November, 1951. At the same time, their commonwealth divisions, i.e. Australia, Canada and New Zealand were using Patrol Dogs quite extensively. The Australian Army's Special Operations Command (SOCOMD) had Special Operations Military Working Dogs (SOMWDs) which provided the specialist sensory detection and protection capabilities to counter numerous threats across a range of environments, both domestically and overseas. This was achieved through highly trained Military Working Dogs and handlers teams. SOMWDs include a variety of breeds, and were sourced directly from breeders or animal rescue organizations. Mixed breeds also proved to be just as effective in Explosive Detection Dogs as pure bred dogs. Experienced dog trainers selected certain traits and tendencies that would ensure the dogs are optimised for particular role rather than selection based on particular breed, age or sex. Selected dogs were then trialed for various roles within SOCOMD and if successful, were posted into SOCOMD units for training and employment. SOMWDs form a very close relationship with their designated handler, and indeed with all members of the units they are posted to and regarded as an integral component of their respective units.

SOMWDs were utilized for detection of explosives, narcotics, tracking the adversary movements in an area of operation, early warning of adversary positions and protection of assets and personnel coupled with the psychological effects of dogs on adversaries.

Most famous and decorated dog of this campaign was York who was recipient of Distinguished Service Award. A brief description is as follows:

York

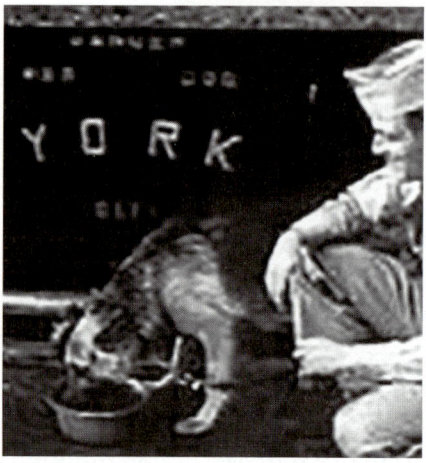

The US Army Scout Dog, York was decorated for outstanding service while serving with the 26th Infantry Scout Dog Platoon in Korea. His silent alerts on enemy locations had saved many American lives. York was awarded the Distinguished Service Award by General Samuel T Williams. York performed 148 combat patrols during the periods of 12th June, 1951 and 26th June, 1953. On 8th May, 1957, York received orders to return to the Dog Training Centre, at Fort Carson, Colorado to be used as a member of a demonstration team. It was felt that York would help to improve public relations by arousing more interest in the recruitment and procurement of dogs for military purpose. When the Army Dog Training Centre, located at Fort Carson was deactivated on 1st July, 1957, York was transferred to Fort Benning, Georgia, and attached to his original platoon, the 26th Infantry Scout Dog Platoon.

26th INFANTRY SCOUT DOG PLATOON

The 26th Infantry Scout Dog Platoon of the US Army, saw plenty of combat actions and their success in saving lives made them invaluable to ground operations in Korea. One regimental Commander remarked that after using a Scout Dog team for a while, the Infantry Patrols did not want to go out without them. 26th Infantry Dog Platoon received a Citation for its outstanding service on 27th February, 1952 vide General Orders 114 Headquarters, Eighth United States Army, Korea, 18th January, 1953. The Citation reads:

"The 26th Infantry Scout Dog Platoon is cited for exceptionally meritorious conduct in the performance of outstanding services in direct support of combat operations in Korea during the period 12th June, 1951 to 15th January, 1953. The full value of the services rendered by the 26th Infantry Scout Dog Platoon is nowhere better understood and more highly recognized than among the members of the patrols with whom the scout dog handlers and their dogs have operated. Throughout its long period of difficult and hazardous service, the 26th Infantry Scout Dog Platoon has never failed those with whom it served; has consistently shown outstanding devotion to duty in the performance of all of its other duties, and has won on the battlefield a degree of respect and admiration which has established it as a unit of the greatest importance to the Eighth United States Army. The outstanding performance of duty proficiency, and esprit de corps invariably exhibited by the personnel of this platoon reflect the greatest credit on themselves and the military service of the United States.

VIETNAM WAR

Vietnam War was fought from 1st November, 1955 to the fall of Saigon on 30th April, 1975, between North Vietnam supported by the Soviet Union, China and other communist allies and the government of South Vietnam supported by the United

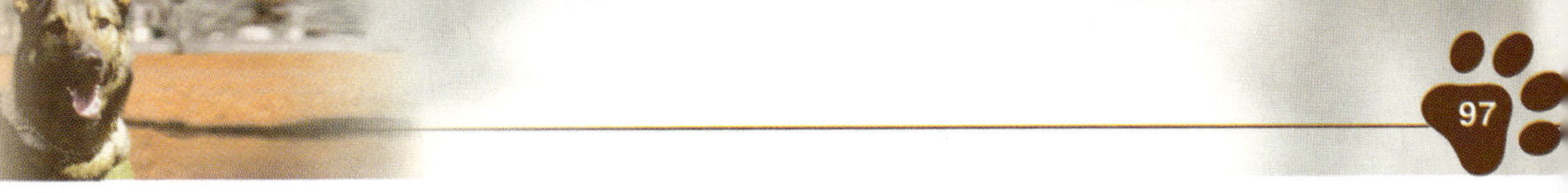

States and other anti-communist allies. The Viet Cong (also known as the National Liberation Front, or NLF), a lightly armed South Vietnamese communist common front aided by the North, fought a guerrilla war against anticommunist forces in the region. The People's Army of Vietnam (aka the North Vietnamese Army) engaged in a more conventional war, at times committing a large number of troops into the battle. The US government viewed American involvement in the war as a way to prevent a communist takeover of South Vietnam. This was part of a wider containment strategy, with the stated aim of stopping the spread of communism. The North Vietnamese government and the Viet Cong were fighting to reunify Vietnam under communist rule. They viewed the conflict as a colonial war, fought initially against forces from France and then America, as France was backed by the US, and later against South Vietnam, which it regarded as a US puppet state.

In 1950, American Military advisers arrived in what was then French-Indo-China. Later, the US involvement escalated in the early 1960s, with troop levels tripling in 1961 and again in 1962. The US involvement escalated further following the 1964 Gulf of Tonkin incident in which the US Destroyer clashed with North Vietnamese fast attack craft. In the US, it was followed by the Gulf of Tonkin Resolution which gave the US President authorization to increase the US Military presence. The regular US combat units were deployed at the beginning of 1965.

In 1961, the American Military Assistance Advisory Group, Vietnam, recommended that the South Vietnamese Army (ARVN) use Military Working Dogs for sentry and scout work. 300 dogs were purchased from Germany and shipped to the ARVN in mid-1962. The German-bred dogs were initially wary of the Vietnamese soldiers and barked or ran away from them. The project did not go well since the Vietnamese as Buddhists, feared that by working with the dogs they would be reincarnated as dogs. They also refused to praise their dogs, which impeded the training practices that US- and German-bred dogs were used to. Finally, the physical condition of the dogs degenerated for several reasons. One was the fact that it would cost an ARVN soldier more to feed his dog each day than his family, so the dogs were often fed rice and many dogs died of malnutrition. In 1964, the ARVN had 327 dogs against their plan to employ over 1000. But by 1966, due to the above conditions, the existing dog strength came down to 130.

In March, 1965, USA approved the use of Military Working Dogs in Vietnam and by 17th July, forty dog teams had been deployed on three bases, i.e. Tan Son Nhut, Ben Hoa and Da Nang. By the end of the year there were 99 dog teams in the country and by September, 1966 more than 500 dog teams were deployed on ten bases. As a result, between July, 1965 and December, 1966, not a single Viet Cong Sapper Team penetrated a base guarded by Sentry Dogs. Between late 1965 and January, 1969, Army Scout Dog Platoons and Marine Scout Dog Platoons were deployed for sentry and tracking duties. Dogs in Vietnam were used for many purposes such as to find dangers like ambushes, booby traps, land mines, caches of weapons, ammunition, and to guard the perimeter of military bases before they claimed lives. Dogs were also used to find downed pilots and runaway ambushers.

The war dogs performed four main tasks in Vietnam.

Scout Dogs: The German Shepherd was the only breed trained for this job. The handler and dog led combat patrols and provided an early silent warning of danger. A Scout Dog team was deployed as "Point man" which is the most vulnerable and dangerous position of a tactical formation moving through enemy territory. Scout

Dogs were trained to give alert on enemy movement, booby traps, land mines, base camps, underground tunnel complexes, and underground caches of weapons, and food and medical supplies. The US Army had the highest number of Infantry Scout Dog Teams deployed throughout South Vietnam and consequently suffered the highest number of casualties amongst dogs and handlers in the war.

Tracker Dogs: The Labrador Retriever was the only breed trained for tracking. Their primary role was to track the enemy's scent or blood trails throughout South Vietnam, so that larger American Forces could re-engage. Black and yellow Labradors were favoured. These dogs were friendly, having a natural instinct for tracking ground scent and took less time to get used to a new handler than a German Shepherd. The Tracker Dog Teams were very effective and relied upon heavily.

Sentry/Patrol Dogs: The German Shepherd was the only breed used for this job. The dog and handler were very effective in defending airfields, supply depots, ammunition dumps, defensive perimeters, and many other strategic military facilities throughout South Vietnam. Sentry Dog Teams were deployed as the first line of defense guarding American base camps day and night.

Mine/Tunnel Dogs: The German Shepherd Dog and handler were generally deployed with the Infantry and Combat Engineer units. They were trained to sniff out mines and booby traps buried in roads, hidden on bridges or in buildings, and sniff out the location of tunnels. After the dog located the tunnel, a soldier would enter the tunnel to investigate.

Water Patrol Dogs: The US Navy successfully used dogs on slow trolling patrol boats operating throughout the American patrolled waterways of South Vietnam. The dogs were deployed to alert on the breath scent of enemy underwater divers breathing through reeds, snorkels and other underwater apparatus. The Water Dogs proved to be quite successful in saving lives and equipment and reduced the enemy's capacity to conduct underwater sabotage operations.

In Vietnam, small, highly-trained units, usually consisting of five men and a Labrador Retriever, called a Combat Tracker Team (CTT) were also deployed. They were a composite group and cross-trained, enabling all members to complete the mission. The purpose of CTT was to re-establish contact with the "elusive enemy", undertake reconnaissance of an area for possible enemy activities and locate lost or missing friendly personnel. The methods used in completing the missions were visual through canine tactical tracking. The unit was usually supported by a platoon or larger force and worked well ahead of them to maintain noise discipline and the element of surprise. The Vietnam War saw a big increase in the use of dogs in direct combat roles whereas jungle patrols were very limited.

The United States' 1st Marine Corps Scout Dog Platoon arrived in Vietnam (30 Marine Scout Dog Teams) in early March, 1966. They were split up and arrived via two C-130 aircraft, 15 teams in each. This was the first time since World War II that Marine Scout Dogs were deployed in combat. The Marines Kennelled their dogs near Da Nang at Camp Kaiser, named after the first Marine Scout Dog killed in action in Vietnam. Between late 1965 and January, 1969 four Marine Scout Dog Platoons were deployed in Vietnam. In 1970, after the army's success, the Marines instituted their own Mine/Tunnel Dog programme.

In October, 1966 the Army planned to provide 14 provisional canine teams to be attached to the most active elements of the infantry, Airborne and Cavalry Divisions and Brigades that were in combat. The deployment of the teams was in groups of four teams (a platoon) to an Infantry Division and groups of two teams (a detachment) to a Brigade. The teams were comprised five men and one dog. Based on the experiences of the British, Black or Yellow Labrador Retrievers were favoured as Tracker Dogs, in contrast to the German Shepherd that filled the ranks of the Scout Dog Platoons. In February, 1968 after training and development at Fort Gordon Georgia, the 60th Infantry Platoon became the first Mine and Tunnel Detector Dog Platoon and was deployed in Vietnam at Cu Chi on 22nd April, 1969 in support of the 25th Infantry Division and the 23rd Infantry Division. Scout Dogs were trained for jungle combat in a twelve-week course that started with obedience and advanced to voice and body signals. They were trained to alert differently for the scent of a living person or an inanimate but unfamiliar object. There was specialized training for daytime or night scouting, detecting tunnels, mines, trip wires and booby traps, and guard duty. Some dogs were specialists in one skill while others were cross-trained.

The buildup of the US forces in Vietnam created large dog sections at the US Air Force Southeast Asia (SEA) bases and eventually 467 dogs were assigned to Bien Hoa, Bien Thuy, Cam Ranh Bay, Da Nang, Nha Trang, Tuy Hoa, Phu Cat, Phan Rang, Tan Son Nhut and Pleiku Air Bases. Within a year of deployment, attacks on several bases had been thwarted when the enemy forces were detected by dog teams. During operations in the Mekong Delta area, Vietnam, the US Navy SEAL teams had to develop a stainless steel pistol called the Hush Puppy, purposely designed to eliminate Viet Cong sentries and their Guard Dogs. The Smith and Wesson model 39 (modified) had a shoulder stock, a locking slide and a suppressor (the slide locked for maximum noise reduction and its suppressor limited the effective range to around 100 yards). Only a few hundreds were made and they were mainly used for disabling sentries, killing Guard Dogs and shattering lights.

The success of Sentry Dogs was determined by the lack of successful penetration of bases and canine units were credited with saving thousands of lives. Between 1964 and 1975, there was a confirmed list of 3,747 dogs identified by ear tattoo who had served in Vietnam as Scout and Sentry dogs, largely German Shepherds. At the end of the conflict, a decision that remains painful even decades later was to euthanise most of the in-country dogs and less than 204 dogs were only returned to the United States or other locations. Handlers were faced with the agonising decision of either euthanising their dog or giving it to the South Vietnamese Army. Black dogs were regarded as bad luck in Vietnam so Labradors had a few prospects. Many handlers today have no idea what ultimately happened to their mates and for some Veterans these are still America's Missing In Action (MIA) canine soldiers.

Australian Combat Units also deployed Tracker Teams in support of operations. These dogs were the core of Combat Tracker Teams that were used from 1967 until the last combat troops left in late 1971. These dogs were trained from the age of about 10 months at the Tracking Wing of the Ingleburn Infantry Centre, NSW, Australia. Two dogs were assigned to each of the Australian Battalions at the Task Force base at Nui Dat, in Phuoc Tuy Province. South Vietnamese soldiers were usually used to set scent trails, so the dogs could get used to following their distinctive smell. Each Tracker Team, consisting of two dogs and their handlers, two visual trackers, and two cover men (a machine-gunner and a signaler) operated on standby out of Nui Dat. Usually called out to follow-up enemy trails or to locate suspected enemy hideouts after a contact, the teams would be airlifted by helicopter

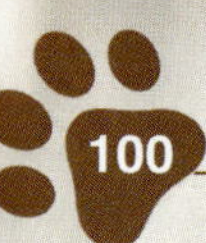

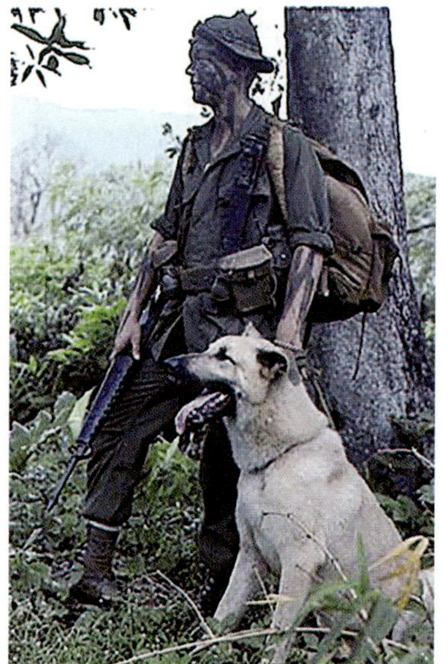

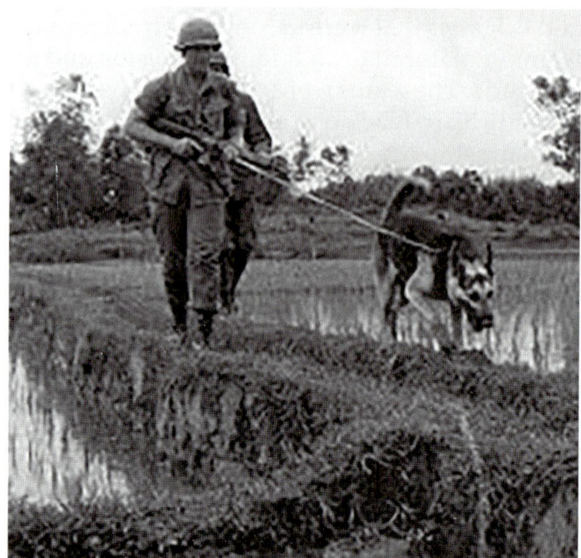

into the area of operation. Once on the ground, the dog would be put on to the scent of retreating enemy. The dog would follow the scent usually at speed until a location was found, when he would stop with nose or paw extended in a 'Point', facing the suspected hideout. The tracker dog would then fall back while the rest of the section searched the area, often finding wounded enemy or recently occupied bunker systems that would otherwise have been missed.

The dogs were outstandingly successful at their combat tasks in Vietnam. Apart from their success in locating enemy and their support systems, the dogs saved the lives of their handlers and team members on many occasions. Although not trained to detect mines (despite recommendations by some soldiers that Mine Dogs be used in Vietnam), the dogs were intelligent and sufficiently well-trained to do so. Handler Peter Haran summed up his dog's worth, Caesar could see, smell and hear Charlie (slang term for Viet Cong, from the military phonetic alphabet for the letters 'V' — Victor and 'C'—Charlie) long before we walked into a firefight. He knew where the mines were, where the trip wires were strung, and he could cover ground chasing the enemy at speeds which literally took your breath away.

The Scout and tracker teams earned high respect for their work. War Dog teams were so effective that Viet Cong began placing bounties on killing the dogs and their handlers. Viet Cong Troops were rewarded for bringing a dog's tattooed ear or a handler's patch back. It has been reported that in Vietnam, the US war dogs were credited with saving up to 10,000 service members' lives. In this war 500 dogs and 294 handlers were killed in action while saving the lives of thousands.

Heroic actions of a few dogs to represent the many Military Working Dogs of the Vietnam War including some whose names have been preserved and some who are remembered only by their handlers and unit buddies are summarized below:

Justin

In November, 1967, Justin, one of two Tracker Dogs with 7th Battalion, the Royal Australian Regiment (7RAR) and his handler, Private Tom Blackhurst of Swansea,

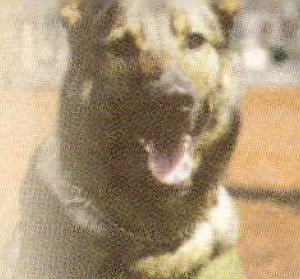

NSW, successfully located a group of Viet Cong during operation Santa Fe in the northeast of the province about 30 yards ahead, a little while after the Viet Cong had withdrawn. The tracker team immediately opened fire and inflicted two fatal casualties.

Kaiser

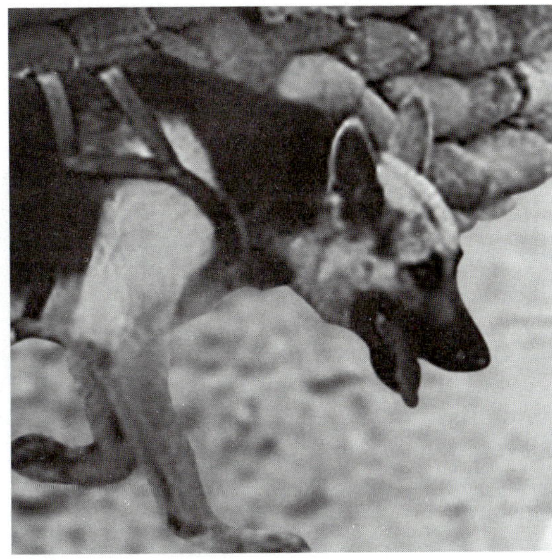

A German Shepherd who served in Vietnam with his handler Marine Lance Corporal. Alfredo Salazar. Kaiser and Salazar did more than 30 combat patrols and participated in 12 major operations together. After the pair joined "D" Company, First Marine Division for a search-and-destroy mission, they were ambushed by enemy forces while on patrol in 1966. Kaiser was hit in the initial barrage and died while trying to lick Salazar's hand. Kaiser was the first Marine Scout Dog Killed in action in the Republic of Vietnam on 6th July, 1966.

Kelly

This dog served and died in Vietnam War in 1971. As a loyal and dedicated member of the 173rd Airborne Brigade, 39th Scout Dog Platoon, 173 Airborne Brigade, US

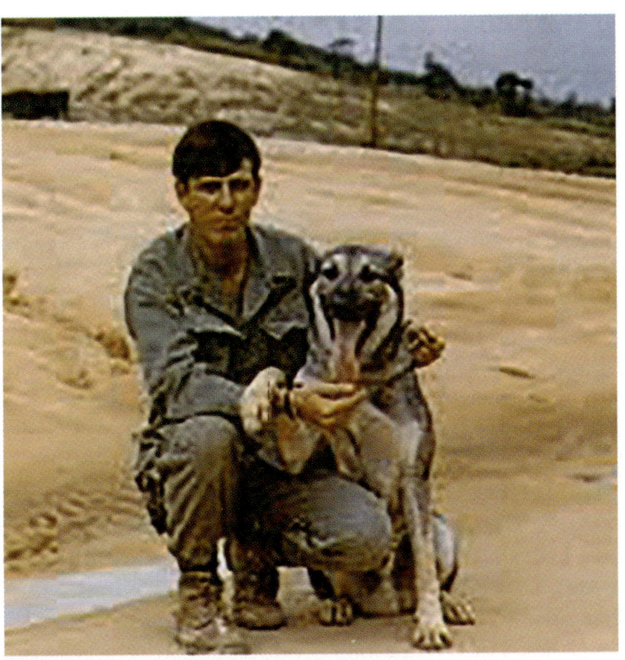

Army. Kelly saved many soldiers from injury and death. He courageously protected his handler when he yanked him up a bank from a rice paddy field, out of the way of mortar fire. His handler Johnny Mayo, 60, now retired and settled in Lexington, South Carolina, USA, fondly remembered his dog Kelly. While visiting the "Vietnam Veterans Memorial" wall in Washington in 2000, he told that once "you go through the war, you always remember the bond you had with the dog". Vietnam War Dog handlers were trained to read and communicate with their canine partners and they will never forget the bond shared and the gratitude and love in their heart for the War Dogs.

Nemo

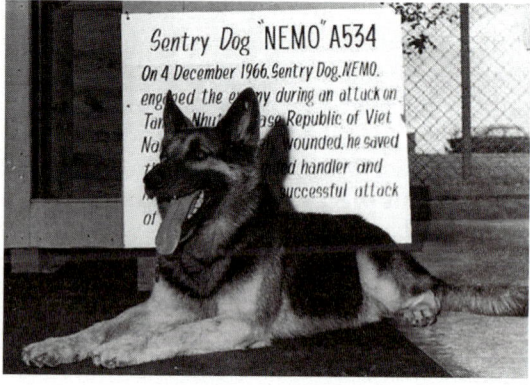

Nemo, a German Shepherd, was born in October, 1962, and was procured by the Air Force in the summer of 1964, from a Sergeant, for training. After completion of eight-week course at Lackland's Sentry Dog Training School, in San Antonio, Texas, Nemo and his handler, Airman Leonard Bryant Jr were assigned to Fairchild AB, Washington, for duty with Strategic Air Command.

In January, 1966, Nemo and Leonard were transferred to the Republic of South Vietnam with a large group of other dog teams, and was assigned to the 377th Security Police Squadron, stationed at Tan Son Nhut Air Base. Six months later, in July, Nemo's original handler rotated back to the States. The dog was then paired with 22-year-old Airman 2nd Class Robert Thorneburg. On December 4th, 1966, during the early morning hours, a group of 60 Viet Cong emerged from the jungle. Several Sentry Dog Teams stationed on preventive perimeter posts gave the initial alert and warning almost simultaneously. Immediately, Rebel, a Sentry Dog on patrol, was released. The response was a hail of bullets that killed the dog. Forty-five minutes later the group was detected by Sentry Dog Cubby. He was released with the same results. It was clear that the VC had learned to handle the Attack Dogs. Another dog, Toby, was killed and several handlers wounded before the attackers were finally driven off. However, as a result of early warning, security forces of the 377th Air Police Squadron successfully repelled the attack, minimizing damage to aircraft and facilities. Meanwhile although wounded, one dog handler notified Central Security Control of their location and direction of travel. Two security policemen in a machine gun bunker were ready and waiting as the Viet Cong approached the main aircraft parking ramp. In a few seconds they stopped the enemy, killing all 13 of the attackers. Security forces rapidly deployed around the perimeter and prevented the infiltrators from escaping, forcing them to hide. Three Airmen and their dogs had died in the brutal fight. By day break, the search patrols believed that all of the remaining Viet Cong were killed or captured. The Sentry Dog Teams deployed that night were quieter than usual. Many of the handlers were thinking about the events of the previous night. They were saddened by the loss of their fellow Dogs. They were also anxious about what awaited them on their patrols. There was a good chance that stragglers from the previous night's attack could still be out there. Airman Bob, Thorneburg and his dog Nemo were assigned duty near an old Vietnamese graveyard about a quarter mile from the Air Base runways. No sooner had they started their patrol, Nemo alerted on something in the cemetery but before Thorneburg could radio the CSC, that "something" opened fire. Thorneburg released his dog and then charged firing into the enemy. Nemo was shot and wounded, the bullet entering under his right eye and exited through his mouth. Thorneburg killed one VC before he too was shot in the shoulder and knocked to the ground. That might have been the sad end of the story but Nemo refused to give in without a fight. Ignoring his serious head wound, the 85 pound dog threw himself at the Viet Cong guerrillas who had opened fire. Nemo's ferocious attack brought Thorneburg the time he needed to call in backup forces. A Quick Reaction Team arrived and swept the area but found no other Viet Cong. However, security forces, using additional Sentry Dog Teams, located and killed four more Viet Cong. A second sweep with the dog teams resulted in discovery of four more Viet Cong who were hiding underground. They, too, were killed. Although severely wounded, Nemo crawled to his master and covered him with his body. Even after help arrived Nemo would not allow anyone to touch Thorneburg. Finally separated, both were taken back to the base for medical attention. Lt Raymond T Hutson, the Base Veterinarian worked diligently to save Nemo's life. Nemo was blinded in one eye and after the Veterinarian felt Nemo was well enough, the dog was put back on perimeter duty.

On 23rd June, 1967, Air Force Headquarters directed that Nemo be returned to the United States with Honours, as the first Sentry Dog to be officially retired from active service. Thorneburg had to be evacuated to the hospital at Tachikawa Air Base in Japan to recuperate. The handler and the dog bid final goodbyes. Airman Thorneburg also fully recovered from his wounds and also returned home with Honours. Nemo flew halfway around the world accompanied by returning Airman Melvin W Bryant. The plane touched down in Japan, Hawaii and California. At each stop, Air Force Veterinarian would examine the brave dog for signs of discomfort, stress and fatigue, after all he was a War Hero! Finally, the C-124 Globemaster touched down at Kelly Air Force Base, Texas, on 22nd July, 1967. Captain Robert M Sullivan, the Officer incharge of the Sentry Dog Training programme was present at Lackland as the head of Nemo's welome home committee. Sullivan said, "I have to keep from getting involved with individual dogs, but I can't help feeling a little emotional about this dog. He shows how valuable a dog is to his handler in staying alive."

Nemo then spent the rest of his retirement at the Department of Defense Dog Centre, Lackland AFB, Texas. He was given a permanent kennel near the Veterinary facility. A sign with his name, serial number, and details of his Vietnam heroic exploit designated his freshly painted home. Nemo died in December, 1972 at Lackland AFB, shortly before the Christmas holiday and the Vietnam War hero was laid to rest at the Dog Centre. His presence at Lackland reminded students, just how important a dog is to his handler and to the entire unit.

Vietnam War Dogs have been belatedly honoured since time immemorial as two War Dog Memorials have been built in the USA during 2000. The inscriptions on the memorial describe **"They protected us on the field of battle. They watch over our eternal rest. We are grateful".**

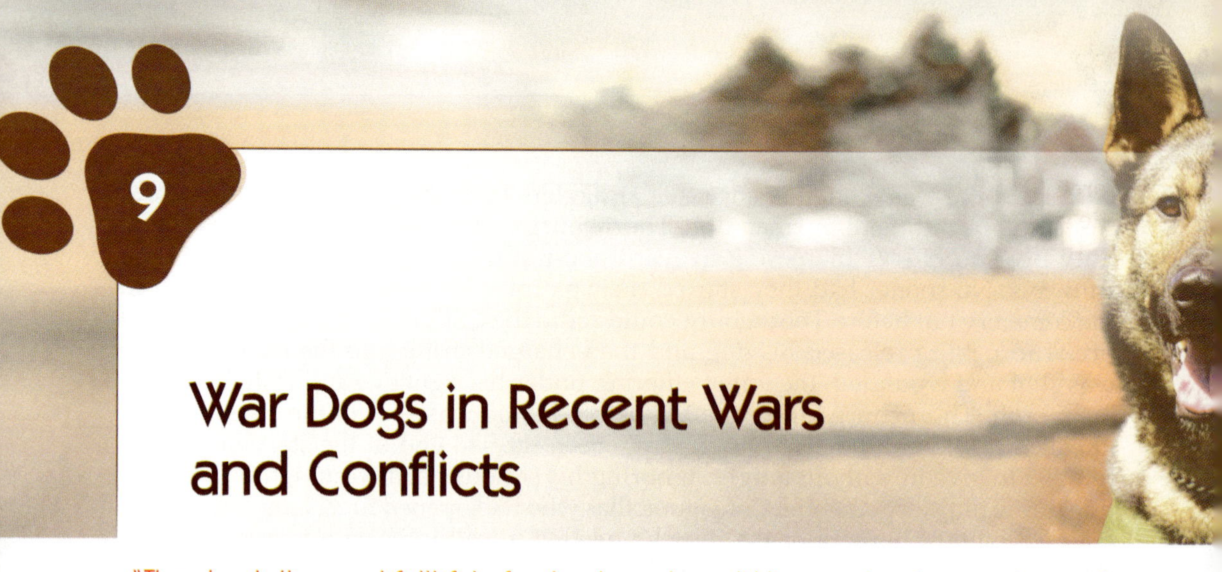

9

War Dogs in Recent Wars and Conflicts

"The dog is the most faithful of animals and would be much esteemed were it not so common. Our Lord God has made His greatest gifts the commonest."

... Martin Luther

During the "Malaya Campaign" from 1949 to 1952, the British Royal Air Force (RAF) Police Anti-Terrorist Tracker Dog Team, comprising four dogs (Bobbie, Jasper, Lassie and Lucky), was attached to the Civil Police and several British Army Regiments including the Coldstream Guards, 2nd Battalion Royal Scots Guards and the Ghurkhas. All the four dogs displayed exceptional determination and life-saving skills during the Malaya Campaign. The dogs and their handlers were an exceptional team, capable of tracking and locating the enemy by scent, despite unrelenting heat and an almost impregnable jungle. Sadly, three of the dogs lost their lives in the line of duty and only Lucky survived to the end of the conflict." "For the outstanding gallantry and devotion to duty, Lucky, a German Shepherd Anti-Terrorist Tracker dog of Royal Air Force Police was awarded PDSA Dickin Medal, posthumously on 6th February, 2007".

In operation "Just Cause," invasion of Panama by the United States in December, 1989, Military Working Dogs (MWDs) were deployed by American Troops and their allies. It was followed by more military operations using MWDs around the globe. "Desert Storm," a war waged by Coalition Forces from 34 nations led by the United States against Iraq in response to Iraq's invasion and annexation of Kuwait, from 19th January, 1991 to 28th February, 1991. Operation "Desert Shield," related to the Iraqi insurgency and Al-Qaeda in Iraq, as a push against American Forces in 2006, Operation "Uphold Democracy", an intervention in Haiti from 19th September, 1994 to 31st March, 1995, designed to remove the Military regime installed by the Haitian Coup that overthrew the elected President Jean-Bertrand Aristide in 1991. Operation " Iraqi Freedom" also known as "Iraq War" from 20th March, 2003 to 15th December, 2011. Operation "Enduring Freedom," the official name initially used by the USA for the war in Afghanistan, together with a number of smaller military actions, under the umbrella of the Global War On Terror (GWOT) from 7th October, 2001. In December, 2001, International Security Assistance Force (ISAF) was established to oversee military operations. In 2003, NATO assumed leadership of ISAF, with troops from 43 countries. NATO members provided the core of the force. One portion of the US Forces in Afghanistan operated under NATO command; the rest remained under direct American Command.

In "Bosnian war" from 6th April, 1992 to 14th December, 1995 and "Kosovo War" from 28th February, 1998 to 11th June, 1999, MWD teams were effectively utilized to enhance the security of critical facilities and areas, as well as bolster force protection and anti-terrorism missions.

Sam, a German Shepherd of Royal Army Veterinary Corps of British Army was awarded PDSA Dickin Medal on 14th January, 2003. The citation reads:

"For outstanding gallantry in April, 1998 while assigned to the Royal Canadian Regiment in Drvar during the conflict in Bosnia-Hertzegovina. On two documented occasions Sam displayed great courage and devotion to duty. On 18th April, Sam successfully brought down an armed man threatening the lives of civilians and service personnel. On 24th April, while guarding a compound harbouring Serbian refugees, Sam's determined approach held off rioters until reinforcements arrived. This dog's true valour saved the lives of many servicemen and civilians during this time of human conflict."

The use of dogs as an auxiliary in war and peace is continuing in the Armed forces of various countries over world. These silent warriors and saviours have established their worth as force multipliers owing to the fact that dogs do save lives, safeguard sensitive installations and further the work of the military service by utilization of inherent powers that human do not possess to the same degree as dogs.

GULF WAR

The Gulf War (2nd August, 1990–28th February, 1991), code named "Operation Desert Shield" (2nd August, 1990–17th January, 1991), for operations leading to the buildup of troops and defense of Saudi Arabia and "Operation Desert Storm" (17th January, 1991–28th February, 1991) was a war waged by Coalition Forces from 34 nations led by the United States against Iraq in response to Iraq's invasion and annexation of Kuwait on 2nd August, 1990. Iraq officially accepted ceasefire terms

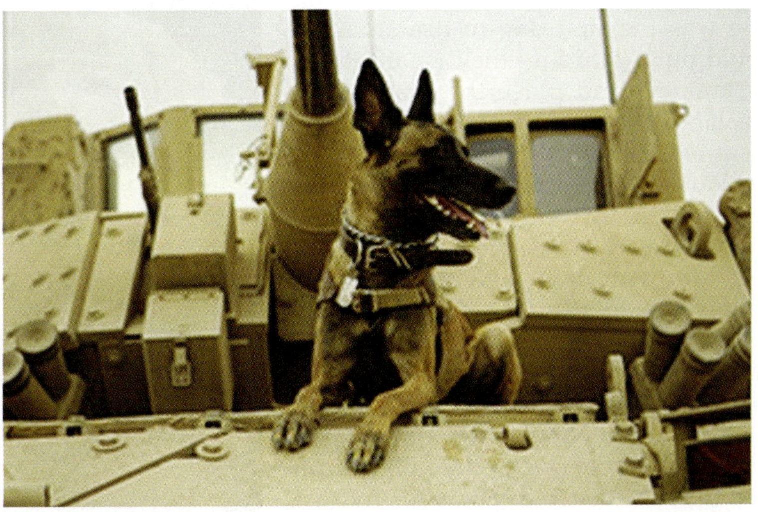

US Air Force dog atop an M2A3 Bradley Fighting Vehicle in Iraq in 2007

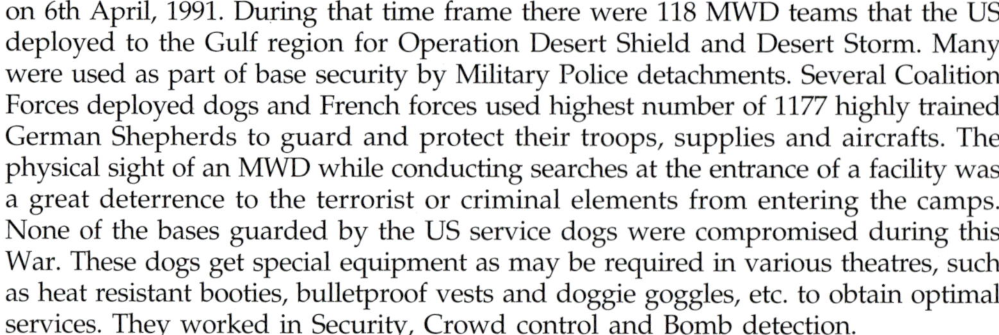

on 6th April, 1991. During that time frame there were 118 MWD teams that the US deployed to the Gulf region for Operation Desert Shield and Desert Storm. Many were used as part of base security by Military Police detachments. Several Coalition Forces deployed dogs and French forces used highest number of 1177 highly trained German Shepherds to guard and protect their troops, supplies and aircrafts. The physical sight of an MWD while conducting searches at the entrance of a facility was a great deterrence to the terrorist or criminal elements from entering the camps. None of the bases guarded by the US service dogs were compromised during this War. These dogs get special equipment as may be required in various theatres, such as heat resistant booties, bulletproof vests and doggie goggles, etc. to obtain optimal services. They worked in Security, Crowd control and Bomb detection.

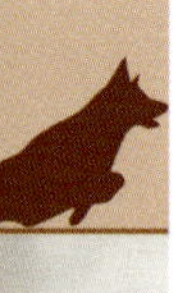

Some heroic deeds of these brave dogs in Gulf War are narrated in succeeding paragraphs.

Buster

Buster, a Spring Spaniel of Royal Army Veterinary corps, British Army, was deployed in Iraq. In March, 2003, while assigned to the Duke of Wellington's Regiment in Safwan, Southern Iraq. Arms and Explosives Search Dog Buster located an arsenal of hidden cache of arms, explosives and bomb making equipment, hidden behind a false wall in a building thought to be the headquarters of extremists responsible for attack on British Forces. Buster is credited for saving the lives of many service personnel and countless civilians and for preventing untold misery for thousands of people. Following the find, all attacks ceased and shortly afterwards troops replaced their steel helmets with berets. Buster was awarded **"PDSA Dickin Medal"** on 9th December, 2003 for outstanding gallantry.

Endal

Endal, a yellow Labrador Retriever was trained as a Fully Operational Assistance Dog. He was able to respond to hundreds of instructions and signed commands. Endal could go shopping, operate electrical switches, run an elevator, and work a washing machine. He was the first dog to use an ATM card and could put a card into the cash machine, retrieve the money, and place the cash into a wallet. In the late 1990s, Endal became the service dog for disabled ex-Royal Navy Chief Petty Officer Allen Parton. Parton suffered serious head injuries during the Gulf War, including a 50% memory loss. Endal was assigned to Parton in order to help him with daily activities. Since he was so intelligent, Endal was featured in multiple television documentaries. He was used as the animal ambassador for service dogs and appeared at training centers and charities. Endal soon became the most decorated dog in the world. He was named the dog of the millennium and awarded the PDSA's Gold Medal for Animal Gallantry "Dickin Medal". During his lifetime,

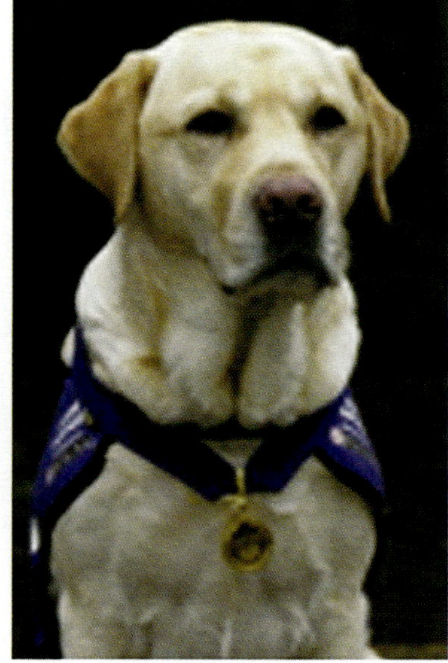

Endal was filmed by over 340 crews and featured on numerous television shows in Japan, Australia, USA, Canada, Europe, and China. He has been called one of the most famous dogs in the history of the UK and was the first dog to ride on the London Eye. In 2001, Endal received worldwide attention when it was reported that he helped save Allen Parton's life. During the event, Parton was knocked out of his wheelchair by a passing car and left unconscious. Endal pulled Allen into the recovery position, retrieved his mobile phone, fetched a blanket, and covered his friend. He then barked for help and ran to a nearby hotel to notify the authorities. It was an amazing act of bravery. Sadly, On 13th March, 2009, Endal died at the age of thirteen. He is remembered as one of the world's greatest Assistance Dogs.

Jack and Benjo

Jack and Benjo both German Shepherd, came to the Joint Base Elmendorf Richardson (JBER), Alaska, USA, on 13th May, 2003 and 24th July, 2004 respectively, after completing more than 100 days of Military Working Dog Training at Lackland Air Force Base, Texas. Like any Military Working Dog, Jack and Benjo were dual-certified as Explosive Detection and Patrol Dog. While assigned at the Elmendorf Air Force Base, they both conducted more than 1,000 hours of search Operations and 400 foot patrols. Tech Sgt Lealofi was Jack's handler during the service whereas Tech Sgt Chad Eagan was the handler of Benjo. They could detect a wide range of explosives and kept JBER safe and secure. Subsequently, Jack and Benjo along with their handlers were deployed in Iraq.

Sgt Lealofi and many other opined that Jack was very laid back and mellow like the lyrics in the Bob Marley song, "Don't worry about a thing cause every little thing gonna be alright". In Iraq, Jack and Lealofi conducted searches of more than 300 vehicles a day in the sandbox, and they both knew it was a magic to come back alive after conducting business. Lealofi knew that Jack would always reassure him with his ears up, big brown eyes, tilt in his head and a just smile. Lealofi reminisced that Jack was more to him and indeed a family member. They had a system that was flawless and it was trust to protect each other till last breath. When all others have left you and the loneliness closes in, I will be at your side. While deployed in Iraq, Jack discovered over 2,000 pounds of explosives in a set-up trap along with a fully armed anti-personnel mine in June, 2006, saving many Soldiers' lives. Upon his return to JBER Jack received a Bronze Star for his Bravery and Exemplary Services.

In 2006, Benjo and his handler, Tech Sgt Chad Eagan were also deployed in Iraq. They braved small arms and sniper fire and explosives to locate 15 weapons caches, 98 mortars and 70 pounds of TNT. Benjo was a great dog and he worked relentlessly with the 140 CAV out of FOB Falcon. Benjo had a great effect on the mission as well as on the morale of the soldiers during hard times there. His handler opined that I handled many dogs during my tenure as a MWD handler but Benjo was always my favourite. Benjo returned to his parent air base, JBER after completing his tenure in Iraq. His achievements were complemented by one and all.

A memorial ceremony was held at Chapel one, Joint Base Elmendorf-Richardson, Alaska, USA, on 15th December, 2012, as the 673rd Security Forces Squadron bid farewell to two of their own-fallen Military Working Dogs, Jack and Benjo, at Chapel 1. On the occasion, Kennelmaster Tech Sgt Christopher Wilson said that "These two warriors will never know how many lives they saved or how many homes they protected. All they did was work, and working was their life". Air Force Lt Col Erick Bruce, Commander, 673 SFS, expressed his sentiments that "They will remain in all our hearts and forever be part of the great long-standing history of Military Working Dogs."

Lex

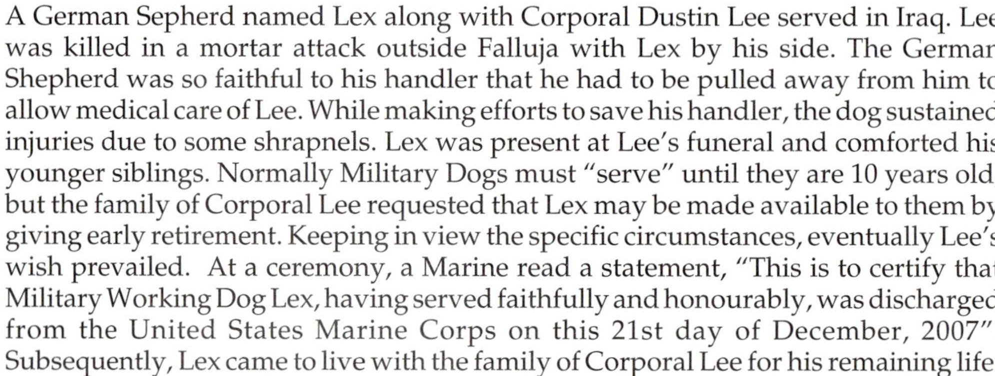

A German Sepherd named Lex along with Corporal Dustin Lee served in Iraq. Lee was killed in a mortar attack outside Falluja with Lex by his side. The German Shepherd was so faithful to his handler that he had to be pulled away from him to allow medical care of Lee. While making efforts to save his handler, the dog sustained injuries due to some shrapnels. Lex was present at Lee's funeral and comforted his younger siblings. Normally Military Dogs must "serve" until they are 10 years old, but the family of Corporal Lee requested that Lex may be made available to them by giving early retirement. Keeping in view the specific circumstances, eventually Lee's wish prevailed. At a ceremony, a Marine read a statement, "This is to certify that Military Working Dog Lex, having served faithfully and honourably, was discharged from the United States Marine Corps on this 21st day of December, 2007". Subsequently, Lex came to live with the family of Corporal Lee for his remaining life.

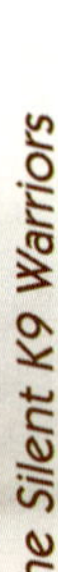

Lucca

Lucca, an eight-year-old Belgian Malinois, an Explosives Detection Dog, alongside Staff Sgt Chris Willingham of the US Army was deployed to Iraq in 2008. Willingham and Lucca headed off to a land in turmoil and constant violence. During the days in Iraq, Lucca and Willingham spent countless hours finding explosives that were designed to kill troops. Their mission was very important one because many lives were in their hands. One mistake could have meant death for them and others following them.

Thankfully, Lucca and Willingham were very good at their job. Their mission was "to alert on the explosives beforehand and have them rendered harmless so the troops can then move out." Once Lucca finds the smell, she will lie down, stare at the scent and communicate the find to Willingham. Willingham is from Tuscaloosa, Alabama and has served in the Corps for ten years. He has been a dog handler for canine and the kennel master of the Camp Echo K9 team. Willingham and Lucca were together for two years on two deployments, one to Iraq and the other to Afghanistan. Willingham credits Lucca with saving his life twice on a previous deployment. He had this to say about the bond he shares with Lucca, who works silently, walking point on a combat patrol, her nose lifted high and then brought low, reading the still air as easily as her handler would read a newspaper. Suddenly, she stops after finding the smell she seeks, and this gifted explosive dog lies down and stares at the scent, communicating the find to her Marine handler. Willingham knows the danger of "choke points", when a convoy approaches points where convoy must slow down or stop, also referred as "choke point", such as a Canal Crossing, intersection or Bend in the Road that gives more time to insurgents to detonate their weapons. During one house to house search, Lucca and Willingham were looking through a TV repair shop, filled with all the typical electrical parts and wiring that one would anticipate finding there. All seemed normal, except the man's composure. In a back room, a box was tucked away under a table, Lucca

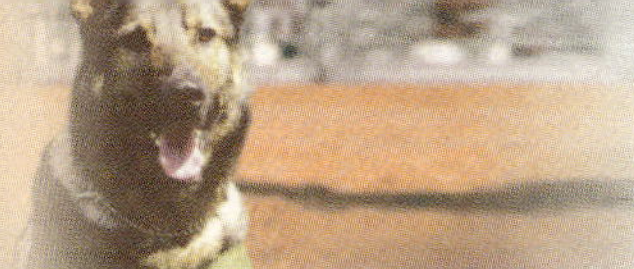

suddenly alerted, and indicaed Willingham that explosives were present. The owner's hands tested positive for residual explosive. One more bomb maker was put out of business in the follow-up action.

Lucca's list of accomplishments is lengthy and includes 2 IEDs, 1 car bomb, caches of homemade explosives, numerous concealed AK-47s with magazines, Dsh-Ks (Vehicle mounted 50 calibre Soviet guns), hidden along the Tigris River and lethal Dsh-K rounds buried in a tomb in a cemetery. Follow-up action ensured arrests of many insurgents.

She has been part of numerous combat patrols, including air assaults. In Willingham's words, "We conducted an air assault one night, and when we hit the house we did not find the "High Value Target," we were looking for. As others were interviewing the witnesses, I took a 4 men team to conduct open area search around the house. Lucca started to show a change, but it was not her normal change of behaviour. I told the team there was something alive out there in the darkness. About 20 yards later, she began to growl, so I alerted the team and they conducted a sweep of the area. About 30 yards away in a canal was the insurgent we were looking for. Although, she is not trained for patrol work, but that's just the dog's natural ability." Lucca spent two tours in Iraq and one in Afghanistan. She has been on 400 patrols and has 40 confirmed finds of explosives, thus saving countless lives. Lucca has definitely established herself as a canine hero among the Marine Corps' Military Working Dogs.

In March, 2008 while on patrol with Cpl Rodriguez in Iraq, Lucca detected a buried explosive, alerted the Marines and kept scouting for more. But the bomb was booby-trapped and as Lucca ran to look for more, a second exploded and she was severely wounded. Cpl Rodriguez heard her squealing and screaming. He went up and gave her first aid, a tourniquet and petted her to keep her calm. It was rough and agonizing moment for both Rodriguez and Lucca. Her wounds were severe and her left front leg had to be amputated.

After her injury, she returned to Camp Pendleton, where she was rehabilitated and subsequently flown from San Diego to Chicago and then to Helsinki via American Airlines, which paid for the flight and bumped the dog to business class.

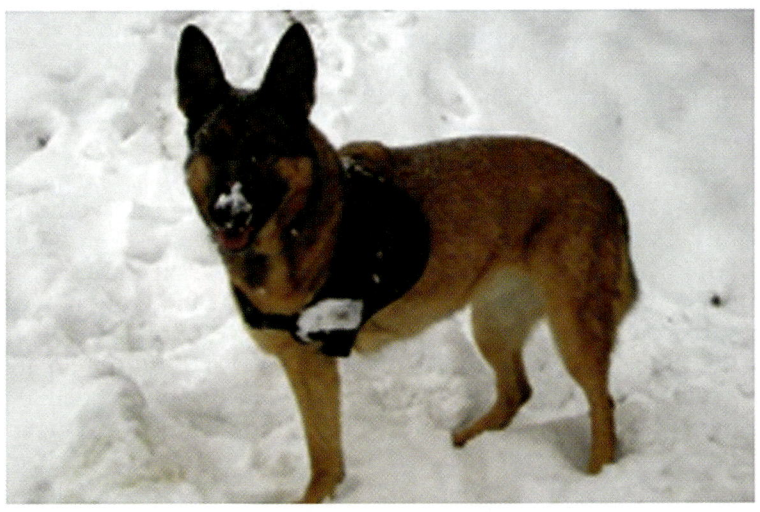

She headed to Helsinki to be reunited with Willingham, who is on embassy duty in Finland. No doubt it will be a happy reunion for both Lucca and Willingham. The Marine Corps Examiner salutes Lucca for her dedicated service to the Marines in Iraq and Afghanistan. She is truly a four-legged heroine in the war on terror.

Rex

A German Shepherd, born in April, 2001 and was trained as an explosive-sniffing dog. His handler was Sergeant Mike Dowling and the duo had unbreakable bond which took them through the scorching heat, the choking dust, and the ever-present threat of violent attack in Iraq's infamous Triangle of Death. In 2004, Rex and his handler were part of the first Marine Corps Military K9 Teams sent to the front lines in Iraq. The team of Rex's and Dowling was employed to sniff out weapons caches, suicide bombers, and IEDs, that wreaked havoc on troops and civilians. The duo always worked into the heart of danger and showed an extraordinary performance in the face of terrible adversity. They saved many lives by detecting explosives, bombs and IEDs as Rex was trained to sniff out nine different explosive materials. After Mike Dowling finished his combat tour, Rex was paired with Marine Corporal Megan leavey. They both made an excellent team and served in two deployments in Iraq, working together to save countless lives as they scoured the war's most dangerous regions. Rex and his handler Megan Leavey were severely injured in 2006 when insurgents detonated an IED at the side of the road they were patrolling. Marine Corporal Leavey was awarded the "Purple Heart" and a "Combat Valor Medal", and the pair spent the next year recovering together from their injuries.

After the duo recovered, Leavey retired from the Marine Corps and tried to adopt Rex, but was unable because he was still considered fit for duty. However, in 2012, Leavey came to know that Sgt Rex was about to retire and she began a new efforts for adoption. She launched a high-profile campaign and received support from Veterans' groups as well as New York Senator Charles Schumer, who started a petition on her behalf called "Saving Sgt Rex", almost 22,000 people signed the petition. Finally, on 7th April, 2012, Sgt Rex retired, and was returned to his old handler, Marine Corporal Megan Leavey who was very happy and said, "Rex and I went through a great deal together and I am just so grateful that we will be reunited again. I will make sure Rex has the best home he could possibly have". Rex lived his remaining life peacefully with Leavy and on 4th January, 2013, Military Working Dog Rex (E168) passed away when he was 11 years old.

AFGHANISTAN WAR

The War in Afghanistan (2001 to present) refers to the intervention by North Atlantic Treaty Organization (NATO) and allied forces in the ongoing Afghan Civil War. The war followed the September 11 attacks in the USA, and its aim was to dismantle Al-Qaeda and denying it a safe basis of operation in Afghanistan by removing the Taliban from power.

The US President George W Bush demanded that the Taliban to handover Osama Bin Laden and to expel Al-Qaeda. The Taliban requested that Bin Laden leave the country, but declined to extradite him without evidence of his involvement in the 9/11 attacks. The United States refused to negotiate and launched Operation Enduring Freedom on 7th October, 2001 with the United Kingdom alongside.

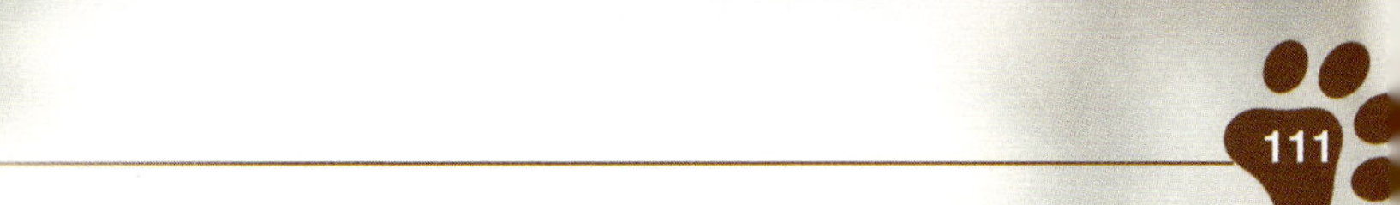

The two were later joined by other forces including the Northern Alliance. The US and its allies drove the Taliban from power and built military bases near major cities across the country. Most Al-Qaeda and Taliban extremists could not be captured as they escaped to neighbouring Pakistan or retreated to rural or remote mountainous regions. In December, 2001, the United Nations Security Council established the International Security Assistance Force (ISAF), to oversee military operations in the country and train Afghan National Security Forces. At the Bonn Conference in December, 2001, Hamid Karzai was selected to head the Afghan Interim Administration, which after a 2002 Loya Jirga in Kabul became the Afghan Transitional Administration. In the popular elections of 2004, Karzai was elected President of the country, now named the Islamic Republic of Afghanistan.

In 2003, the NATO assumed leadership of ISAF, with troops from 43 Countries. The NATO members provided the core of the force. One portion of the US Forces in Afghanistan operated under the NATO Command and the rest remained under direct American Command. Taliban leader Mullah Omar reorganized the movement and in 2003 launched an insurgency against the government and ISAF.

In Afghanistan, the American marines began a pilot project with nine Bomb-Sniffing Dogs in 2007. Over a period of time this number increased to 350 and reached 650 by the end of 2011. Similarly, the British Army raised its first ever Military Working Dog Regiment in 2010 and assigned primary role to support the lead Brigade in Afghanistan with the provision of specialist Military Working Dogs (MWDs) and Veterinary support to Command. Quoting the words of Gen David Petraeus, Commander of the US forces in Afghanistan, "The capability they (the dogs) bring to the fight cannot be replicated by man or machine. By all measures of performance, their yield outperforms any asset we have in our industry. Our army would be remiss if we failed to invest more in this incredibly valuable resource." The dogs are a fighting force on four legs that are able to parachute into action, rappel into combat and swim into a skirmish. They are outfitted with protective body armour and a powerful bite. According to the US Air Force, the bite from a German Shepherd, has a force between 400 and 700 pounds. Infact a dog and a handler outperform any technology on the ground today. At a remote location in the north-eastern mountains of Afghanistan, near the Pakistan border, sits the US Army Forward Operating Base having four Dog Teams with a mission to support the Infantry as they flush out and eliminate the Taliban and other terrorists during the fiercest fighting.

Australian Defence Force (ADF) has also provisioned Special Operations Military Working Dogs (SOMWDs) to support its Special Air Service Regiment deployed in Afghanistan. As on 21st August, 2012, the ADF had 13 Working Dogs in Afghanistan. Explosive Detection Dogs (EDDs) share the dangers of the ADF personnel they work with. Eight EDDs have been killed by improvised explosive devices (IEDs) or small arms fire. The dogs and their handlers undertake patrol to an enemy fighting position, saving human lives while heroically giving their own. Whilst deployed in Afghanistan as a part of Mentoring Task Force 4 (MTF 4), they find Improvise Explosive Devices (IEDs) more commonly known as "roadside bombs", weapons, and ammunition caches. This is to stop the Insurgents (Taliban) from injuring not only Australian and Coalition Forces but ordinary men, women and children who are just trying to live a normal life. Special Operation Task Group (SOTG) personnel credit the dogs with saving the lives of their handlers and patrol members with their actions during countless missions.

In 2008, some of Australia's unsung military heroes have finally been recognized for their bravery. For the first time, unofficial medals have been awarded to the country's courageous canines by the Australian Defence Force Trackers and War Dogs Association (ADFTWDA).

The Taliban has also noticed the value of the dogs and they have wisened to the fact that these dogs are very successful at uncovering IEDs. Accordingly, they are actually a target and if these dogs are out on a lead or often go in front of the unit, they attract sniper fire.

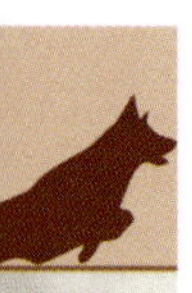

The US SEALs bought four tactical vests for their dogs at a cost of more than $20,000 per unit. The vests are reported to have infrared and night-vision cameras that allow handlers to use a monitor from up to 1,000 yards away to see what the dog sees. The handler is also able to communicate with the dog through a speaker on the vest.

Some of the famous dogs are only described here as a representatives of all the heroic dogs deployed in Afghanistan War:

Brando

Brando, six-year-old male German Shepherd, is a Patrol Dog of Italian Army deployed in Afghanistan. He was trained to perform in territorial control operations in high-intensity scenarios. Brando may infact be considered a true sensor and thanks to his extraordinary olfactory and auditory abilities, he could be used both for searching any type of explosive and for the supervision of points and sensitive areas. In Afghanistan, while seconded for two weeks at the Base Delaram in Farah province, he identified a dangerous explosive device that was readily neutralized. For this reason he was awarded a medal in Rome in the presence of the president of the Republic of Itlay.

Cairo

When the SEAL DevGru team landed at Osama bin Laden's compound in Pakistan on 2nd May, 2011, Cairo's feet would have been the first on the ground. Cairo, a Malinois (Belgian Shepherd), was wearing superstrong, flexible body armour and outfitted with hightech equipment that included "doggles" (specially designed and fitted dog goggles with night-vision and infrared capability) that would even allow Cairo to see human heat forms through concrete walls. The SEAL dogs are generally twice as fast as a fit human, so anyone trying to escape is not likely to outrun them.

Cairo was part of the team that patrolled outside the compound to prevent fighters running out to engage the Americans, Suicide Bombers and Squirters.

During the visit of the US President Barack Obama to Fort Campbell, Kentucky, while meeting the Commando Team that killed Osama Bin Laden, only one of the 81 members of the supersecret SEAL DevGru unit was identified by name, i.e. Cairo, the War Dog, a canine member of the elite US Navy SEAL. "I want to meet that dog." The was President Obama's response upon hearing that a Belgian Malinois named Cairo was on the raid. The President was told that Cairo was in an adjoining room, muzzled, at the request of the Secret Service.

"If you want to meet the dog, Mr President, I advise you to bring treats, the Navy Seal Squadron Commander joked as Obama went over to pet Cairo".

The New Yorker magazine gave details of the raid, including Cairo's role. Inside the two helicopters on the raid were twenty-three Navy SEALs from Team Six, which

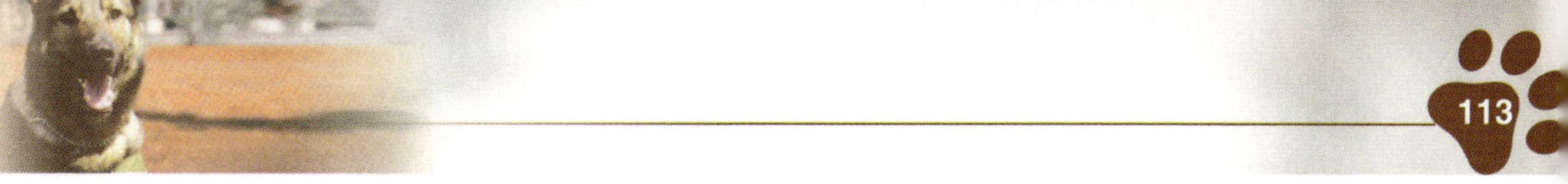

is officially known as the Naval Special Warfare Development Group, or DEVGRU. A Pakistani-American translator, and Cairo, a Belgian Malinois, highly intelligent and fearless breed increasingly used by the Military.

The two Black Hawks, each of which had two Pilots and a Crewman from the 160th Special Operations Aviation Regiment, "Night Stalkers", had been modified to mask heat, noise, and movement. The copters' exteriors had sharp, flat angles and were covered with radar-dampening "skin".

Twelve SEALs, including Mark, boarded "Helo One". Eleven SEALs, Ahmed, and Cairo boarded "Helo two".

"Cairo's role was a help to clear the buildings, sniff for bombs and booby-traps, search for false walls or hidden doors where Bin Laden could be hiding, or help to keep curious neighbours at bay".

As it turned out, after one of the helicopters crashed outside the compound's walls. Cairo, a translator named Ahmed, and four SEALs were responsible for closing off the perimeter of the house while six other SEALs, the contingent that was supposed to have dropped onto the roof, moved inside. For the team patrolling the perimeter, the first fifteen minutes passed without incident. Neighbours undoubtedly heard the low-flying helicopters, the sound of one crashing, and the sporadic explosions and gunfire that ensued, but nobody came outside.

Eventually, a few curious Pakistanis approached to enquire about the commotion on the other side of the wall. "Go back to your houses," Ahmed said in Pashto, as Cairo and his Seal Team stood on watch. "There is a security operation under way." The locals went home, none of them suspecting that they had talked to an American.

When the Squadron Commander, spoke at the ceremony honouring the Seal Team Six, he started by citing all the forward operating bases in Eastern Afghanistan that had been named for SEALs killed in combat.

"Everything we have done for the last ten years, prepared us for this," he told Obama. The President was "in awe of these guys," Ben Rhodes, the Deputy National-Security Adviser, who travelled with Obama, said. "It was an extraordinary base visit," he added. "They knew he had staked his Presidency on this. He knew they staked their lives on it."

And Cairo, the brave Belgian Malinois, trained to slide down a rope or jump 5,000 feet to help protect our troops and country, was there.

Cougar

Cougar, a SAS Patrol Dog of Australian Army, was deployed in Afghanistan along with his handler SAS Trooper Mark Donaldson. The dog participated in an Operation with Donaldson. During the operation, Cougar was shot in the face, leg and had three rounds into his chest. Notwithstanding his wounds, he managed to swim across a river, back to his handler but could not survive.

Cougar was among five who died during service in Afghanistan over the past decade. On 12th August, 2008, Corporal Mark Donaldson (then Trooper) was also wounded in action whilst conducting nighttime operations in Uruzgan Province, Afghanistan. He recovered from his minor wounds and continued on the deployment.

On 2nd September, 2008, he was involved in an incident in Uruzgan Province, Afghanistan, when a five-car Coalition convoy has been ambushed, 13 men are wounded. He saw an Afghan terp who had been shot in the head lying face down in the dust behind. While a mate advised him to stay, Donaldson stubbornly took off. As he dragged the interpreter 80 metres back to the car, the incoming fire was so heavy that the rounds created an effect like a thunderstorm and he never experienced anything like it. This gallant action in the face of enemy, resulted in award of the "Victoria Cross" to Corporal Mark Donaldson and he become the first Australian in almost 40 years to be awarded the nation's highest military honour. He was invested by her Excellency the Governor General of Australia at Government House, Canberra on 16th January, 2009.

Donaldson admits that he has been inspired by the SASR's combat assault dogs, which have been shot attacking terrorists, and seeing mates run across roofs, knowing enemy inside are firing at them. Watching guys dodging bullets while trying to drop grenades down a funnel pipe, and then do it over again and again – that's amazing.

At a ceremony held at the Australian War Memorial in Canberra on 23rd February, 2014 to recognize the animals that have served in Australia's war efforts, Cougar, the former SAS Patrol Dog belonging to Trooper Mark Donaldson, VC. was honoured. On this ceremonial occasion, Memorial Director, Brendan Nelson said "We as Australians who are civilians, too often we forget that the animals are involved."

Devil

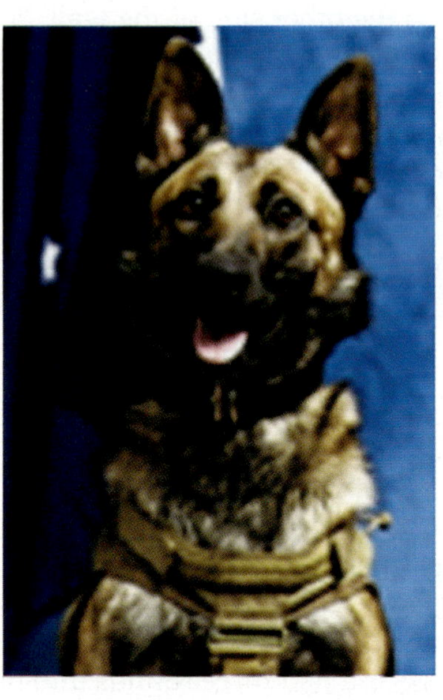

Special Operations Military Working Dog (SOMWD), Devil, a Belgian Shepherd, was born on April 14, 2009. He was raised and trained by a civilian breeder until 2010. In late-mid 2010, Devil was posted to the SASR after performance trial and was deployed to Afghanistan in February, 2011. He returned to Australia after completion of tour. With SOTG rotation, he was deployed again to Afghanistan in February, 2012. During the mission, Devil provided early warning of an enemy fighting position. A firefight ensued between the SOTG patrol and the insurgents, during which Devil was targeted by an insurgent at close range which killed Devil instantly on 2nd July, 2012, while he was on his second tour to Afghanistan with a new handler.

During the same mission, SASR's Sgt Blaine Diddams was also killed.

At the time of the dogs' deaths, Commanding Officer SOTG said, "Their loss would have a big impact on the task group. Personnel who work closely with our dogs form extremely close bonds with them so these deaths will affect them. These dogs were much loved members of the SOTG and they will be surely missed."

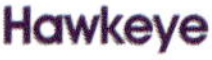

Hawkeye

On 6th August, 2011, the dog of the slain US Navy SEAL remained loyal even in death. Petty Officer Jon Tumelson was killed in Afghanistan when the US Chinook helicopter was shot down by Taliban insurgents. During the funeral service which was attended by 1,500 people, his Labrador Hawkeye walked up to the casket, heaved a sigh and lay down in front of it for the entire duration of memorial. Hawkeye was highly trained, highly skilled, highly motivated Special Ops Experts, able to perform extraordinary military missions by Sea, Air and Land (thus the acronym). He carried out wide range of specialized duties such as to detect and identify explosive material and hostiles or hiding humans, for the military teams to which he was attached.

Herbie

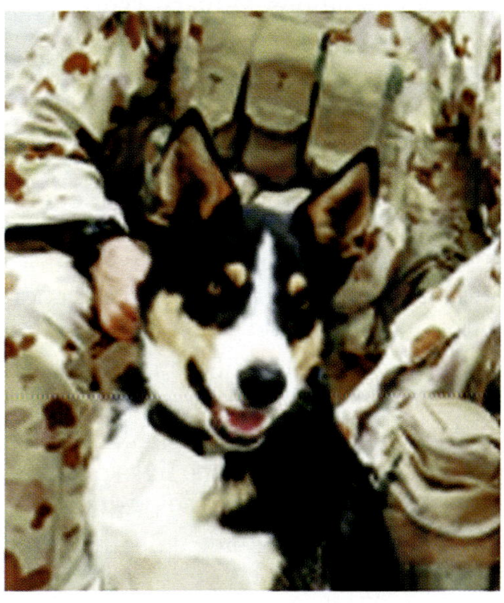

Herbie, a Border Collie, Explosive Detection Dog along with Sappers Darren Smith and Jacob Moerland, conducted a route clearance ahead of an Australian Patrol in the Mirabad Valley region of Oruzgan province in Afghanistan on 7th June, 2010. Sapper Smith and the Sniffer Dog Herbie had detected an enemy bomb and as the two soldiers from the Brisbane-based 2nd Combat Engineer Regiment approached the improvised explosive device (IED), the still summer morning was rocked by a massive explosion. A Taliban insurgent had detonated the device by remote control killing Sapper Smith and Herbie and severely wounding Sapper Jacob Moerland who died later from his wounds. Acting Chief of the Defence Force Lieutenant General David Hurley described it as a "tough day".

Sapper Darren Smith is the first Australian Defence Force Military Working Dog handler to be killed in action while working with an Australian Miltiary Working Dog on the battlefield. Herbie was not buried in Afghanistan, like other explosive detection dogs before but her body was returned to Australian soil where she was cremated. During a small ceremony at Gallipoli Barracks (Enoggera, Brisbane, Queensland). Herbies ashes and medals were presented to Sapper Darren Smith's wife, Mrs Angila Smith.

In memory of Sapper Darren Smith and his explosive detection dog "Herbie" who, together with Sapper Jacob Moerland, were killed in action by an Improvised Explosive Device in Afghanistan on 7th June, 2010, a memorial was dedicated by the Australian Defence Force Trackers and War Dogs Association at 139 Wacol Station Road, RSPCA Animal Campus, Wacol, 4076, Queensland, Australia.

Megane

Megane, a seven-year-old female German Shepherd was the first dog to have been qualified as an Italian Military Mine Detection Dog. She is very exuberant with a great desire to play but when there is a job to do, she is transformed. She has an exceptional sense of smell and probably no technology can compete with her in this regard. She is able to reclaim areas and potentially dangerous routes in no time, avoiding the risks of mine accidents. Her professional career has included many missions abroad, such as Enduring Freedom in 2004. Posted in Khost Province in Afghanistan, she has been widely used in the reconnaissance of routes in one of the highest-density landmine area in the world.

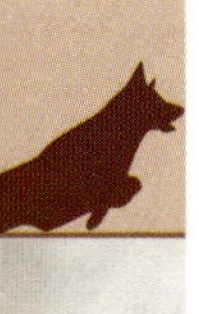

Quake

Special Operations Military Working Dog Quake, a Belgian Shepherd, was born on 9th March, 2008. He was inducted into the RAAF puppy programme, raised and mentored by an Air Force dog handler until 2011. Trialed in early-mid 2011, the dog was posted to the SASR after satisfactory performance in trial. The dog was deployed to Afghanistan with Special Operations Task Group (SOTG) from September to December, 2011 to replace another SOMWD that was wounded in action. After the successful completion of his tour, Quake returned to Australia in December, 2011. He was redeployed for his second tour to Afghanistan in February, 2012. Quake was instrumental in informing the SOTG patrol of insurgent actions and also supported SOTG tactical action with great distinction, allowing the SOTG patrol to engage and kill several enemy personnel.

During an SOTG mission on 25th June, 2012, he provided early warning of an enemy sentry position.

The insurgent engaged Quake at close range with small-arms fire and killed him. Quake's actions saved the lives of his handler and the other members of the patrol who were approaching the position.

At the time of the dog's death, Commanding Officer SOTG said that personnel who work closely with our dogs form extremely close bonds with them so these deaths will affect them. These dogs were much loved members of the SOTG and they will be surely missed and their loss would have a big impact on the task group.

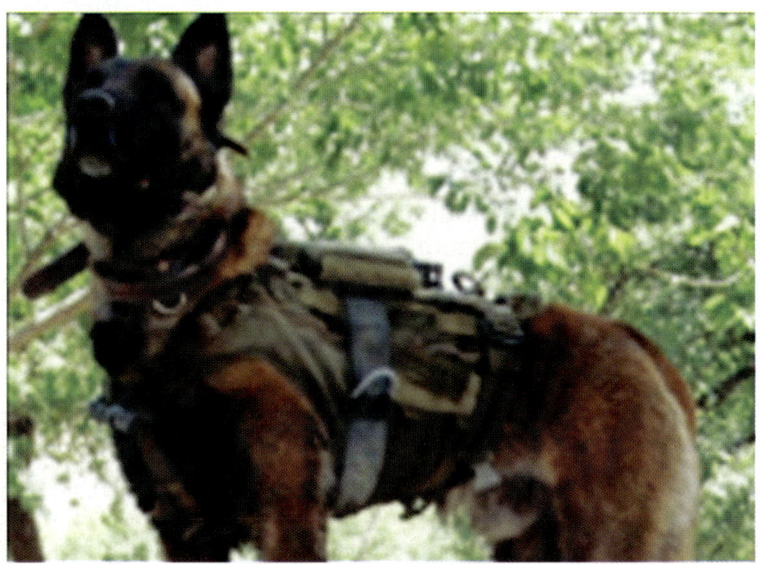

Razz

Razz, was an Explosive Detection Dog of mentoring Task Force (MTF) of Australian Defence Force in Afghanistan. On 21st September, 2007, a Special Task Force (SOTG) vehicle was hit by an IED in Oruzgan Province in which two soldiers were wounded. On 24th September, 2007, Razz and his handler were deployed on the road clearance task. During the search, Razz discovered a large roadside bomb (IED) and he moved into sit position. Moments before Australian troops moved in to try to defuse the IED but in the process the device was detonated and Razz was vapourized. He saved not only his handler's life but the lives of the troops around him.

Razz was the first ever Military Working Dog in the history of the Australian Defence Force to be killed in action (KIA) on the battlefield.

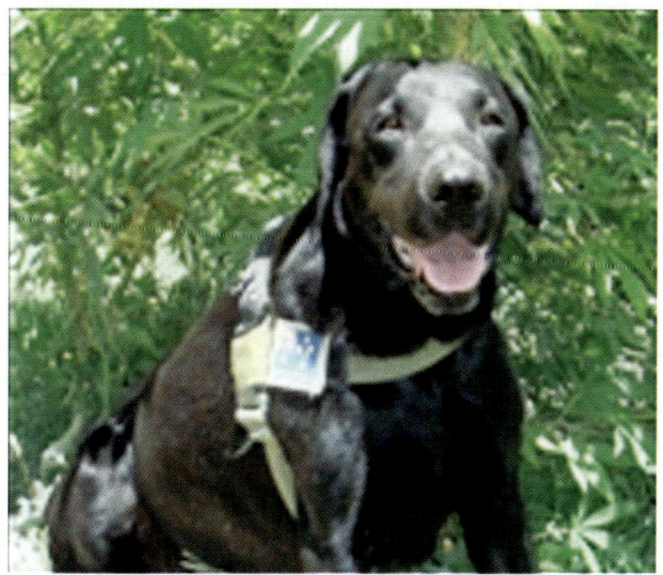

Sarbi

Sarbi, a female black Labrador/Newfoundland cross dog of Australian Army, was trained in explosives detection. Sarbi was deployed in Afghanistan with her handler Corporal David Simpson as part of the Australian Army's "Operation Slipper" which is the name of Australian Military's role into the ongoing War in Afghanistan. She was trained to detect Improvised Explosive Devices (IEDs) in Oruzgan Province. Previously she was used by the Incident Response Regiment during the 2006 Commonwealth Games held in Melbourne, Australia. It was her second tour of duty in Afghanistan, having been deployed in 2007 also. Sarbi went missing after a Joint Australian, American and Afghan vehicle convoy was ambushed by insurgents on 2nd September, 2008 during the Battle of Khaz Oruzgan. Sarbi's handler was Corporal David Simpson, who was also one of nine Australian soldiers injured in the ambush.

Sarbi disappeared 'in the heat of battle' when a rocket exploded near her during the ambush. It was the same action in which SAS Trooper Mark Donaldson became the first recipient of the Victoria Cross for Australia, since 1969. Sarbi was declared missing in action (MIA) in September, 2008, and the Special Operations Task Group had made repeated attempts to find out her.

She was rediscovered by an American Soldier in North-Eastern Oruzgan province, when he noticed her accompanying a local man. The soldier, only identified as 'John', was aware that the Australian Forces were missing a dog, and determined through the use of voice commands that this was indeed a trained Military Dog. After being flown back to her Australian base in Tarin Kowt, handlers confirmed the dog was Sarbi.

The news of Sarbi's return was released by the Department of Defence on 11th November, 2009 (Remembrance Day), and generated worldwide media attention. More so, the Australian Prime Minister Kevin Rudd and the ISAF head General Stanley A McChrystal were making a surprise visit to the Tarin Kowt base on the same day. Brigadier Brian Dawson, Head of Defence Public Affairs, held a press conference about Sarbi and said that the military would probably never know what had happened to Sarbi while she was missing, but her good health indicated that somebody had been looking after her. However, "The Australian", a broadsheet newspaper published in Australia from Monday to Saturday each week since 14th July, 1964, reported on 13th November that, according to a senior Australian Military Officer who asked not to be named, Sarbi, was wounded in the ambush, did return to a nearby ISAF forward operating base, but was chased away by Afghan guards.

Prime Minister Rudd said of Sarbi's rediscovery:

"Things like that, may seem quite small, but in fact the symbolism is quite strong, and the symbolism of it is us, out there doing a job. We haven't awarded any Australian Victoria Cross for 40 years. Trooper Donaldson stands out there as an Australian Hero, and now his dog Sarbi is back home in one piece and a genuinely nice pooch as well".

Sarbi's handler Corporal David Simpson, expressed that he had never given up hope of finding her, and was profoundly relieved at her recovery. The trainer who confirmed Sarbi's identity described her as "an exceptionally good worker, very gritty dog and has found many improvised Explosive Devices and saved quite a few lives in her work". "It's amazing, just incredible, to have her back."

Trooper Donaldson, who was in London to meet the Queen at the time of Sarbi's rediscovery, said that it "closed a chapter in their shared history" and "She's the last piece of the puzzle, having Sarbi back gives some closure for the handler and the rest of us that served with her in 2008. It's a fantastic morale booster."

Sarbi was required to undergo a period of quarantine, and be assessed for exposure to diseases, before a return date to Australia could be set. Under AQIS rules, dogs would not normally be allowed entry to Australia directly from Afghanistan, but would rather have to spend six months in an intermediate approved country. Sarbi passed initial Veterinary checks and would be retired on her return to Australia. Prime Minister Kevin Rudd stated that he would be working with the Australian Quarantine and Inspection Service (AQIS) to "ensure Sabi's eventual return to Australia."

On 5th April, 2011, Sarbi was awarded a Royal Society for the Prevention of Cruelty to Animals (RSPCA) "Purple Cross Award" at the Australian War Memorial. The RSPCA Australia Purple Cross Award recognizes the deeds of animals that have shown outstanding service to humans, particularly if they showed exceptional courage while risking their own safety or life to save a person from injury or death.

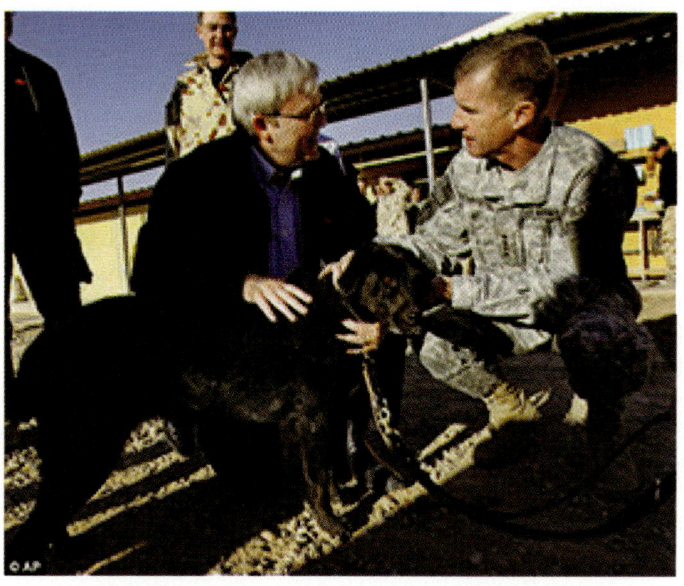

Australian Prime Minister Kevin Rudd with Sarbi

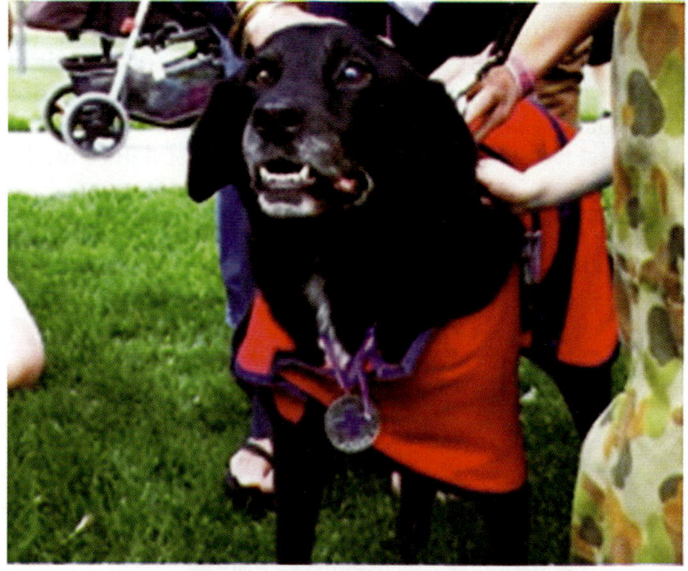

Veteran war dog Sarbi at war memorial event

Sasha

Sasha, a four-year-old yellow Labrador who was trained to hunt out explosives, is credited with saving the lives of scores of soldiers and civilians in Afghanistan. Sasha was deployed with handlers from the British Royal Army Veterinary Corps, attached to the 2nd Battalion, The Parachute Regiment. Alongside her handler, she was tasked with carrying out advance patrols to find safe routes for soldiers and sniffing out weapons and IEDs. Sasha's determination to search and push forward despite grueling conditions and relentless Taliban attacks, was a morale boost to the soldiers who entrusted their lives to her weapon-finding capability. On one occasion recalled by regimental colleagues, Sasha was searching a building in Garmsir when she detected two mortars and a large quantity of weaponry, including explosives and mines. This find alone undoubtedly saved the lives of many soldiers and civilians. In 2008, she was assigned to 24-year-old L/Cpl Rowe and the pair was considered the best in the Kandahar region. Sasha had 15 confirmed finds of Improvised Explosive Devices (IEDs), mortars and hidden weaponry. Sasha and Rowe died together on 24th July, 2008 when their routine patrol was ambushed by a rocket-propelled grenade attack by Taliban. She was awarded the **"PDSA Dickin Medal"** on 29th April, 2014.

"This prestigious award is the recognition of her devotion and skills that undoubtedly saved the lives of many troops in Afghanistan, also acknowledge the excellent work and the immeasurable contributions to military operations by Military Working Dogs and their handlers".

Target, Rufus and Sasha

Target and two other dogs, Rufus and Sasha were stray dogs who befriended American soldiers stationed at Afghanistan Military Base Dand Patan. Soldiers started to feed them as pets and would play with them while they were free, got bored and remembered their homes. One night in February, 2010, these three proved to be more than just a remedy for the soldiers' homesickness, when they detected a suicide bomber who came to the base in the middle of the night, wearing 25 pounds of explosives with an intent to kill Americans. The three dogs frightened, barked at and also bit the bomber so as to scare him and waking up the sleeping soldiers in the process. Deterred by the dogs, the terrorist detonated himself outside instead of coming in the barracks where soldiers were sleeping. As a result of the

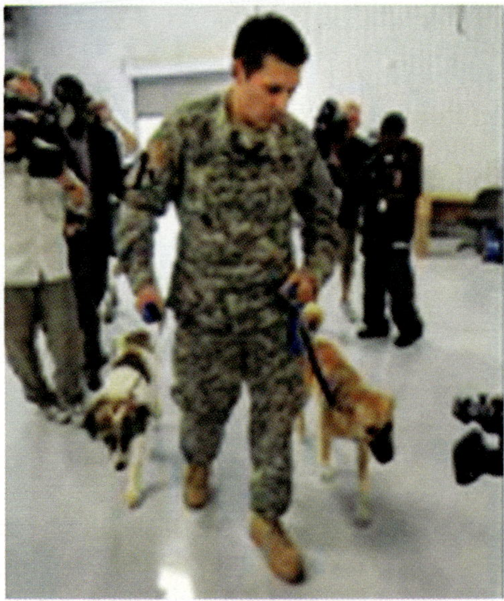

Sgt Terry Young with Target and Rufus

heroic acts of these dogs, the lives of 50 soldiers were saved and only five soldiers sustained minor injuries from which all of them recovered. In the explosion one of the three dogs, Sasha was killed on the spot. Rufus and Target were injured and subsequently saved due to timely treatment and care of these dogs. Sgt Terry Young with the help of an aid group was allowed to take remaining two dogs with him to America in August, 2010 when he returned from his tour on duty. Rufus and Target received a Hero's welcome when they landed and Target even appeared on Oprah show about amazing animals in September, 2010.

Sadie

A Labrador, Arms and Explosive Search Dog of Royal Army Veterinary Corps of British Army, was deployed in Kabul, Afghanistan in November, 2005. On 14th November, 2005, military personnel serving with NATO's International Security Assistance Force in Kabul were involved in two separate attacks. Sadie and Lance Corporal Yardley were deployed to search for secondary explosive devices.

Sadie gave a positive indication near a concrete blast wall and multinational personnel were moved to a safe distance. Despite the obvious danger, Sadie and Lance Corporal Yardley completed their search and at the site of Sadie's indication, they found an explosive device which was later made safe by Bomb disposal team. The bomb was designed to inflict maximum injury. Sadie's actions undoubtedly saved the lives of many civilians and soldiers. Sadie was awarded "**PDSA Dickin Medal**" on 6 February, 2007 "For outstanding gallantry and devotion to duty while assigned to the Royal Gloucestershire, Berkshire and Wiltshire Light Infantry during conflict in Afghanistan in 2005".

Theo

Theo, a Springer Spaniel, served with the British Royal Army Veterinary Corps as an Arms and Explosives Search Dog. While deployed with 104th Military Working Dog (MWD) Squadron during conflict in Afghanistan", Theo's handler, Lance Corporal Liam Tasker was killed during an exchange of fire with insurgents in March, 2011 but the dog survived and subsequently suffered with a fatal seizure just hours later and died. Theo was awarded **"PDSA Dickin Medal"** posthumously on 25th October, 2012 "For outstanding gallantry and devotion to duty while deployed with 104th Military Working Dog (MWD) Squadron during conflict in Afghanistan from September, 2010 to March, 2011."

After the award ceremony, Lance Corporal Tasker's mother, Jane Duffy, said that she is so proud of the award. It is like they were a team. One couldn't have worked without the other and she is sure that Theo died of a broken heart. Laura Tasker, sister of Lance Corporal, said Theo helped her brother who received a posthumous **"Mention in Despatches" (MID)** while he was serving in Afghanistan. I don't think people realize how close they actually were, "they were completely made for each other."

Treo

The eight-year-old black Labrador along with handler Sergeant Dave Heyhoe of Royal Army Veterinary Corps, British Army, was deployed in Afghanistan in March, 2008. Sgt Heyhoe and Treo started their military career together in Northern Ireland, then moved to North Luffenham and then to Afghanistan in 2008. Treo was one of the 25 dogs in Afghanistan, supporting British Troops on patrol. His work involved searching for arms and explosives as part and parcel of the search element which may not the ultimate answer but definitely an aid to search. The duo was working as a Forward Detection Dog Team tasked with searching for weapons and ammunitions concealed by the Taliban. On 15th August, 2008, while acting as forward protection for 8 Platoon, The Royal Irish Regiment in the town of Sangin, Helmand Province, Treo located a daisy chain IED, an improvised explosive device designed to trigger a series of bombs, on a roadside where soldiers were about to pass. It was subsequently confirmed that the device recovered would have inflicted significant casualties. On 3rd and 4th September, 2008, Treo's actions were reported as "Saving 7 Platoon from guaranteed casualties", as the result of timely detection of another IED. Treo's actions and devotion to his duties, while in the thick of conflict, saved many lives. Army authorities recommended him for the award to PDSA in recognition of Treo's heroism which saved soldiers and civilians from death and serious injury.

The black labrador, accompanied by his handler, Sergeant Dave Heyhoe, was presented with the **"PDSA Dickin Medal"** by Princess Alexandra at the Imperial War Museum in London on 24th February, 2010. Sgt Heyhoe dedicated the award to every dog and their handler working in Afghanistan and Iraq.

The pair of Treo and Heyhoe have worked together for five years and after their Military tenure, Treo has now become a family pet of Sgt Heyhoe. Everyone will say that Treo is just a Military Working Dog—yes, he is, but he is also a very good friend of Heyhoe and they look after each other.

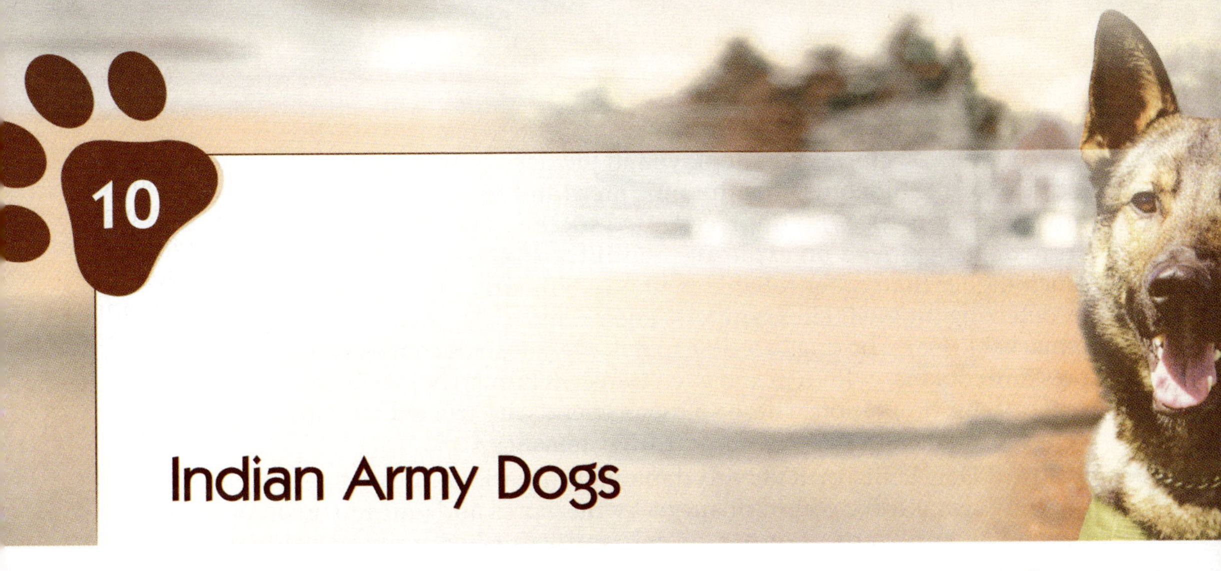

10 Indian Army Dogs

"People leave imprints on our lives, shaping who we become in much the same way that a symbol is pressed into the page of a book to tell you who it comes from. Dogs, however, leave paw prints on our lives and our souls, which are as unique as fingerprints in every way."

... Ashly Lorenzana

In India, during pre-independence era, the Indian Army Veterinary Corps (IAVC) commenced its war dog training in 1943 at Babugarh (near Hapur) to train Mine Detection Dogs, however, this facility was closed on culmination of World War II. In the post-independence era, Remount Veterinary Corps (RVC) of Indian Army started training of army dogs at Dog Training Wing of RVC Centre and college on 1st march, 1960. The Corps was entrusted with the responsibility of the procurement, breeding, training and issuance of dogs to meet requirements of the Army, Air Force, National Security Guards (NSG) and Special Frontier Force (SFF). This training module consistently progressed and metamorphosed into state-of-the-art 'Dog Training Faculty' as of today. Initially the training was focused on guard and tracker dogs, subsequently, the 1965 and 1971 Indo-Pak wars necessitated training of Infantry Patrol and avalanche rescue operation dogs. With the winds of terrorism setting roots in the country in eighties, highly specialized dogs for explosive detection, mine detection, narcotic detection and search and rescue operation dogs were trained to deploy in the counterinsurgency and counterterrorism role. The predominant breeds of dogs being labradors, German Shepherds and Belgian Malinois. However, trials are conducted from time to time to find out the suitability of other breeds as per the defined role.

Right from introduction of dogs till present scenario, these silent warriors have rendered invaluable service in tracking saboteurs, guarding vital installations, explosive and mine detection, augmenting Infantry patrols, saving the lives of troops in avalanche disaster and other natural calamities. The success rate against the militants, terrorists and anti-national elements increased many-fold with the use of army dogs, and now virtually every unit deployed in counterinsurgency operations requested the services of these dogs in their endeavours. Dogs have proved lifesavers for the forces in many instances, as they have led patrols safely through the thick jungles, deeply buried explosives, IEDs and old mine fields in the northeast as well as in northern sector. When deployed in the deep jungles in Naxal affected areas to locate Naxalite hideouts, their training areas and ammunition caches, these saviours proved their mettle with unprecedented success. The effectivity and success rate of army dogs deployed on explosive and IEDs detection jobs, is 84 per cent which is much higher than other reliable methods. Similarly, the services rendered by dogs in detecting ambush sites, snipers, enemy hideouts, and infiltration, have been a remarkable feat. The dogs are able to detect explosives concealed in suitcases, boxes, pressure cookers, cylinders and even transient human bombs because of their higher sense of discrimination. These soldier's friends are trusted for sanitizing buildings, vehicles, roads and helipads in sensitive areas.

Army Dog Units of RVC are deployed in various theaters to employ dogs in boosting war efforts, counterinsurgency measures and anti-terrorism operations as per the requirement. Regular on job and refresher training of dogs and their handlers/trainers along with their fitness for duty and adequate veterinary cover is integral part of the unit. Area specific advanced veterinary facilities are also provisioned so as to ensure that the dogs continue to work at specific location. Well-equipped veterinary hospitals with latest facilities are available to provide advanced treatment to canines hurt and wounded in combat.

In July, 1965, one legendary army dog Alex, a golden Labrador, along with Lance Dfr (ADT) Mangal Singh created history by successful tracking for three miles on two days old sent, and the culprits who attempted to assassinate the King of Bhutan were apprehended. Army dogs have been most frequently used in counter-insurgency operations in eastern and northern theatres. The Infantry patrol dogs resolutely led many columns in thick jungles, difficult terrain, snow-bound areas as well as other strategically important trails and guided the troops befittingly about the presence of enemy in close vicinity. Similarly, tracker dogs led own troops to hideouts of hostiles and camps of anti-national elements for the appropriate military action. During the Indo-Pak wars in 1965 and 1971, army dogs proved their usefulness and rendered valuable services for security of vital installations, and also Prisoners of War (POW) camps, after the end of 1971 war.

The canine saviours have done wonders not only in war scenario but in peace times too. The exceptional performance of these army dogs in various national calamities and disasters, e.g. Bhuj earthquake, Tsunami in Andaman and Nicobar Islands, J&K earthquake and cloud burst at Leh, etc. have won accolades from one and all. When deployed in search and rescue work after the deadly earthquake of October, 2005 in the Kashmir Valley, these dogs played a heroic role in search of survivors and detection of dead bodies in the vicinity of earthquake site. Similarly, the avalanche rescue operation dogs of Indian Army have earned an enviable reputation in avalanche-prone areas. These dogs have saved many lives of soldiers who got trapped in severe avalanches in snow-bound areas. One such army dog Ashok, a Labrador, deployed at Zozila pass in northern theatre in November, 1986, with his handler Dfr (ADT) Gyan Singh, successfully rescued several casualties and saved the lives of many, buried in heaps of snow. This heroic dog draws some parallel to life-saving ability of "Berry" one of the most famous dogs in the world whose stuffed body now forms part of the Natural History Museum in Bern, Germany. Berry, a St Bernard, while serving as a search dog for St Bernard Monastery from 1800 to 1812 saved more than 40 human lives on the pass between Mont Balsas and the Dallier Apes. The St Bernard was trained by monks to help them rescue people who got lost in the Alps. His most famous rescue was when he found a child in the snow.

He licked on the child to keep him warm and kept barking to signal the monks of their location. When the monks couldn't reach them because of the snow, the boy wrapped his arms around Barry and the dog carried him to safety. He retired from his rescue career in 1812 and was cared for the remaining life by one of the monks.

The unparalleled excellence of army dogs in detecting explosives and improvised explosive devices has saved thousands of lives of soldiers as well as civilians. The performances of mine detection dogs have been exemplary in de-mining the mine fields during and after various military operations/conflicts. They were uniquely successful in detecting the plastic mines and the leftover mines from the fields after being screened with metal detectors. The above elaboration is a drop in the vast ocean of heroism of Army dogs in various fields. The last decade has seen an ever-increasing demand of these silent warriors owing to the fact that Army dogs have proved their worth and they are now being considered a valuable asset in furthering the cause of troops deployed. With the ongoing low intensity conflicts and counter-insurgency operations, these selfless, dedicated heroes are contributing a great deal in achieving success against the evil designs of militants and anti-national elements.

The brave, courageous, reliable and indispensable Army dogs along with their trainers/handlers have thus earned their most deserving existence in Indian Army with tremendous appreciation and a plethora of honours and awards at various levels in recognition of the distinguished services rendered.

The vital contribution of these dogs has been recognized time and again which gives them pride of place in public displays at the prestigious Army Day and Republic Day Parade.

HEROIC INDIAN ARMY DOGS

From the times of Mahabharata and Campaigns of Persians, Conquest of Roman Empire, World Wars, Sino-Indian and Indo-Pak Wars, dogs have gone into battle in direct or indirect support of operations. These canine heroes have been referred as "Force Multipliers". Picking up threads from the history, Indian Army Dogs have etched a glorious chapter in the annals of the Indian Army and earned a mark of grudging respect of one and all. The phrase "Heroism of Army Dogs" includes the bravery and distinguished acts of the team of duo, i.e. Army dogs and Army Dog Trainers (ADTs)/Handlers. The recognition of good job done and honours and awards conferred on either depict the joint effort and efficient functioning of the team.

The tally of medals awarded to army dogs and their handlers, complied up to 15th August, 2013, includes Shaurya Chakra (1), Sena Medal Gallantry (6), Mention in Dispatch (1), Chief of the Army Staff Commendation Cards (136), Vice Chief of the Army Staff Commendation Cards (4), General Officer Commanding in Chief Commendation Cards (408), Chief of the Army Staff (COAS) Unit Citation to Army Dog Units (2) and General Officer Commanding in Chief (GOC-in-C) Unit citation to Army Dog Units (5), speaks volumes about the heroism of these silent warriors.

The details of all gallant actions and distinguished performance of heroic dogs and their handlers in war and peace is a vast field, and practically not possible to include each and every detail in this text. However, the unique and exemplary acts which should make us feel proud of army dogs are being reproduced here as representatives of these silent warriors.

A136 Alex: The Legendary Army Dog

An attempt on the life of King Jigme Doji Wangchuk of Bhutan was made on 31st July, 1965 during a celebration to offer 1,000 butter lamps at Kyushu Monastery on the occasion of 4th day of the 6th month of Bhutanese calendar where the King had gone to offer 1,000 butter lamps. The King was suddenly attacked by an enemy, who threw a hand grenade and also fired shots. On the request of Bhutanese Government, Army Dog Alex, a Tracker Dog of 3 Army Dog Unit along with Swr/ADT Mangat Singh was employed on 2nd August, 1965 to track down the assailant. The dog team was flown to PARO by a helicopter. It commenced tracking from the scene of crime on a scent, which was already two days old, from the only article left by the assailant, "a Grenade lever". Nevertheless, Alex put his nose down and commenced his long and tortuous track along the grassy forest slopes and crisscrossed footpaths. After tracking for 3 miles, the track winded into a house where the assassin had taken shelter. From this site, Alex pursued further on another track leading to a hill feature and after a mile long run entered a temple where the culprit was caught hiding in one of the temple rooms. The King of Bhutan rewarded Alex and his trainer with a cash award, a gold ring and a certificate for their undeterred performance.

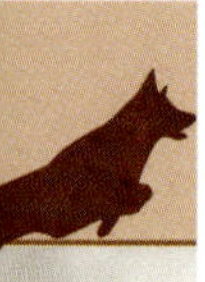

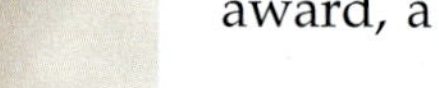

Certificate

English translation of certificate awarded by the King of Bhutan under his seal read:

"On the occasion of the celebration of the 4th day of the 6th month of the Bhutanese calendar, I had gone to offer thousand butter lamps at the Kyushu Monastery. On the eve of the celebration, an enemy rascal made an attempt on my life by throwing a hand grenade and firing a few shots. By the grace of God I escaped unharmed. My worthy friend, the Government of India as well as Army authorities at Siliguri were very kind in aiding me with the loan of their well-trained dog Alex and its trainer ADT Mangat Singh. The latter with his dog underwent a lot of trouble in tracing the culprit and finally succeeded in capturing him. It was wonderful and I was exceedingly grateful."

51A9 Amit

On 20th December, 2000, Amit, a Tracker Dog along with trainer L/Dfr (ADT) B Mohanty of 16 Army Dog Unit was assigned to a column of 95 Field Regiment in eastern sector for counterinsurgency operations named "OP RED HERRING". Amit covered a distance of 30 km in thick jungle terrain towards assigned objective. The hideout of Undergrounds (UGs) was finally cordoned off. The early morning of 21st December, 2000, witnessed the sudden heavy firing from the UGs on the Indian Troops. Thick jungle made it easy for the militants to run away and hide there. Amit picked up the scent from the leftover footwear of the UGs and tracking at a fast pace, led troops to a nearby house which has been used by militants the previous night. Search of this house resulted in recovery of one AK-56 rifle, certain incriminating documents pertaining to National Socialist Council of Nagaland (NSCN), and articles of routine uses. Amit was immediately given carting scent in that house and quickly followed the trail of fleeing militants for about 2 km and entered in a small ditch from where Amit pulled out one pouch which contained one hand grenade, one AK-47 magazine and 90 live rounds of AK-47 rifle. In recognition of this daring performance, Army Dog Amit was awarded **GOC-in-C Eastern Command Commendation Card** on 26th January, 2002.

65A7 Babli

Babli, a black Labrador, the name, every person of 15 Army Dog Unit cheered with utmost honour and pride. Babli, a Tracker Dog was associated with a number of search operations carried out by Infantry Troops. The award winning performance was on 23rd September, 2002, when Babli with handler ALD (ADT) Ajay Kumar was employed with 41 RR Battalion to track down the escaped terrorist in general area Gulgam in District Kupwara. Babli picked up the scent in hazardous and inhospitable terrain conditions. This courageous, reliable and indispensable force multiplier swiftly led the search party on scent trail at a very fast pace. At about 1240 hours, the search party suddenly came under fire and in the ensuing gun fight three terrorists were killed. They were later identified as Shauquat War, Rehmat Ali Khan and Abdul Aziz Rehman, most wanted trio and a prized catch by the security forces. The action also led to recovery of three AK-47 rifles, 5 Chinese grenades and large quantity of ammunition. In recognition of exemplary performance, Army Dog 65A7 Babli was awarded **Chief of the Army Staff Commendation Card** in 2003.

68A9 Balraj

On 5th August, 2000 at 0430 hours, based on specific information, Balraj, a Tracker Dog of 15 Army Dog Unit was pressed into the search operation along with Dfr (ADT) Suresh Chandra to assist an Infantry Battalion in Northern Sector. Balraj picked up the casting scent from the site and followed the track on a difficult terrain. The operation resulted in killing of one dreaded militant and discovery of a well-established underground natural hideout measuring 8 ft × 6 ft. The other important achievement was recovery of a Kalakop Rifle, a new weapon not recovered earlier, along with a large quantity of ammunition and operational stores. For the act of courage and excellent performance of the team of Army Dog and its handler, Dfr (ADT) Suresh Chandra was awarded **GOC-in-C Northern Command Commendation Card**.

Once again on 6th July, 2001, Balraj and his handler ALD (ADT) Md Manirul Islam were pressed into the search operation by an Infantry Battalion. Balraj picked up the scent from the footmarks effectively and followed more than two kilometres trail in difficult terrain and led the column to hide out of terrorists. In the ensuing firing, two terrorists, a District Commander and a Company Commander, were killed. Huge quantity of arms and ammunition was also recovered during the search operation. In yet another repeat performance, on 12th July, 2003, Balraj with handler Swr/ADT AK Khan, while deployed with 41 RR Battalion led the party through mountainous track to a terrorist, who was killed in the ensuing gunfight. One AK-47 rifle, three magazines and four hand grenades were recovered.

To top it up, on 17th July, 2003, Balraj and Khan duo were deployed with 18-JAK rifles, in a search operation in general area Hamnag. He picked up the scent from the water bottle left behind by fleeing terrorists in jungle. He followed the trail skillfully and led the search party towards a natural water stream (nullah) with dense undergrowth. On seeing the search party, the terrorist named Farooq Ahmad Mughal of JUM voluntarily surrendered to the troops. One AK-47 rifle, three magazines, two hand grenades and 47 rounds of AK-47 were recovered from the surrendered terrorist. Balraj and his handler ALD (ADT) DD Magar were again deployed with 41 RR Battalion on 27th July, 2003 in general area Khumarial. During this search operation, three Lashkar-e-Tayeba (LET) terrorists were detected and killed. A large quantity of arms and ammunition was also recovered from their possession.

114A Balram

On 30th June, 2006, Balram, an Explosive Detection Dog of 14 Army Dog Unit and handler ALD (ADT) Dhanvate Adinath were detailed on Road Opening Patrol (ROP) duty with 23 RR Battalion to sanitize the road National Highway-1A (NH-1A) under their area of responsibility. The handler deployed Balram and searched in detail the assigned area. While near a culvert, he pointed towards an unshapely object and the handler understood the signal. On close examination, it was an IED located under the culvert at kilometre stone 80 concealed in a ghee tin and wrapped in gunny bag. The Bomb Disposal Team further examined the IED and destroyed it *in situ*. The IED was a potent threat to convey of holy Amaranth Yatra which was averted. In recognition of the professional skill of very high order and excellent performance with courage and dedication, ALD (ADT) Dhanvate Adinath and Army Dog Balram were individually awarded **GOC-in-C Northern Command Commendation Card** in 2007.

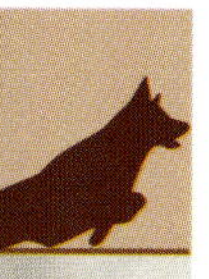

Similarly, on 24th June, 2007, Balram and handler ALD (ADT) SK Kumawat were deployed on Road Opening Patrol (ROP) duty again with 23 RR at general area Ralmandu (MZ0039). The handler employed Balram and searched the area of responsibility very carefully and diligently. Balram detected and pointed a gunny bag lying in the vicinity filled with explosive material. Immediately Bomb Disposal Team was requisitioned which undertook the detailed examination of the explosive material and confirmed it to be RDX. The bag contained 10 kg of RDX which had the potential of causing immense damage to men and material. For this achievement, excellent performance and devotion to duty, Army Dog Balram was awarded **Chief of the Army Staff Commendation Card** in 2008.

BO86 Banu

Banu, an Explosive Detection Dog of 27 Army Dog Unit was deployed alongside his handler with 60 RR Battalion for counterinsurgency/counterterrorism operations. On 8th January, 2010, based on input by own sources, the handler and the dog were deployed along with a party of 66 RR at a strategically significant culvert on Kotranka Road in Kandi location. The dog was employed to search any explosive material at and nearby the culvert. On careful and thorough sniffing of the area displaying high standards of professional skill, Banu pointed out a site indicating the presence of explosives. On getting the sign the dog handler examined the area and confirmed the presence of IED placed in a steel box and two wires of IED were protruding outside. The IED was removed safely saving the lives of troops and civilians which had the potential to damage the bridge, Banu's efforts had been successful in ensuring smooth flow of traffic on the road and continuity of supply chain and logistics of army. In recognition of the outstanding performance and devotion to duty Army Dog Banu was awarded **GOC-in-C Northern Command Commendation Card** on 15th August, 2011.

64AO Barkha

Barkha, an Explosive Detection Dog of 14 Army Dog Unit and her handler ALD (ADT) Kiran Kumar Tadaka were deployed to sanitize the road NH-1A, life line of J&K, on 10th August, 2004 between kilometre stone 171 to 183 with ROP column of 47 AD Regiment. Barkha detected and indicated an Improvised Explosive Device (IED) weighing approx 5 kg in a metal canister and hidden in a gunny bag which was placed off the road at kilometre stone 172.9. Barkha displayed exceptional courage and devotion to duty by detecting IED laid by the Anti-National Elements (ANEs) thus preventing loss of precious human lives and property as also ensuring uninterrupted flow of traffic on NH-1A.

Other notable achievements of Barkha on National Highway-1A also include detection of an IED on 9th January, 2002 at kilometre 174.5, when deployed with ALD (ADT) Anoop R. Again on 17th October, 2003, Barkha with handler L/Dfr (ADT) Vikram Singh detected an IED at kilometre 191.5 NH-1A. and on 5th February, 2004, Barkha with ALD (ADT) Manoj Kumar brought glory to her unit after she detected an IED at kilometre 174.5 on NH-1A. This commendable role of Army Dog Barkha assisting ROPs to ensure the National Highway-1A remains safe for traffic and speedy movement of one and all in that sector, won her the laurels, accolades of one and all. For her heroism and devotion to duty, Army dog 64AO was awarded **GOC-in-C Northern Command Commendation Card.**

664A Baru

On 12th October, 2010, ALD (ADT) Md Mofizul Islam and Baru, a Tracker Dog of 27 Army Dog Unit were participating in "OP KATORISAR" with 60 RR Battalion in general area Katorisar (MY5744). During the search in their area of responsibility (AOR) at about 1750 hours, two terrorists were spotted by the column and exchange of fire followed. By the time last light firing stopped and outer cordon was established to seal the escape routes. On 13th October at 0600 hours, the dog team was deployed for the deliberate search. The handler cast the dog intelligently and carried out search carefully and minutely with perseverance in rugged terrain. The dog Baru pointed towards a small heap of leftover articles which were identified as 34 fired cases of ammunition, one live round of AK-47 and one cleaning rod of AK-47 rifle. Baru was again cast on the scent of these leftover stores and soon the duo found out the route taken by the fleeing terrorists. The team of Mofizul and Baru tracked the trail relentlessly and finally lead the column towards the hideout of the terrorists. In the ensuing exchange of fire both the terrorists were killed and a cache of arms, ammunition and war equipment which included one AK-56 rifle, one AK-47 rifle, 43 rounds of ammunition, Thuraya radio sets, GPS Garmin, RSI Com, Mobile phones, etc. were recovered. For the outstanding performance, professional skill, courage and devotion to duty, ALD (ADT) Md Mofizul Islam was awarded **GOC-in-C Northern Command Commendation Card** on 26th January, 2012.

66A4 Bazz

Bazz, a Tracker Dog of of 4 Army Dog Unit with handler ALD (ADT) NK Verma was deployed with 18 RR Battalion on 18th January, 2006 and tasked to track the injured militant who had escaped after an encounter with troops. The dog was cast on the scent available at the site and tracking the trail reached a village. Bazz repeatedly pointed the presence of the injured militant in the village. As such a cordon and search operation was undertaken which finally culminated in the killing of militant and recovery of one AK-47 rifle, three AK-47 magazines, one UBGL and one radio set. For this act of bravery and professionalism, ALD (ADT) NK Verma was awarded **GOC-in-C Northern Command Commendation Card** on 15th August, 2008. In a repeat performance of similar type, Bazz was paired with handler ALD (ADT) Pintu Kumar and deployed again with 18 Rashtriya Rifles (RR) Battalion as part of Quick Reaction Team (QRT). On 12th June, 2007, the duo while being part of an operation to chase the terrorists in the given area of responsibility were tasked to track the trail of escaped militants. The dog took scent from the site which had footprints and some blood spots of fleeing militants. Bazz was cast on the trail and finally led the QRT team to a hideout of militants. Subsequent engagement with troops led to elimination of three militants and recovery of large cache of arms and ammunition including AK-47 rifles and hand grenades. In recognition of exemplary professionalism and devotion to duty, Bazz and his handler, ALD (ADT) Pintu Kumar were individually awarded **Chief of the Army Staff Commendation Card** on 15th January, 2008.

Similarly, on 14th September, 2007, Army Dog Bazz was paired with handler Dfr (ADT) Dharmender Singh. The duo was deployed with 8 Rashtriya Rifles (RR) as a part of QRT ex Varnua COB at the site from where some anti national elements involved in an incident, were required to be tracked. The handler familiarized the dog with the site and the scent available at the spot and cast Bazz on the trail. The duo followed the trail vigorously. The dog indicated a place from where arms and ammunition were recovered which included one UBCL, one UBCL grenade, one AK-47 rifle with magazine and 8 rounds. From here, the dog took fresh scent from the foot marks of fled terrorists and followed the trail swiftly. After tracking for quite sometime in darkness and covering a long distance the dog team lead the QRT in morning hours to one hideout covered with black tarpaulin of size 15′ × 7′. On thorough search of the hideout, 2 magazine of AK-47 rifle and 34 rounds of ammunition were recovered.

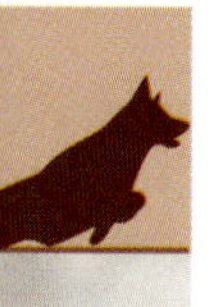

For the exemplary performance and dedication to duty Dfr (ADT) Dharmender Singh was awarded **Chief of the Army Staff Commendation Card** on 15th August, 2008.

416A Beagle

Beagle, an Explosive Detection Dog of 16 Army Dog Unit along with handler ALD (ADT) SK Sahu was deployed for duty with 9 Para-Field Regiment. On 8th July, 2005 while on duty to detect explosives and IEDs in area of responsibility at Jirivam, detected one powerful IED, thereby avoided immense loss of lives of troops and civilians in the area. Beagle was bestowed with **Chief of the Army Staff Commendation Card** on 15th January, 2006.

78A2 Bhawana

On 25th May, 2002, Swr (ADT) Shiv Lal along with Bhawana of 23 Army Dog Unit, a Mine Detection Dog, was detailed on the Road Opening Patrol (ROP) duty for sanitizing the road. During the process Swr/ADT Shiv Lal judiciously checked all the suspect points on the road for Improvised Explosive Device (IED) with Bhawana. At around 0800 hours, a broken patch was noticed by the Road Opening Patrol party. Swr (ADT) Shiv Lal guided Bhawana to the hill feature to check for any planted explosive. She successfully detected the buried explosive site but destiny had something else for this heroic duo. While the IED was being removed from the site, the terrorists hidden in the vicinity detonated it and the IED exploded. The Dog died on the spot. Swr (ADT) Shiv Lal was severely injured and evacuated to Command Hospital, Udhampur, where he succumbed to multiple splinter injuries. The team of the Bhawana and her handler gave their supreme sacrifice and saved many lives. No word of appreciation, compliments, laurels or honours and awards can match the heroism and bravery shown by the duo.

"Humble salute to Shiv Lal and Bhawana"

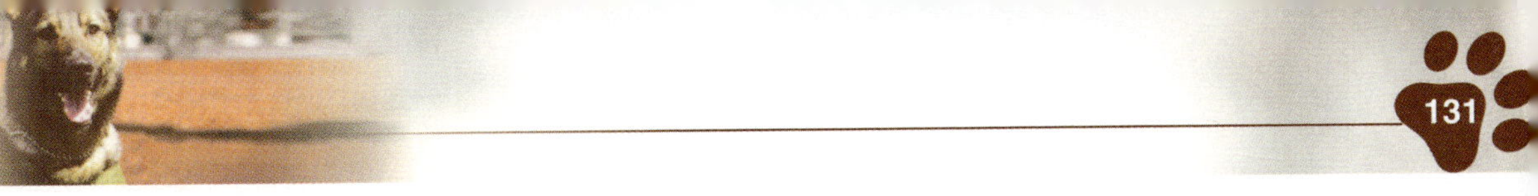

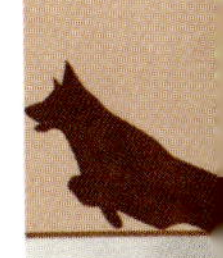

80AO Bingo

Army dog Bingo, an Explosive Detection Dog of 8 Army Dog Unit along with handler Dfr (ADT) Dharam Singh was deployed with 4 Jat Regiment at North Lakhimpur, Assam. While sanitizing the area of responsibility prior to 26th January, 2005 (Republic day) celebrations, the team of Dharam Singh and Bingo detected IEDs planted by extremists on four different places which were subsequently deactivated carefully.

This act thwarted the nefarious design of ULFA extremists to disrupt the Republic day celebrations 2005 at North Lakhimpur and avoided loss of lives of a large number of civilians and troops. In recognition of professionalism of very high order and devotion to duty, Bingo was awarded **Chief of the Army Staff Commendation Card** on 15th January, 2006.

628A Birender

An operation was launched by 33 RR Battalion on 26th January, 2007 at Shehlal in J&K against two terrorists identified in that area. In a brief fight one terrorist was killed whereas the second terrorist though injured but escaped leaving a blood trail behind. Birender, a Tracker Dog and ALD (ADT) Basudev Panja, of 4 Army Dog Unit were deployed to track the fleeing terrorist. The dog was cast on the blood trail successfully by the handler and the duo followed the scent trail with great courage, speed and zeal. The fleeing injured terrorist was soon spotted enabling the troops to encircle him. Caught in a bind, the terrorist lobbed a grenade on the party which somehow did not explode. The action was retaliated by the troops and the terrorist was eliminated in exchange of fire. On closer identification, he was found to be Mohd Akbar Bhatt, radio code Tahir, a dreaded Hizbul Mujahideen terrorist. Two AK-47 rifles, seven AK-47 magazines and 70 rounds of ammunition were recovered from his possession. The bravery and devotion to duty depicted by duo of Punja and Birender in tracking the terrorist and in recognition of their dedication to service, ALD (ADT) Basudev Panja was awarded **Chief of the Army Staff Commendation Card** on 15th January, 2008.

563A Bittu

On 26th October, 2008, at 1230 hours, an encounter took place between troops of 2 Maratha Light Infantry (MLI) and suspected terrorists who fled away in general area Bichwal, leaving a rucksack behind. The duo of Bittu, a Tracker Dog along with handler ALD (ADT) KS Vishwas of 15 Army Dog Unit were tasked to track the fleeing terrorists. The dog took the scent from the rucksack and the handler cast the dog on the scent trail. After successfully tracking the trail for approximately 2 km, they came across a hand glove suspected to have been of fled terrorists. The dog was again cast on the scent of hand glove which further strengthened the track scent. The track continued on undulating terrain and varying heights till they successfully noticed a hideout. On seeing the movement of the troops, the hidden terrorists opened fire in which the dog handler was also shot in his left shin but it did not deter him and he along with his dog Bittu continued on the mission. Subsequent exchange of fire between troops and the terrorists led to killing of three terrorists and recovery of huge cache of arms and ammunition. In recognition of the exemplary bravery and professionalism of Bittu and Vishwas, ALD (ADT) Khilare Sagar Vishwas was awarded **Chief of the Army Staff Commendation Card** on 15th January, 2008.

65A6 Bobby

A Mechanized Infantry Battalion while carrying out search operation on 8th November, 2000 was successful in elimination of two terrorists. Further, search for remaining Anti-National Elements (ANEs) was launched by the Battalion. Army Dog Bobby, a Tracker Dog of 18 Army Dog Unit, with handler ALD/ADT Kumar Das N, was deployed to assist the column in the given task. Bobby took the scent from the footprints of fleeing ANEs and tracked them down to a house. In the ensuing gunfight, the handler not only saved his dog but returned effective fire. In fierce encounter both terrorists were killed and a large cache of arms/ammunition was recovered. In recognition of the exemplary bravery and extreme dedication of the team of Bobby and his handler, ALD/ADT Kumar Das was awarded **Chief of the Army Staff Commendation Card** in 2001.

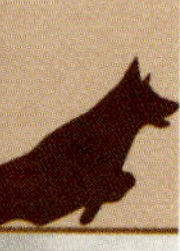

A062 Bolo

Bolo, an Avalanche Rescue Operation (ARO) Dog of 19 Army Dog Unit was attached with 29 Mob Fd Vet Hospital under 17 Mtn Div for operational role. On 28th February, 2003, at around 1740 hours, MFVH intimation was received to move the ARO Dog to Yalka Base of 5 Assam Battalion where two OR of the Battalion were buried in snow during an avalanche. OC 29 MFVH along with Bolo and his handler ALD (ADT) Sunil Das left for the destination at about 1800 hours. The team reached 5 Mile Transit Camp at around 0300 hours on 1st March, 2003 and halted for night. Next day, early morning, the team left the camp and finally reached the Yalka base of 'B' Coy of 5 Assam Battalion at about 1130 hours. The team along with the guide of 5 Assam left for the Sapat Base, at a height of 14432 feet, and reached the Base at around 1500 hours on foot. Keeping in view the inclement weather condition, exhaustion due to distance covered on foot and lack of acclimatization, the team was made to halt for night at Sapat Base.

On 2nd March, 2003 at around 0700 hours the dog team further moved to another location called Choti Post along with the guide party of 5 Assam Battalion. On reaching the site, the dog was given sufficient rest before deploying for the task. Subsequently, the dog was given the scent of clothes of the two OR buried in the avalanche. The dog swiftly moved forward sniffing the avalanche area. On reaching the exact location, Bolo gave indication by vigorous sniffing and pawing the snow out. The snow was removed and finally both the bodies which were about 10 feet under snow were recovered. For this admirable performance, Bolo, the Avalanche Rescue Operation Dog, was awarded **GOC-in-C Eastern Command Commendation Card.**

51A1 Borris

During September, 2000, an operation was launched by an Infantry Batallion against the terrorists who indiscriminately fired at the search party and fled away into the fields. Dfr (ADT) Lakhbinder Singh and Borris, a Tracker Dog of 13 Army Dog Unit, were deployed to track the militants. Borris took scent from the footprints of fleeing persons and the duo followed the trail. Borris and Lakhbinder successfully led the search party up to a wounded terrorist. The follow-up action resulted in killing of three terrorists and recovery of large cache of arms and ammunition. In recognition of this gallant act both Dfr (ADT) Lakhbinder Singh and Borris were individually awarded **Chief of the Army Staff Commendation Card** in 2001.

B021 Bulli

On 2nd June, 2010, subsequent to firing by terrorists on area dominance patrol ex 22 Rashtriya Rifles (RR) and return firing by the patrol on unidentified terrorists at Bhagatpura location in Sopor, terrorists got injured but escaped leaving a blood trail. Bulli and handler L/Dfr (ADT) Godse Dhiraj Sitaram of 26 Army Dog Unit were deployed to track the fled terrorists. The dog was cast on the blood trail which was only few hours old but got faded due to exposure to direct sunlight and heat. The duo exhibited exceptional courage, pinnacle of professional acumen and disregarding their personal safety, tracked a zig zag trail in built up area which involved jumping the boundaries and fences made of tin sheets. In the process the dog had to be redeployed/ recast six times on the far end of the fence which was not fully sanitized and also partially occupied by own troops. The dog and the handler duo continued the track with full zeal and enthusiasm and lead the column unrelentlessly in almost hostile environment. Finally the dog indicated a house in which suspected injured terrorists were hiding. A cordon search operation was launched and the hidden injured terrorists were killed in the encounter. The valiant act and professionalism of highest order of the duo Bulli and Godse was duly recognized by awarding L/Dfr (ADT) Godse Dhiraj Sitaram with **Chief of The Army Staff Commendation Card** in 2011 and Bulli was awarded **GOC-in-C Northern Command Commendation Card.**

7A15 Dalvi

Dalvi, a Tracker Dog and his handler ALD (ADT) KSS Rao of 5 Army Dog Unit were deployed with an Infantry Battalion for a cordon and search operation near a village on 30th November, 1992. The duo located two AK-56 rifles buried under ground. Dalvi was given scent from the butt of a rifle and he identified two Anti-National Elements (ANEs) from the village successfully. In another search operation, the team of Dalvi and Rao was deployed with another Infantry Battalion. Dalvi was cast on the scent from an ammunition pouch found by the search party in a house. The dog tracked the trail and got one suspected ANE apprehended. Based on the lead provided by the ANE, one hand grenade was recovered from the nearby orchard. In another cordon and search operation, an Infantry Battalion had arrested six ANEs and recovered some weapons from them. One ANE during interrogation confessed that he had hidden some more arms and ammunition but refused to give the location. The duo of Dalvi and Rao were deployed, Dalvi took scent of the ANE and followed the trail. He pointed towards a stone wall. On deep search, two AK-47 magazines filled with 60 rounds and two hand grenades were recovered from within the stone wall. On 29th November, 1993, Army Dog Dalvi and ALD (ADT) KSS Rao were deployed at a place where the ROP party had noticed an IED wire. Dalvi was given scent from the wire, which led the party to a site near main road from where IEDs weighing 10 kg and 2 detonators were recovered. On giving the scent from recovered IED, the dog led the party to a shop from where terrorists had bought the wire, which was used in making IEDs. The duo proceeded further 300–400 metres and identified 4 suspected men hidden in a house who were associated with the crime. The dog was again given scent from the IED and made to identify the people who had handled the IED. Out of 25 suspected persons, Dalvi identified 6 persons who were apprehended. The ROP party recognized two of these six who had run away after being sighted by them. The success of operation was the result of professional handling and functional competence of Army Dog Dalvi. In recognition of the exemplary services and devotion to duty, 7A15 Army dog Dalvi was awarded **GOC-in-C Northern Command Commendation Card** in 1994.

On 31st October, 1995, at around 1900 hours, few shots of AK-47 rifle were heard in the area adjoining an Infantry Battalion. 'A Quick Reaction Team' (QRT) along with Army dog Dalvi and handler ALD/ADT Babloo Kumar was pressed into action. The incident was a case of murder by a terrorist, who, by the time the QRT reached had made an escape. Dalvi picked up the scent from some footprints at the site and led to the apprehension of four terrorists including their two prominent leaders along with recovery of weapons. In recognition of courage, professional competence and devotion to duty ALD (ADT) Bablu kumar was awarded **GOC-in-C Northern Command Commendation Card** in 1996.

Once again, on 26th September, 1996 at 1530 hours Army Dog Dalvi and handler L/Dfr (ADT) CP Sharma were deployed to track the trail of a suspected ANE who escaped leaving his shoe behind. Dalvi was given the scent from the leftover shoe belonging to a suspected ANE and was cast on trail by the handler. Dalvi and Sharma tracked down for 250 yards and led to a house where terrorists were hiding. On seeing the dog and L/Dfr (ADT) CP Sharma approaching towards them, the ANEs fired at them. Immediately the area was cordoned off. The exchange of fire followed till 0200 hours and taking the advantage of darkness, the ANEs escaped from the house and hid in a heap of paddy in surrounding fields. Dalvi was redeployed on the track used by ANEs to escape. After a successful trail, the ANEs were located and four militants including one self-styled Battalion Commander were killed in exchange of fire. In recognition of excellent work, distinguished service and bravery of very high order, Dalvi was again awarded **GOC-in-C Northern Command Commendation Card** in 1997.

Yet again on 27th August, 1997 at 0630 hours, Army Dog Dalvi was deployed by handler ALD/ADT SPS Rathore for search operation. After taking scent from articles recovered from the dead militants, Dalvi picked up the trail and after tracking through fields and undulating area, he reached a spot near an open scrub and indicated at a spot where huge quantity of arms and ammunitions were hidden under a boulder. It became a common saying that with Army Dogs like Dalvi on trail, terrorists can run for a while but they cannot escape. In recognition of exemplary service, courage and professional competence, 7A15 Army Dog Dalvi was once again awarded **GOC-in-C Northern Command Commendation Card** in 1998.

Bravo Dalvi!

31A6 David

Explosive Detection Dog David and ALD (ADT) PS Patni of 18 Army Dog Unit recovered an Improvised Explosive Device (IED) near a village panchayat on 27th July, 1998, while on Road Opening Patrol duty with a Paramilitary Force Battalion (PMF Bn). The IED weighing 5 kg and wrapped in a cloth was planted by Anti-National Elements (ANEs) to disrupt a religious procession. This was concealed under a heap of stones and tied to a pressure cum release device with a string extending to a house. Identification and removal of IED saved many precious lives and enhanced the image of security forces amongst the civilian society. Once again On 30th July, 1998, based on specific information, the duo of Army Dog David and handler ALD (ADT) PS Patni while on Road Opening Patrol (ROP) duty recovered an IED concealed behind a boulder next to a road. The IED weighed approximately 2 kg, elliptical in shape, 1.6 feet long and 8 inches broad and was wrapped in insulation tape. In addition, one remote control and one 9 volt battery with wire were recovered from the site which, if not detected, would have caused immense damage to lives of soldiers and civilians passing through this area. In recognition of the excellent professional services and dedication to duty David was awarded **GOC-in-C Northern Command Commendation Card**.

25A7 Deepti

The Transit Camp Guwahati, located close to railway station is the 'life line' for movement of troops in the eastern sector. Army Dog Deepti and Dfr (ADT) Jitendra Pradhan of 19 Army Dog Unit were deployed at this transit camp for search operations. The dog, besides being a deterrent to the extremists, was a source of confidence building amongst all the passengers at Guwahati Railway Station. On 7th May, 2001 at about 1030 hours an unattended package was noticed in railway reservation complex located opposite Guwahati Transit Camp. Deepti, an Explosive Detection Dog, was brought to the site along with handler to detect if anything explosive material was kept in the unattended package. Deepti when brought near the package registered the smell and indicated the presence of the explosives. The device had a hightech circuit and contained 28 gelatin sticks timed to explode two hours after recovery. This IED was then safely taken away and was defused by the experts. Thus a major tragedy was averted. In recognition of the dedication and professionalism of highest order depicted by the duo enabling timely detection of dangerous and life-threatening IED, which could have been catastrophic, Army Dog Deepti was awarded **GOC-in-C Eastern Command Commendation Card** on 26th January, 2002.

Subsequently on 15th February, 2003, Deepti along with handler Swr (ADT) Dharmendra Giri was deployed with 28 Punjab Regiment for providing support in Counterinsurgency Operations (CI Ops). Based on specific information that some objects have been placed by the United National Front of Assam (ULFA), Quick Reaction Team (QRT) along with the duo of Deepti and her handler was immediately rushed to the location at Chengalijan village of Dibrugarh District. The search of the area resulted in the recovery of a cylindrical iron object filled with nuts and bolts and covered with wax targeting the nearby oil pipeline. The well-trained and experienced Army Dog Deepti was cast on the smell of this device and she took no time in giving clear indication that ibid object was indeed an IED which was recovered safely and destroyed. Thus Deepti was instrumental in averting a major catastrophe to the oil pipeline and also saved valuable human lives. Once again for exhibiting high sense of professionalism and devotion to duty, Deepti was conferred with **GOC-in-C Eastern Command Commendation Card** on 15th August, 2003.

Again, on 26th June, the same year, Deepti with handler L/Dfr (ADT) Subhash Prasad Singh formed a part of the search party of 28 Punjab Battalion for Counter Insurgency Operations. Based on specific information, the team was to sanitize the general area, Gabrupathar of Dibrugarh District. After two hours of thorough scanning, the Army Dog indicated the presence of explosive material among the animal hides lying in a heap. The cache included a black plastic bag containing 2.5 kg of explosive with primer, electric detonator with electric wire, six rounds of 9 mm and seven rounds of AK-47. The detection of explosives and live ammunition in spite of the presence of extraneous, strong animal hide odour, which could easily mask the explosive scent, was a grand feat. In recognition of exceptional devotion to duty and working proficiency. Deepti was once more awarded **GOC-in-C Eastern Command Commendation Card** on 26th January, 2004.

" Great achievement"

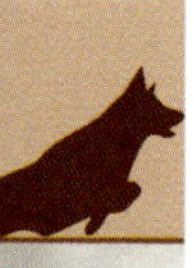

1A16 Deep and 4A31 Dhiman

A murder took place at the location of a HQ Mountain Division and nobody owned up the crime. All possible investigations were carried out but they could not give any indication about the motive of murder and also the whereabouts of the culprit who committed the crime. Three days passed in various efforts to solve the mystery of the murder but still no clue was in sight. At this belated stage, on 28th October, 1986, it was decided to take the help of Army Dogs. Accordingly, ALD (ADT) AN Sharma and ALD (ADT) Balbir Singh along with Deep and Dhiman of 11 Army Dog Unit were deployed under the supervision of Dfr (ADT) NS Rawat. The handlers cast their respective dogs on the scent available at the site of the murder, which was already three days old. Both dogs along with their handlers skillfully followed the trail under the guidance of Dfr (ADT) NS Rawat and finally nabbed the culprit. For the exemplary performance, Dfr (ADT) NS Rawat, ALD (ADT) AN Sharma and ALD (ADT) Balbir Singh were individually awarded **GOC-in-C Northern Command Commendation Card.**

36AO Delta

Delta, a Mine Detection Dog, initially posted to 12 Army Dog Unit, was subsequently transferred to 20 Army Dog Unit on 14th September, 2001. A sincere and dedicated Labrador, he brought many laurels to the unit. On 2nd November, 2002, Automatic Grenade Launcher Detachment (AGD) Commander noticed a freshly dug earth near the piquet at around 0830 hours. Deep Search Metal Detector (DSMD) was brought to check, but it was not effective. Delta, who was on Road Opening Patrol (ROP) duty with 27 RR Battalion was requisitioned and put into action. The dog took the scent from the loose earth and immediately gave clear indication of the presence of the explosive. On detailed search, the explosive was found in a polythene bag, buried underground with two wires coming out which were likely to be used for detonation. On the same day while deployed on another search mission, Delta indicated one more battery operated improvised explosive device (IED) hidden in a bush which was also directed towards same AGD. Valuable lives of many soldiers were saved and damage to Government property avoided by sensible application of senses by Army dog Delta. For this gallant act and dedication, Delta was awarded **Chief of the Army Staff Commendation Card** in 2003.

36A8 Diana

On 4th February, 1998, an army patrol was ambushed by militants and in the cross fire, two culprits were killed. Army Dog Diana, a Tracker Dog of 3 Army Dog Unit, along with its handler Dfr (ADT) PK Kurian were deployed on 5th February, by giving scent from magazine pouches of dead persons. The dog followed the trail enthusiastically and led the column to a place where illegal weapons were being manufactured in a big way. The place was immediately cordoned off. The search of this so-called local arms manufacturing factory led to the recovery of large quantities of war-like material. Similarly, on 25th January, 1999, Diana with handler Swr/ADT

AK Mishra was deployed with an Infantry Battalion to track a suspected Anti-National Elements (ANEs), the duo of Diana and Mishra successfully assisted in apprehension of ANEs hiding under thick undergrowth.

On 28th December, 2000, Diana with her handler ALD (ADT) Dilip Kumar was deployed to track underground ANEs after an aborted ambush with troops of 15 JAT Battalion. Diana registered the scent and the duo started chasing the fleeing extremists with great speed. While tracking, the dog detected one empty magazine of AK-47 and a Kukhri. Diana freshened up the scent by sniffing the recovered objects and started moving with aggressive spirit towards a village named Tamenglong. Suddenly the undergrounds hiding in the village, started firing and throwing grenades at the search party indiscriminately. In the ensuing exchange of fire, two hardcore militant of National Socialist Council of Nagaland-Isak Muivah (NSCN-IM) were killed and one 12 bore double barrel gun, one Chinese rifle, one revolver and two grenades were recovered. For this act of devotion, bravery and excellent teamwork of the duo, Army Dog Diana was awarded **Chief of the Army Staff Commendation Card** in 2001.

31A8 Diwya

On 12th August, 2000, Diwya, an Explosive Detection Dog of 20 Army Dog Unit was deployed by her handler Dfr (ADT) BC Singh for a routine search. The Army Dog confirmed the presence of an IED hidden in a landslide covered with a heavy boulder of 30–40 kg. A week later on 19th August, 2000, the duo of Diwya and BC Singh confirmed the presence of an IED in a gas cylinder. The dog proved extremely useful to avert a major disaster. Again, on 2nd November, 2000, while on ROP duty Army Dog Diwya with handler Dfr (ADT) BC Singh was instrumental in detection of a powerful IED weighing about 4 kg. Similarly, On 1st July, 2000 at 0645 hours, while on Road Opening Patrol (ROP) duty, Army Dog Diwya and handler G Anandam confirmed the presence of one powerful IED. This remote-controlled device contained 20 kg of RDX explosive and was concealed in an aluminum container which has the potential of devastating explosion. The IED was later destroyed *in situ* and Diwya was successful in averting a major catastrophe which could have resulted into loss of many innocent lives and public property. The brave and efficient Army dog Diwya brought laurels to her unit and was awarded **GOC-in-C Northern Command Commendation Card**.

"Fantastic Track Record"

7A47 Drona

Drona, a Tracker Dog of 4 Army Dog Unit was deployed in militancy hit valley in March, 1994. His achievements not only in the field of his specialization but also as a "Rescue Dog" speak volumes of the unlimited potential this wonderful creature has. Drona was instrumental in apprehending more than 125 Anti National Elements (ANEs) in about forty cordon and search operations carried out by troops in different areas of South Kashmir. L/Dfr (ADT) SC Mishra and later ALD (ADT) Vijay Shankar formed an awesome team with Drona to assist the troops in their fight against militancy. Drona was put to an acid test on 18th January, 1995, when his handler L/Dfr (ADT) Dilip Nikam volunteered for an Avalanche Rescue Operation. It was near village Wujur, where in an unexpected avalanche, Rifleman Abdul Hamid was buried deep under snow. The dog was given the scent of the lost soldier's bedding by his handler. The duo searched the area with utmost dedication in adverse climatic conditions and finally pin pointed the spot where the body of Rifleman Abdul Hamid was burried under 10 feet of snow for the past two days. "A unique feat indeed," since Drona was not an Avalanche Rescue Operation (ARO) Dog but still completed the arduous task successfully. In recognition of timely initiative and exemplary performance of the handler along with Army Dog Drona, L/Dfr (ADT) Dilip Nikam was awarded **Chief of the Army Staff Commendation Card** in 2004.

8A95 Dusky

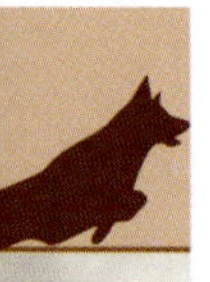

Army dog Dusky, a Tracker Dog of 2 Army Dog Unit and her handler Swr (ADT) Santhil Kumar M were deployed with 15 Kumaon Battalion in "OP MALHAR". On 16th November, 1993, a search operation was launched based on the intelligence input about undergrounds (UGs), a word then used for Anti-National Elements. Santhil and Dusky were leading the column so as to locate the exact location of the UGs. At about 1115 hours, suddenly the column came under intense fire. It seemed to be a fortified LMG position. As the duo moved little ahead, Santhil Kumar noticed an UGs camp and AK-47 fire coming from beyond the cover. While protecting his dog, Santhil charged the UGs camp and in the course, he was hit on his head by AK-47 burst killing him instantaneously. In the follow-up exchange of fire, all UGs were eliminated.

In recognition of his gallant act, exemplary courage beyond the call of his duty and bravery of highest order, Swr (ADT) Santhil Kumar M was awarded the prestigious **Sena Medal (Posthumously)** on 26th January, 1995.

252A Genny

It was 31st January, 2004 and the winter was at its peak in J&K. Genny, a Mine Detection Dog of 28 Army Dog Unit and ALD/ADT Anirudh Kumar with a team of 44 RR Battalion were out on routine Road Opening Patrol (ROP) duty on Balapur, Pulwama Road, since 0700 hours. At around 0835 hours, Genny indicated an Improvised Explosive Device (IED) near 42 km at Kigam on side of the road bend. However, any such device was not visible on the site. After initial search without success, the dog was again cast tactically in the vicinity of earlier indicated spot by handler ALD/ADT Anirudh Kumar. Once again Genny indicated the presence of IED by pawing action on a site which was covered with thick snow. On intensive search and finally digging the indicated spot carefully, a 5 kg gas cylinder was visible. Further examination revealed that it was filled with RDX to make it a remote-controlled IED. The device was very dangerous and considered unsafe to remove from the site. Accordingly, it was decided to blast the IED *in situ* by team of 44 RR Battalion. Surely, but for Genny's dedicated efforts and Anirudh's devotion to duty, such remote-controlled IED would have caused enormous damage to men and material. In recognition of the exemplary performance, Genny was awarded **Chief of the Army Staff Commendation Card** in 2005.

504A Hema

On 31st July, 2005, Army Dog Hema, a Mine Detection Dog of 19 Army Dog Unit along with handler L/Dfr (ADT) SP Singh were part of a special operation launched by 2/9 Gorkha Regiment. While sanitizing the area of responsibility, Hema detected a powerful IED weighing approximately 10 kg. The IED had a devastating potential and was subsequently deactivated, thus saving the valuable lives of many soldiers.

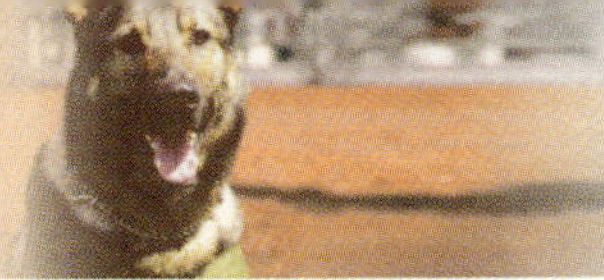

In recognition of the high standard of professionalism, courage and devotion to duty, Hema was awarded **Chief of the Army Staff Commendation Card** on 15th January, 2006.

322A Hirani

The successful Counterinsurgency Operations one after another at rapid pace in which Hirani, a Tracker Dog of 18 Army Dog Unit took part, justifies the name "English Deer" given to this dog. On 8th April, 2004, Army Dog Hirani and her handler ALD (ADT) YMK Rao while deployed with troops of 36 RR, 5 PARA and STF Battalions at Anantnag, assisted in a search operation. The dog and handler's duo successfully tracked the hideouts of suspected Anti-National Elements (ANEs) without caring for their safety. The subsequent exchange of fire resulted in killing of two militants and recovery of one AK-47 rifle, three magazines and 68 rounds of AK-47. On 14th July, 2005, Hirani with her new handler ALD (ADT) Vijay Fernandes was deployed with 9 RR Battalion to lay a cordon and search operation at village Sheikhgund. At 0400 hours contact was established with three terrorists who somehow managed to escape. Immediately the dog team was pressed into action and Fernandes gave scent of the footprints of escaped terrorists to Hirani and the duo followed the trail carefully and tactically. They tracked for about 2.5 km and sighted an orchard near a nullah. Hirani indicated the presence of terrorists with precision. Alert was given to the troops and in the follow-up action, three militants were killed at about 0800 hours. These militants were identified as Saqlain @ Lukman (HM) resident of Pak, Abdul Rashid resident of Naidpura and Md Yusuf Dar resident of Sopor (HM). Recovery of two AK-47 rifles, one SLR, one mobile, eight hand grenades, 8 AK-47 magazines and a lot of ammunition of AK-47 and SLR was made. Ten days later, on 24th July, 2005 the duo of Hirani and Fernandes were again part of 9 RR Battalion Search Operation. The Tracker Dog was instrumental in elimination of two militants and recovery of two AK-47 rifles, 8 hand grenades, two RC IED Box and 158 rounds of AK-47 ammunition. It is for the Army Dogs like Hirani that an English Daily has written **"Militants fear dogs more than soldiers."** In recognition of her excellent performance, courage and devotion to duty, Army Dog Hirani was awarded **GOC-in-C Northern Command Commendation Card**.

413A Hitesh

On 9th July, 2005, based on intelligence input on the presence of terrorist in a particular area, a Column was launched by F-Coy of 42 RR Battalion at Trail in J&K. It was dark night and after a small engagement with exchange of fire, the terrorist took the advantage of darkness and escaped from the scene. Army Dog Hitesh, an Explosive Detection Dog along with his handler Swr (ADT) Lakshmanudu Magapu of 13 Army Dog Unit was deployed to track the escaped Anti-National Elements. The dog handler while examining the area noticed blood spots on a site and he cast the tracker dog Hitesh on the blood trail. Hitesh picked up the scent from the site and started tracking with full zeal and enthusiasm. Despite the darkness all around, Hitesh and Magapu duo remained focused on their task with full determination. They tracked through difficult terrain passing through various fields. Finally, they lead the column to a group of small houses where the terrorists were holed in. Subsequently, a fierce encounter took place and in exchange of fire, the dreaded terrorists were eliminated. The valour, courage and professionalism of very high order as depicted by the Hitesh and

Lakshmanudu duo was aptly recognized by awarding Army Dog Hitesh with **GOC-in-C Northern Command Commendation Card** and the handler Swr (ADT) Lakshmanudu Magapu with **Chief of the Army Staff Commendation Card** in 2006.

B327 Holi

Holi, a Tracker Dog of 26 Army Dog Unit and handler ALD (ADT) Kadam Jairam Ramdas were deployed on 17th October, 2010 with 3 Madras. At about 1900 hours based on intelligence input about the presence of terrorists in general area Barzula (MT-5048), a search operation was launched and contact was established with the terrorists. In the exchange of fire one terrorist was killed whereas another terrorist was injured but managed to escape, taking advantage of darkness in the jungle and mountainous terrain. Holi and her handler Kadam were pressed into action at 0730 hours on 18th October, 2010 for tracking the injured terrorist who escaped previous night in unknown direction. The handler cast the dog for taking scent on the telltale signs in the area and the duo followed the trail vigorously. While tracking they passed through unknown areas including non-sanitized jungle terrain and they could see some built up areas having small houses. On careful searching in and around this area, Holi finally pointed towards a building which happened to be a religious pace, a mosque. Further, cordon and search of the mosque was undertaken by the troops and the injured terrorist was caught. In recognition of the excellent performance, indomitable courage, dedication and highest degree of professional skill, ALD (ADT) Kadam Jairam Ramdas was awarded **GOC-in-C Northern Command Commendation Card.**

11A1 Icker

On 26th July, 2001, during a search operation "OP CHAKRAZAQ KHAN," Icker, a Tracker Dog of 4 Army Dog Unit along with ALD/ADT Khem Karan Lal led the search party into a field where the militant was hiding. Heavy exchange of fire followed in which the militant, later identified as Tauheedul Islam of Karachi and belonging to Al-Badar group, was eliminated. The operation also led to recovery of 2 AK-47 rifles, 4 hand grenades and large quantity of ammunition. On 16th November, 2001, during a combined operation named "OP DAS BARAH," launched by HQ 10 Sector RR and HQ 12 Sector RR to apprehend three fleeing militants. Army Dog Icker and handler L/Dfr (ADT) Bhagwan Singh were deployed to track the militants. Some footprints were noticed in the area and Icker was cast on the scent of these foot marks. The track successfully led the search party into a house where three militants were hiding. On intensive search of the house, one militant was apprehended. However, other two militants managed to escape leaving behind a cap of one of the escaped militants. Icker was again cast on the scent of the cap and the duo of Icker and Bhagwan Singh swiftly followed the trail. The second militant was tracked successfully and caught. Subsequent interrogation of the two apprehended militants led to the capture of the third militant. This operation also resulted in recovery of huge quantity of arms and ammunition.

On 12th December, 2001 Icker along with handler ALD/ADT PK Singh was deployed in a search operation (OP PINYUR) to track down the militants who escaped the troops leaving behind weapons. The dog was cast on the scent of recovered weapons. The smart German Shepherd Icker, lead the search party to a village where the assailant was hiding. The dog identified the culprit whose name

was Ghulam Navi Vani, a serving police constable of J&K Police. He was apprehended and handed over to the police for further interrogation. Two AK-47 rifles, one 7.62 SLR and huge quantity of ammunition were recovered in this operation. It is true that when police catch a suspect it is no big deal, but when an Army Dog catch a police constable, it is big news! In recognition of the exemplary performance, Army Dog Icker was awarded **Chief of the Army Staff Commendation Card** in 2002.

502A Kimi

Army Dog Kimi, an Explosive Detection Dog of 16 Army Dog Unit and handler ALD (ADT) Manoj Kumar Singh were detailed on duty with 306 Medium Regiment on 2nd September, 2006 to detect explosives and IEDs in the area of responsibility. Kimi indicated eight IEDs tied to the 132 KVA Pylons of PGCIL near Jirivam Sribar railway track and avoided enormous loss of lives of troops and civilians passing through the area. Army Dog Kimi was awarded **Chief of the Army staff Commendation Card** on 15th August, 2007.

34A4 Lobo

In a bizarre incident during October, 1999, some terrorists ambushed Army's search party and took away their weapons. In the counteraction launched by the troops, Dfr (ADT) Raj Kumar and Army Dog Lobo, a Tracker Dog of 11 Army Dog Unit, were deployed with an Infantry Battalion to track down the terrorists. The dog registered the scent and following the trail relentlessly, led the search party in the correct direction and identified the hideout. Consequently, the stolen weapons were recovered and nine militants were killed. Similarly, in the night of 27/28th November, 1999, militants attacked the HQ of an Infantry Battalion with rockets. Next morning Lobo along with ALD (ADT) RL Patil was deployed to track the militants. Lobo picked up the scent from footprints and led the column to the site from where a large quantity of ammunition, rockets, command RPG ammunition and electronic device, left behind by terrorists were recovered.

Again on 18th June, 2000, Lobo and handler Dfr (ADT) SP Rana, deployed with an Infantry Column were tasked to track down terrorists in a forest area. After tracking 4 km, the dog led the team to a deep gorge, where they were fired upon by terrorists. Despite being in the range of fire, Dfr Rana and Lobo depicting exemplary courage and highest standard of professionalism, kept the terrorists engaged. This enabled cordon to get established. In subsequent gun fight three terrorists were killed. Just two days later, on 22nd June, 2000, Lobo was yet again deployed by Dfr (ADT) SP Rana and picked up the scent from footprints of a militant who had visited a village for carrying food. The duo led the search team to militant's hideout. In the exchange of fire that followed, three militants were killed. Subsequently, on 16th September, 2000, the team of Lobo and handler ALD (ADT) DN Nath was tasked to track down terrorists in a forest. The team led the search party to a location where terrorists were resting. In ensuing gun battle ten terrorists were killed. Once again, on 18th September, 2000, Lobo with ALD (ADT) DN Nath was tasked to track down terrorists from the scent of hand gloves recovered in a search operation. Lobo and Nath followed the trail for 4 km and led the column to the terrorists' hideout. In subsequent exchange of fire 13 terrorists were killed. In recognition of his exemplary performance, courage and dedication to assigned task, Army Dog Lobo was awarded **GOC-in-C Northern Command Commendation Card**.

163A Mahesh

Avalanche Rescue Operation (ARO) Dog Mahesh of 5 Army Dog Unit was deployed with High Altitude Warfare School (HAWS) for rescue operations. On 18th February, 2003, an avalanche struck the Taj Loading Point of 5 Bihar Battalion under 17 Infantry Brigade. The avalanche washed away the soldiers' living accommodation along with a lot of controlled stores. Ten personnel were reported missing including one civilian porter. The search and rescue operation could not commence till 23rd February, 2003 due to continuous heavy snowfall and avalanche warning. On 24th February, 2003, search and rescue operations commenced at about 0800 hours. Mahesh and handler No. 7240192W L/Dfr (ADT) SS Ranga were part of the HAWS team and were specially flown in from Gulmarg. The duo of Mahesh and his handler relentlessly searched in the icy cold wind and bone chilling temp for hours and pinpointed the buried mortal remains of two personnel who were washed away down the slope. One soldier and one civilian porter were rescued alive. The mortal remains of remaining six along with controlled stores were also recovered during the subsequent search operations. Working on six days old scent and indicating the exact site of buried persons, was a great achievement for Mahesh and Ranga.

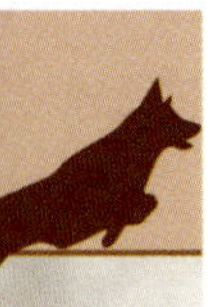

Army Dog Mahesh exhibited a very high standard of professionalism, determination to work relentlessly and devotion to duty in the face of adversities and was bestowed with **Chief of the Army Staff Commendation Card** in 2004.

31A2 Mala

On 1st March, 2002 Mala, a Mine Detection Dog of 3 Army Dog Unit and handler ALD (ADT) Amrendra Kumar were deployed on Road Opening Patrol (ROP) duty with 8 Assam Rifles. While moving on the Imphal Road, the party noticed freshly dug up suspicious area at village Nangda. Amrendra Kumar, a fearless dog handler, on being entrusted to sanitize the area employed Mala to sniff the area carefully. The dog indicated the presence of two IEDs. After pointing the exact location to the party Commander and sensing the danger, the dog team started moving away from the IEDs. The militants, who were probably watching the movements, triggered off the IED but the alert handler jumped off along with the dog to a safe distance, avoiding threat to their lives. For this act of bravery, dedication to duty and exemplary performance, Army Dog Mala was awarded **Chief of the Army Staff Commendation Card.**

Similarly, on 11th September, 2002, Mala now paired with handler L/Dfr (ADT) Mangal Swarup, while on ROP duties with 7 Mahar Battalion was deployed to sanitize an area on the Leimakhong to Pledinga route. When the duo reached near Khurkul (Senapati, Dist, Manipur), Mala gave accurate indication about the presence of Improvised Explosive Device (IED) which contained 7.5 kg of PEK explosive and detonator. The device was later destroyed *in situ* by the experts, thus avoiding heavy loss of lives and property. For this act of devotion, excellent teamwork and exemplary performance, Mala was once more awarded **Chief of the Army Staff Commendation Card.**

Yet again on 23rd February, 2003, when deployed on the road Koirengi-Seikmai, Mala, this time with handler L/Dfr (ADT) Bheem Yadav was assisting 71 Field Company of 55 Engineer Regiment for ROP duty. A power source and a remote control device were recovered from two slain militants. Additional intelligence input was suggestive of more explosives in the vicinity. On being entrusted to sanitize the area, Mala searched the area thoroughly and indicated the presence of main charge of the IED which was buried along with the electronic detonator, weighing 1.5 kg, in the middle of the road. The IED was later destroyed *in situ* by the Bomb Disposal Team. In recognition of her exemplary performance, dedicated services and devotion to duty, **Chief of the Army Staff Commendation Card** was awarded to Army Dog Mala for the **third time.**

Indeed a great hatrick and big salute to Mala's heroism

158A Mini

Mini, a black Labrador, an Explosive Detection Dog and her handler ALD (ADT) Devi Dayal of 20 Army Dog Unit were deployed on duty with 38 RR. On 13th march, 2009, based on intelligence input, a search and destroy operation was launched at 0600 hours at Haryana Ridge MY 2148/Belni forest. During the search, Mini was successful in detecting two (one cylindrical and one conical) metallic IEDs weighing about 1.5 kg each and containing 500 gm explosive each. In addition, the team also detected one NMM-14 land mine wrapped in a polythene and planted underground. These explosive devices had the potential to cause great harm to the troops, if remained undetected. Although, Mini does not carry a gun, nor does she speak but she has a nose unlike others in the battlefield and her heroics during a counter-terrorism operation saved many precious lives.

Mini's bravery and exemplary performance, for sniffing out two IEDs in the jungles of the Poonch district, Jammu and Kashmir, during a counterterrorism operation in 2009, resulted in award of **"Chief of the Army Staff's Commendation Card"** on Independence Day, 15th August, 2010.

32A5 Nandi

Nandi, a Tracker Dog of 5 Army Dog Unit was known to give her best in tracking the militants. On 30th August, 1999, 2/9 Gorkha Rifles Battalion killed three militants in the 'OP CHHATARNAR'. The remaining militants managed to escape in the forest. Due to bad weather and thick forest, the search party had no hope of tracking the fled militants. Next day, Nandi and ALD (ADT) Vijay Kumar Gaji of 5 Army Dog Unit were pressed into action. Nandi was given the scent of footprints of the fled militants and started tracking in the treacherous terrain in the forest. The dog along with her handler tracked about 5–6 km in the forest and led the party to a spot where militants were hiding. Suddenly the militants started firing towards the dog and handler. The handler ALD/ADT Vijay Kumar Gaji gave silent indication to the search party about the direction of fire and the hiding place of the militants. In the heavy exchange of fire, three militants were killed and a large quantity of arms and ammunitions were recovered. For this exceptionally commendable act, Army Dog Nandi was conferred with **Chief of the Army Staff Commendation Card** in 2000.

9A60 Nalani

It was the Independence Day, 15th August, 1997, Army Dog Nalani, a Mine Detection Dog, of 15 Army Dog Unit and handler ALD/ADT Shakil Ahmed were part of the Road Opening Patrol (ROP) party along with a platoon of the Engineers Regiment. At 0830 hours, an Infantry Battalion requested the services of a Mine Detection Dog for sniffing the suspected areas on the road falling in their Area Of Responsibility (AOR). The ibid team left for the suspected site on foot and simultaneously opening road stretch of 8 km. On reaching the suspected area, Shakil Ahmed along with Nalani started searching the area carefully, displaying perfect harmony and excellent man–animal relationship. Exploiting her full potential of sense of smell, the dog indicated first IED buried underground with no visible signs. Nalani indicated second IED at a distance of 7 feet from first IED and third IED was only 6 feet away from second. Subsequently, all the three IEDs were destroyed *in situ*. In recognition of the exemplary performances of the handler ALD/ADT Shakil Ahmed and Army Dog Nalani, they both were individually awarded **GOC-in-C Northern Command Commendation Card.**

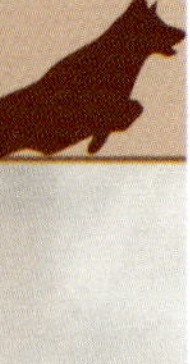

9A16 Neeta

On 31st July, 1996, some suspicious footmarks were observed by one of the patrol parties in their vicinity and it was decided to track down the suspected persons. Army Dog Neeta, a Tracker Dog of 13 Army Dog Unit along with her handler ALD (ADT) Diwan Singh was deployed for the purpose. Neeta was cast on the scent of footmarks and the duo of Diwan and Neeta followed the trail carefully leading the search party to a hideout where four militants were hiding. In the ensuing action militants were killed and a huge cache of arms and ammunitions were also recovered. In recognition of the gallant act and excellent performance ALD (ADT) Diwan Singh was awarded **Chief of the Army Staff Commendation Card** in 1996.

7A97 Neetu

While deployed on the Road Opening Patrol (ROP) duty on National Highway-1A, between Lethapur to Panthachowk, on 22nd August, 1995 at 0715 hours, Army Dog 7A97 Neetu, a Mine Detection Dog of 12 Army Dog Unit with handler L/Dfr ADT Akhilanand Rai confirmed the presence of two Improvised Explosive Devices (IEDs) weighing 2.5 kg at the BSF post at Panthachowk. These devices were encased in rectangular iron casing fitted with watch timer. The recovery saved the life of a whole section of BSF (1 JCO and 6 OR), deployed at that post. Earlier, on 11th August, 1995, Neetu and L/Dfr (ADT) Akhilanand Rai during the ROP duty recovered one IED at the sentry post of 93 Field Regiment. There were no "tell tale" marks of any IED and it would have gone unnoticed. Noticing the reaction of the dog, the handler L/Dfr Rai assessed the presence of an IED in the area. On thorough search the "IED" was found to be buried four feet deep and cleverly camouflaged. Subsequently, in September, 2000, a search operation was launched by an Infantry Battalion against the terrorists, who had fired at the search party and fled into the fields. Once again Neetu was pressed into action. She successfully tracked down a wounded terrorist and recovery of large catch of arms and ammunitions was made. In recognition of the exemplary performance, Army Dog Neetu was awarded **Chief of the Army Staff Commendation Card** in 2000.

7A82 Nimi

Nimi, a Tracker Dog of 2 Army Dog Unit and her handler Swr (ADT) Dev Narain were deployed with 12 Assam Rifles (AR) in "OP PRINDA". On 12th October, 1992, a search operation was launched based on the intelligence input about the activity of UGs in the area of responsibility. At about 2040 hours, the handler cast the dog on the trail and led the column to a village called Sains and indicated a house belonging to D Khel. Before the column could organize themselves, UGs started firing with automatic weapons. The column returned the fire effectively leading to killing of three UGs. During the exchange of fire, the dog handler Dev Narain was hit by a bullet and got wounded. Despite his injured state, the handler successfully deployed Nimi on trail which lead to the recovery of huge quantity of arms, ammunition and some cash. Swr (ADT) Dev Narain later succumbed to the bullet injury and died. His act of gallantry, highest standard of professionalism, courage and devotion to duty, earned him the coveted **Sena Medal (posthumously**).

16A7 Pinki

On 11th December, 1998, Pinki, a Mine Detection Dog of 18 Army Dog Unit, when deployed by her handler ALD (ADT) Anirudh Kumar on Road Opening Patrol (ROP) duty, detected one powerful IED planted on roadside near a village. The IED comprised four bottles of 750 ml capacity filled with approx 3 kg of explosives and was capable of a big catastrophe. Pinki and Anirudh duo, without caring for their personal safety recovered the IED. For this gallant act and exemplary performance, the handler ALD (ADT) Anirudh Kumar was awarded **GOC-in-C Northern Command Commendation Card.**

On 1st September, 2000, while operating with an Infantry Battalion, Army Dog Pinki and handler ALD (ADT) BN Mondal participated in a search operation. After initial contact with the search party, the Anti-National Elements (ANEs) escaped. Pinki was deployed by her handler to track the fleeing ANEs. She took the scent from the site and following the trail led the search team to a paddy field where terrorists were hiding. In the ensuing action two hard core terrorists were killed and a large cache of arms and ammunitions were recovered. Once again on 24th August, 2001, Pinki and ALD (ADT) Bansi Lal led the search team of an Infantry Battalion to the backyard of a house in the centre of a maize field from where a huge dump of arms and ammunitions buried was recovered. In recognition of her exemplary performance, courage and devotion to duty, Army Dog Pinki was awarded **Chief of the Army Staff Commendation Card** in 2002.

9A75 Racer

During May, 1994, a case of loss of pistol of one of the Post Commanders of an Infantry Battalion was reported. The Officer had handed over the pistol to his sahayak for depositing it in the kote. The sahayak kept the pistol in his bag and someone removed it from the bag when left unattended for some time. After about 20 days, the pistol was found hanging near unit lines. Dfr (ADT) C Chennapan along with Army Dog Racer, a Tracker Dog of 13 Army Dog Unit, were tasked to track down the miscreant. The dog was cast on the scent of fingerprints on the pistol and an identification parade of all the unit personnel was carried out. Normally the tracker dog follows the scent of one human being only, but in this rare case, it identified and indicated four individuals. All these four individuals later confessed that though one of them had removed the pistol from bag but all of them had handled it at one stage or the other. Dfr (ADT) C Chennapan displayed exceptional professional ability and devotion to his duty in training and deployment of Army dog Racer, as a result the mystery of the lost pistol was solved so appropriately. For this act of professionalism and utmost devotion to duty, No. 7238273 X Dfr (ADT) C Chennapan and Army dog No. 9A75 Racer were individually awarded **GOC-in-C Northern Command Commendation Card**.

Again on 7th August, 1994, Racer along with ALD (ADT) Hakim Singh Yadav was deployed with an Infantry Battalion to track down the militants. The dog was given scent from a haversack recovered after ambush of ANEs near a post in the Brigade Sector. ALD (ADT) Hakim Singh Yadav deployed the Army Dog and followed the scent in the most difficult terrain and led the search party to a hideout from where a huge catch of arms and ammunitions were recovered. On 15th September, 1994, the Infantry Battalion again recovered one haversack after laying ambush of ANEs near a post in the Brigade Sector. ALD (ADT) Hakim Singh Yadav deployed Racer in most appropriate way and tracked down the scent in a difficult and hilly terrain. This led to the recovery of two AK-47 rifles, two pistols, two grenades, four mines and 30 rounds of ammunition. ALD (ADT) Hakim Singh Yadav of 13 Army Dog Unit displayed exemplary courage and devotion to duty while deploying Army Dog Racer in the most hostile and inhospitable terrain. He was awarded **Chief of the Army Staff Commendation Card** in 1996.

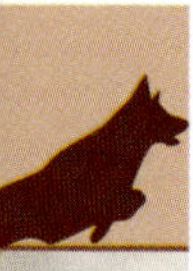

683A Rag

On 30th November, 2007, special operation was launched by the column of 10 JAK LI, in general area of their responsibility based on the intelligence input. Army Dog Rag, an Explosive Detection Dog of 3 Army Dog Unit and handler ALD (ADT) Naushad NP were deployed to assist in the operation. The motivated, alert and fearless duo of Naushad and Rag moved upfront the column. During the course, Army dog Rag indicated the presence of four IEDs at different locations, each weighing approximately 500 gm. The area was immediately cordoned off and all the four IEDs were destroyed at their respective location, thus saving many precious lives of troops and civilians. For the high standard of professionalism and devotion to duty, Army Dog Rag was awarded **Chief of the Army Staff Commendation Card** on 15th August, 2008.

09A9 Ram

Ram, a Tracker Dog of 16 Army Dog Unit was instrumental in many success stories during Counterinsurgency Operations (CI Ops). His first notable act was on 5th February, 1998, when deployed with 22 Assam Rifle Battalion, he helped in apprehension of three hard core ANEs of National Liberation Front of Tripura (NLFT) at Gatichandra Chars, who were later handed over to police at Manu, Tripura. On 11th February, 1998, the dog tracked the scent trail successfully to recover one 9 mm Carbine Machine, two country-made SBML rifles and ammunition. Once again on 18th March, 1998, Ram helped in apprehension of two NLFT hard cores with arms at Doganga, Tripura. For the remarkable canine efforts in the successful missions, Army Dog Ram was awarded **GOC-in-C Eastern Command Commendation Card** on 26th January, 1999.

Subsequently, on 16th July, 2002, Ram when deployed with 14 Jat Battalion was tasked to track down the Undergrounds (UGs) responsible for the ambush of the Army troops. The dog was given the smell from the ambush site and after tracking through dense forest busted the hideout of the culprits. The ensuing encounter resulted in recovery of dead bodies of two Anti-National Elements (ANEs), one grenade launcher, AK-56 ammunition and various other war stores. On 19th–20th February, 2003 again, Ram was deployed with 17 Punjab Battalion to track down the culprits responsible for laying ambush which occurred in their Area of Responsibility (AOR). The dog took the scent from the ambush site and after tracking through dense forest, the party led by Ram and his handler busted the hideout of Undergrounds responsible for the ambush. The encounter that followed resulted in recovery of one UMG and its ammunition, leftover by the fleeing culprits. In recognition of the exemplary performance, 09A9 Army Dog Ram was awarded **GOC-in-C Eastern Command Commendation Card** second time on 15th August, 2003.

09A7 Ramesh

On 13th August, 1995, ALD (ADT) Surender Singh and Ramesh, an Explosive Detection Dog of 15 Army Dog Unit, were detailed with the search party and tasked to locate the rocket site from where rockets have been fired on the location of an HQ Infantry Division on 12th August, 1995. After registering the scent, Ramesh and handler Surender tracked the trail successfully and located the site and further led the Army column to the point where the rockets were planted. Without caring for personal safety ALD (ADT) Surender Singh dismantled the battery connections of two live rockets and four other rockets tied to the tree trunk. Further, on 2nd September and again on 12th September, 1995, Surender and Ramesh foiled the devious attempts of ANEs by timely detection of IEDs. For the gallant act, courage and utmost dedication to the assigned task ALD (ADT) Surender Singh was awarded **Chief of the Army Staff Commendation Card** in 1996.

Yet again on 1st September, 1996, Dfr (ADT) RN Singh and Tracker Dog Ramesh formed a part of the Road Opening Patrol (ROP) along with an Infantry Battalion troop and IED team of Engineers Regiment. While searching in detail, RN Singh and Ramesh duo detected an IED concealed in a fruit stall near the local bus stand. On subsequent interrogation it was revealed that the IED was planted with intention to cause panic amongst local people on the eve of visit of the Election Commissioner of India to that place. In recognition of the act of bravery and outstanding performance, ALD (ADT) RN Singh was awarded **GOC-in-C Northern Command Commendation Card** in 1996.

15AO RAMMAR

On 6th August, 1997, Rammar, a Tracker dog of 8 Army Dog Unit, was deployed with Maratha Light Infantry Battalion (Double First) along with his handler ALD (ADT) Ved Prakash to assist in search operations. The team covered a distance of approx 10 km at night, for the cordon and search operation being conducted by the Double First. After the cordon was established by first light on 7th August, the search commenced and the trail led to one abandoned hut on the fringes of the village. The hut seemed to have been abandoned in a hurry leaving behind some clothing items and bedding. Soon the extremists who were hiding in the vicinity started firing on the search party. In the ensuing fierce encounter, 8 hard core militants including two self-styled group commanders were killed. Despite being tired after the long march and firing taking place between the Army and the militants of National Democratic Front of Bodoland (NDFB) at various places in the village, Rammar was again deployed to search the remaining hideouts if any. To the surprise of all, Ved Prakash and Rammar duo recovered one sack containing a ready to use Improvised Explosive Device, and also found some very important documents of the NDFB and one M-20 magazine and ammunition. For the above commendable act and exemplary performance, Army Dog Rammar was awarded **GOC-in C Eastern Command Commendation Card** and the handler ALD (ADT) Ved Prakash was awarded **Chief of the Army Staff Commendation Card.**

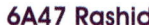

6A47 Rashid

On 17th January, 1993, Dfr/ADT Sanjeevi and Rashid, a Tracker Dog of of 11 Army Dog Unit were deployed to search militants in a given area. Their dedicated efforts led to apprehension of a militant leader. On 5th April, 1993, during a sanitizing operation, the duo were again instrumental in the recovery of a grenade and a pistol from the site where the Governor was to visit in a village. On 27th April, 1993, this duo proved their mettle and facilitated apprehension of two suspected militants after tracking down a distance of 5 km. Similarly, on 5th May, 1993 in an intensive search operation Rashid and Sanjeevi helped in the recovery of 4 LMGs magazines and 100 rounds of ammunition.

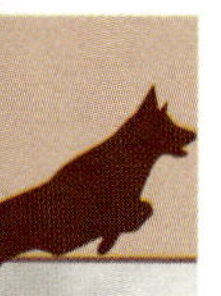

On 1st October, 1999, Military Hospital reported theft of medicines costing approximately ₹ 2 lacs. Dfr/ADT Bhupendra Prakash and Army Dog Rashid were tasked to track down the culprits who were involved in the theft. Registered with the scent from fingerprints and footprints, the dog was tasked to screen all the suspected 25 staff members who were lined up for the purpose. After thorough screening of each individual, Rashid was able to identify two staff members who admitted their guilt. **GOC-in-C Northern Command Commendation Card** was awarded to Army Dog Rashid for this excellent performance. On 8th February, 1995, ALD/ADT Mangal Swaroop along with Rashid was deployed to find out the culprits involved in three consecutive blasts, which took place at an Infantry Battalion (Inf Bn) location. No visible source of scent material was seen. However, ALD/ADT Mangal Swaroop noticed faint marks at the blast site and the dog was given the scent from these marks. While searching the area Rashid sustained fracture in left hind leg. However, the handler lifted the dog and followed the trail. Finally the search operation was concluded successfully and led to the recovery of a blanket used by the militant, which gave valuable information regarding the extremist and resulted in his subsequent apprehension. For this exemplary performance and dedication to duty, ALD (ADT) Mangal Swaroop was awarded **GOC-in-C Northern Command Commendation Card.**

24A6 Ravi

On 25th October, 1999, specific information was received that an IED has been placed in the local market through which army convoy passes. During a search operation by the troops, a sand bag was noticed on a heap of stones and when the sand bag was pushed aside with the help of a bamboo, a polythene bag was seen which led to the suspicion of an explosive device. Immediately, an Explosive Detection dog Ravi, of 18 Army Dog Unit, along with his handler L/Dfr (ADT) SR Baba Singh was pressed into action. Ravi and Baba Singh swiftly and carefully examined the area while approaching the suspected device. The dog sniffed the subject article and confirmed it to be an Improvised Explosive Device (IED). Thus a major mishap was averted on an important convoy route. To recognize the outstanding performance of the brave Army Dog Ravi and equally brave handler L/Dfr (ADT) SR Baba Singh, they both were individually awarded **GOC-in-C Northern Command Commendation Card.**

9A92 Rex

Rex, a golden Labrador, Tracker Dog of 14 Army Dog Unit under Delta Force was deployed in the areas adjoining the town of Bhaderwah, to help troops in trailing and tracking militants. On 24th May, 1995, operating with troops of 25 RR in jungles of Badrot, South of Bhaderwah, he tracked a militant injured in an encounter who had escaped leaving his slippers behind. Rex took sent from the slippers and followed the trail for over 3 km in the thick of militant fire. In a chase that lasted for over four hours, the militant was apprehended along with one AK-56 rifles and a haversack containing 92 rounds. On 18th–19th April, 1998, while on a patrol, in area Gulgandhar, along with his handler ALD (ADT) Satish Kumar, and employed to track an injured militant who escaped after the security forces killed two dreaded militants and badly injured one. Picking up the scent of his blood, 'Rex' went hot on the trail and moved speedily and stealthily over strenuous undulating mountains. After tracking over 2 km, he succeeded in tracing out the body of the militant in a hideout where he had succumbed to his injuries. On 4th May, 1998, Rex and Satish Kumar were deployed to locate the bodies of two militants killed in exchange of fire at the height of 11,500 feet. The team successfully traced the bodies of two militants buried under snow and also a hideout with blankets, dry ration and cooking utensils. On yet another trail with the QRT of CO 25 RR in Daraba near Rajouri, Rex suffered an unfortunate fall and sustained serious intestinal injuries. He was evacuated to the nearest Army Veterinary Hospital where he finally succumbed to his injuries on 22nd September, 1999. Rex was awarded **"GOC-in-C Northern Command Commendation Card"** for his outstanding and exemplary performance.

7A31 Ricky

On 2nd December, 1992, Ricky, a Tracker Dog of 4 Army Dog Unit, along with handler L/Dfr (ADT) JD Thakur, was deployed with an Infantry Battalion in cordon and search operation of a village. The dog was cast on the available scent to track down the suspected militants. Ricky and Thakur duo were successful in leading the party to a hard core militant, who was killed in the encounter and recovery of large quantity of arms and ammunition.

On 26th August, 1995, while carrying out search operation at village Mongehal, in Northern Theatre some abandoned 'pherans' and shoes were located nuar a nullah. Ricky and his handler L/Dfr (ADT) Sukh Dev Ghosh were pressed into service. The dog showed extreme swiftness and coupled with the handler's tremendous skill, the duo quickly led the party to a paddy field where three militants were hiding. On closing in, one militant started firing on the search team and shot dead the dog Ricky. L/Dfr Ghosh showed exceptional courage and presence of mind and bravely returned fire, shooting the militant dead. The other two militants were also killed in the ensuing gunfight with the search party. L/Dfr Sukh Dev Ghosh showed professional skill of very high order, exemplary courage, determination and devotion to duty. In recognition of this unique act of gallantry L/Dfr Sukh Dev Ghosh was awarded the prestigious **SENA MEDAL** on 26th January, 1996.

Long live Ricky!

07A5 Rimpi

An Improvised Explosive Device (IED) blast was reported near a Mobile Field Veterinary Hospital (MFVH) on 15th May, 1997. ALD (ADT) Des Raj, along with Army Dog Rimpi of 11 Army Dog Unit was tasked to track down the militants involved in the blast. There was no article which could provide scent to the dog. However, some footprints were observed by her handler Des Raj. Rimpi picked up

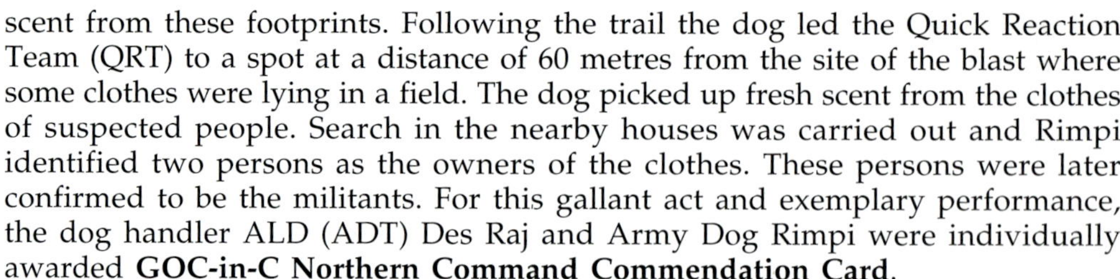

scent from these footprints. Following the trail the dog led the Quick Reaction Team (QRT) to a spot at a distance of 60 metres from the site of the blast where some clothes were lying in a field. The dog picked up fresh scent from the clothes of suspected people. Search in the nearby houses was carried out and Rimpi identified two persons as the owners of the clothes. These persons were later confirmed to be the militants. For this gallant act and exemplary performance, the dog handler ALD (ADT) Des Raj and Army Dog Rimpi were individually awarded **GOC-in-C Northern Command Commendation Card**.

7A49 Robert

On 2nd August, 1996, Robert, a Tracker Dog of 11 Army Dog unit along with handler ALD (ADT) BG Gopal was deployed after an Improvised Explosive Device (IED) blast in the area of an Infantry Brigade (Inf Bde). The dog took scent from the site and searched the area meticulously leading to the apprehension of the culprits involved in the blast. The great effort and the result-oriented approach of Robert and Gopal was appreciated by one and all. Later, Army dog Robert paired with Dfr (ADT) PR Bhai Ganesh Bhai was deployed with an Infantry Battalion (Inf Bn) for a search operation. On 4th October, 1997 at 1630 hours the duo were tasked to track down three militants, who ran out of a house during combing operations. After tracking down for a distance of 2.5 km, some items belonging to one of the militants were recovered. After giving scent from these recovered objects, the dog led the team to a house, where the militants were hiding. For this commendable performance both Drf (ADT) PR Bhai and Robert were awarded **GOC-in-C Northern Command Commendation Card**.

Once again on 11th March, 1999, after receiving specific information of a militant hiding in a village, a cordon was laid around. By then the militant managed to escape leaving behind his blanket. Dfr (ADT) Ramanuj Choubey along with Army dog Robert was tasked to track down the militant. Robert, after having obtained the militant's scent from the blanket moved fast on the trail. In spite of difficult terrain, adverse climate and enemy threat, Robert led the search party to the militant hideout and after exchange of heavy fire, the dreaded militant was killed. For this exemplary performance and devotion to duty, Army Dog Robert and Dfr (ADT) Ramanuj Choubey were individually awarded **GOC-in-C Northern Command Commendation Card.**

12A3 Rocket

Rocket, a Tracker Dog of 16 Army Dog Unit has done proud to his name by tracking militants like a rocket. On 8th February, 2000, the dog along with his handler deployed with 95 Field Regiment in "OP-NISHANA" and tasked to track the fleeing militants and their hideout. The dog and handler followed the trail with great speed and after covering a long distance quickly, the duo achieved success in their untiring efforts. The outcome was rewarding, leading to killing of one militant and apprehension of another along with recovery of two weapons. Similarly, on 5th March, 2000, Rocket when deployed in "OP-TANDEV", to search a wanted militant completed the trail quickly and successfully. In the follow-up encounter, the culprit was killed and one pistol, one AK-47 rifle and Chinese hand grenades were recovered. On 11th October, 2000 while deployed with 17 Para Battalion, Rocket played an important role in apprehension of extremist leader named Sher Ali Barbhuyia with weapon and ammunition during a search operation at Tarapore Power Plant on NH-53. Again on 12th October, 2000, Rocket was instrumental in apprehension of another extremist leader named Ishaq Ali Miya with weapon and ammunition during a search operation at Naga Punji on NH-53.

On 20th February, 2001, Army dog Rocket, during a specific search operation identified escape route of culprits, who had killed two women at Silchar town. Further careful tracking lead to the arrest of one of the culprits in presence of many people and the culprit confessed his crime. For the invaluable services and exemplary performance, Army Dog Rocket was awarded **Chief of the Army Staff Commendation Card** in the year 2001.

9A66 Roshan

On 16th August, 1994, Roshan, a Tracker Dog of 13 Army Dog Unit along with his handler ALD (ADT) Jitendra Pradhan was deployed with an Infantry Battalion for selective search operations. In the process the Army dog and his handler followed the defined trail and led the search party to an Anti-National Element (ANE) who on further interrogation disclosed a hideout of large cache of arms and ammunition. On 20th July, 1996, Roshan along with handler L/Dfr (ADT) MP Das was deployed with an Infantry Battalion. Suddenly an encounter took place with militants but they managed to flee. Das and Roshan were pressed into action and registering the scent effectively, the duo followed the trail of fleeing militants relentlessly and led the search party to the hideout of the militants successfully. In the ensuing firing one militant was killed and one AK-47 rifle was recovered.

For the exemplary performance leading to success of mission, L/Dfr (ADT) MP Das was awarded **GOC-in-C Northern Command Commendation Card.**

Once again, Army dog Roshan and handler ALD (ADT) Satyabrata Samal were deployed with an Infantry Battalion. On 28th October, 1997, Roshan and Satyabrata were pressed into action to track the militants from their last known location. Accordingly, the dog was cast on the scent and the duo followed the trail skillfully till Roshan indicated the presence of militants in Rishipur area. In the ensuing action by search party one hard core militant was killed and large cache of arms and ammunition was recovered. In recognition of the outstanding performance ALD (ADT) Satyabrata Samal was awarded **GOC-in-C Northern Command Commendation Card.**

02A2 Rudali

On 1st April, 1999, during a road clearance operation a freshly dug patch of earth was observed, while sanitizing the area. Army Dog Rudali, an Explosive Detection Dog of 14 Army Dog Unit with ALD (ADT) Raj Kumar were pressed into action. Within no time, the dog detected an Improvised Explosive Device (IED) weighing approx 3.5 kg buried under the ground. Timely detection of this IED saved many lives as well as military equipments and hardware. On 11th October, 2000, Rudali and handler L/Dfr (ADT) Lekh Raj were deployed for Road Opening Patrol (ROP) duty with Armourd Regiment. Thorough search made by Rudali and Lekh Raj led to detection of an IED placed on 'retaining wall' about four and half feet from the road. The IED was half dug inside the ground and covered by grass. Such device if explodes leads to a large number of casualties and heavy loss of equipment. The Army's bomb disposal team later destroyed the IED *in situ*. For displaying exemplary performance and devotion to duty, Rudali was awarded **GOC-in-C Northern Command Commendation Card.**

O77A Sabu

On 13th August, 2005, Sabu, an Explosive Detection Dog of 27 Army Dog Unit and the handler ALD (ADT) Raj Kumar were deployed to sanitize a specific area along with 59 RR Battalion (Assam). Based on intelligence input, obtained in an intercept of terrorist communication between call sign 313 (HUJI) and 47 (Zulkami Huji), it was suspected that a powerful IED has been planted in this area. The handler employed the dog Sabu and the duo screened carefully and minutely all over the defined area, using their professional skill, courage and at times ignoring their own safety. Finally, the dog pointed out the location of IED and true to Sabu's verdict, an IED weighing approximately 4.5 kg was found inside a steel vessel which has the potential of causing severe damage to lives and property. In recognition of the outstanding performance, courage and devotion to duty, ALD (ADT) Raj Kumar and the brave dog Sabu were individually awarded **GOC-in-C Northern Command Commendation Card**.

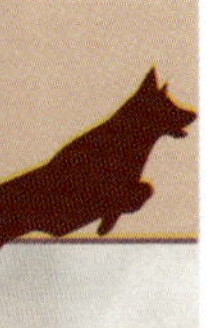

A858 Shekhar

During January, 1983, a BSF Jawan was trapped in an avalanche. Army Dog Shekhar, an Avalanche Rescue Operation Dog of 5 Army Dog Unit, along with ALD (ADT) Shiv Dhari Yadav was deployed to trace the victim. The duo without caring for their own safety and bearing the bone chilling cold, successfully traced the body of BSF Jawan. In recognition of exemplary courage and devotion to duty, ALD (ADT) Shiv Dhari Yadav was awarded the **Chief of the Army Staff Commendation Card** in 1985.

On 21st December, 1983, one officer and one NCO of an Infantry Battalion along with one civil porter were trapped in an avalanche. ARO Dogs Shekhar and Ashok with their handlers ALD (ADT) Nahar Singh and ALD (ADT) Kadar Singh respectively were pressed into action. The handlers deployed their dogs in the most difficult terrain. During the course of their deployment both handlers along with their dogs were also swept away by a subsequent avalanche. They, however, had a providential escape and managed to come out of the snow alive along with their dogs. In spite of the injuries and shock, they continued their task undaunted and were successful in tracing all the bodies by 25th December, 1983. For this gallantry act, courage and dedication to duty, ALD (ADT) Nahar Singh was awarded **Chief of the Army Staff Commendation Card** in 1984 and ALD (ADT) Kadar Singh was awarded **GOC-in-C Northern Command Commendation Card**.

O69A Shilpi

Shilpi, a Mine Detection Dog of 27 Army Dog Unit and her handler ALD (ADT) Ravinder Kumar were deployed in "OP AATISH." On 11th August, 2007, outbreak of a major fire was reported at 21 Field Ammunition Depot (FAD) Kundroo and thorough search of the area visually as well as by metal detector failed to detect any unexploded explosive in and around the Depot. At this stage, Shilpi and Ravinder were tasked to detect leftover unexploded explosive material in the area. Ravinder familiarized Shilpi with the kind of explosives she was required to detect so as to register the proper scent. Thereafter, the duo started searching the vicinity and especially the thickly forested area of FAD. The team of Ravinder and Shilpi undertook intensive search and without caring for their own safety, toiled day and night to accomplish the assigned task. The dog and the handler displaying high standards of physical endurance, professional skill and mental robustness were successful in detecting 12 Shells, 55 fuses and 6 Cargo bomblets with a tally of 73 recoveries from the area declared free earlier by visual search and using metal detector. For the exceptional courage and dedication to duty, ALD (ADT) Ravinder and Shilpi were individually awarded **GOC-in-C Northern Command Commendation Card**.

032A Sultan and 009A Chelesey

As part of confidence building measures between India and Pakistan, Government of India decided to start bus service between Srinagar and Muzaffarabad. This bus service was opposed by many militant outfits. Troops were given the responsibility to sanitize the National Highway-1A (NH-1A). Army Dog Sultan, a Mine Detection Dog and his handler Dfr (ADT) Kedar Pradhan of 26 Army Dog Unit were deployed with 29 RR Bn for this mission. On 5th April, 2005 while sanitizing NH-1A in general area Palhalan before commencement of first ever Srinagar–Muzaffarabad bus service, an IED comprising 25 kg gun powder, plastic can containing 40–50 litre of liquid explosive, metal shrapnels, two detonators and one Remote-Controlled Improvised Explosive Device (RCIED) were detected. The brave and timely act by Sultan, contributed significantly in defeating the evil designs of militants opposed to the bus service. The '**Peace Bus**' crossed the **Aman Setu** as scheduled. Again on 21st April, 2005, before commencement of second Srinagar–Muzaffarabad bus service, an attempt was made by militants to interrupt the process by placing an IED. This time the credit to foil the nefarious design went to Army dog Chelesey who along with her handler ALD (ADT) Kavinder Kumar was deployed with 2 RR Battalion for sanitizing NH-1A at Chainabal. The duo of Chelesey and Kavinder detected the powerful IED well in time, thus saving precious human lives and the peace process too.

A820 Sundri

The prestigious Gallantry Award "Shaura Chakra" was earned for the first time in the history of Remount Veterinary Corps by an Army Dog Trainer in the year 1977. L/Dfr (ADT) Gurbachan Singh was bestowed this honour, while deployed with Army Dog Sundri, for his outstanding performance, conspicuous gallantry and comradeship of highest order. The citation reads:

"Lance Dafadar (ADT) Gurbachan Singh with his dog formed part of a team to track culprits who had cut underground cables of Army Headquarters Receiver Station. In the dark night, though got detached from the team, Sundri led her master to the culprit hide out who attacked him. Single handedly he grappled with him and subdued him in spite of being wounded on his head. In this action Lance Dafadar Gurbachan Singh along with his dog displayed professional skill of a very high order, exemplary courage, determination and devotion to duty". In recognition of the unique act of gallantry and dedication to duty, L/Dfr (ADT) Gurbachan Singh was awarded the prestigious **Shaura Chakra.**

"A big round of applause for Gurbachan and Sundri"

378A Sundari

On 28th July, 2005, Army dog Sundari, an Explosive Detection (ED) Dog of 19 Army Dog Unit was deployed along with handler to assist 115 Engineers Regiment at Rangiya Railway Station in Assam. The sanitizing operation, conducted carefully and minutely, lead to the detection of four bags containing 30–35 kg of narcotic material. It was a unique feat and a severe dent to the smuggling of such products by undesirable elements. In recognition of professionalism of very high order and devotion to duty, Army Dog Sundari was awarded **Chief of the Army Staff Commendation Card** on 15th August, 2006.

371A Sushil

Sushil, an Explosive Detection Dog of 16 Army Dog Unit and the handler ALD (ADT) SK Tiwari were deployed with 12 Grenadiers. On 26th October, 2004 while on duty to detect explosives and IEDs in area of responsibility, the duo detected one powerful IED, thus saving many lives of troops. In recognition of the high order of professionalism and devotion to duty, Army Dog Sushil was awarded **Chief of the Army Staff Commendation Card** on 15th January, 2006.

4A46 Tango

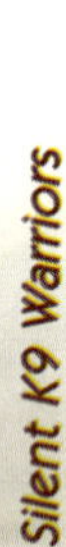

L/Dfr (ADT) SB Naik and Tango, a Tracker Dog of 4 Army Dog Unit were deployed with an Infantry Battalion for counterinsurgency operations. On 13th August, 1993, the team was tasked to track down the infiltrators who escaped the troops. On being cast on the scent from leftover belongings, Tango and Naik tracked relentlessly on difficult trail in high altitude area for 8 hours and finally reached a place where twenty-two heavily armed infiltrators were hiding. In the ensuing firing between the Anti-National Elements and Army troops all the 22 infiltrators were killed.

In recognition of the conspicuous bravery and professionalism of very high order, No. 7238661F L/Dfr (ADT) SB Naik was awarded **Chief of the Army Staff Commendation Card** in 1994.

38A3 Uma

Uma, a Tracker Dog of 5 Army Dog Unit and handler ALD (ADT) AK Dehury were deployed in a specific search operation based on intelligence input about the activity of some militants in the area of responsibility on 15th August, 1998. The duo of Uma and Dehury, disregarding their personal safety, led the column successfully to the hide out of militants. In the follow-up exchange of fire, two militants were killed. For the courage and professional skill of very high order as depicted by the dog and the handler team, ALD (ADT) AK Dehury was awarded **GOC-in-C Northern Command Commendation Card** and Uma was bestowed with **Chief of the Army Staff Commendation Card** in 2000.

On 19th June, 2001, Uma and handler Dfr (ADT) Ram Das Arjun Gawde were part of search team of 5 Mahar. On specific information, the team conducted a cordon and search operation in the village Lacshipura and in a fierce encounter six militants were killed. Further, with an aim to search remaining militants and their arms/ammunitions, Uma was given scent of the 'hand gloves' of a killed militant and the duo of Gawde and Uma started tracking on the treacherous terrain in thick forest. They tracked about a kilometre in the jungle and down the hill to a spot from where a large cache of arms, ammunitions and equipment was recovered. Uma along with Dfr (ADT) Gawde displayed professionalism and unfailing determination leading to success of the operation named "OP MAHESH". For this commendable act, Dfr (ADT) RA Gawde was awarded **Chief of the Army Staff Commendation Card** in 2002.

ARMY DOGS IN MINE FIELD SANITIZATION

95A8 Dimpy and 76AO Binky

From being sentinel for Napoleon troops to Mine Sniffing in Vietnam, the progress has been remarkable. Many a times, more accurate than many metal detectors, Mine Detection Dogs have been successfully employed in "UN Demining Operations" in Equador, Namibia, Cambodia, Mozambique and Bosnia. Accordingly, importance and utility of these dogs is rapidly increasing, thereby keeping a pace with humanitarian demining efforts. In India, the exceptional olfactory capabilities of Mine Detection (MD) dogs were put to utmost use in the largest mine recovery operation during the year 2003 in "OP PARAKRAM". The highly specialized and trained Dogs were used to sanitize the mine fields so as to ensure that all the mines have been detected and recovered by the mine/explosive detectors used for the purpose. The dogs and their handlers/trainers were deployed in forward areas under Western Command and they proved their mettle by detecting a large number of missing mines which were left undetected by other means. The tally of various types of mines recovered were NMM-14 Anti-Personal (139), NDMK-1 Anti-Tank (26) and one NDMIK-III (Anti-Tank).

This speaks volumes about the efficacy of dogs and also proves their superiority over other methods of mine detection. If such large number of mines would have remained undetected after the operations are over than we can well imagine the likely devastating effects to life and property of local population habiting in and around those areas. Local farmers and others civilian population imposed great faith and confidence in the capabilities of these silent warriors and they willingly took over their fields declared safe by the Army Dogs. The key players in this notable feat were Mine Detection Dogs Dimpy, Binky, Borg, Balbir, Charu and Ravi along with their handlers who performed the most arduous task with courage and determination.

In recognition of the courageous, gutsy and daredevil act during Demining Operation, ALD (ADT) SK Mondal and bravest of the brave Army dogs Dimpy and Binky of 2 Army Dog Unit, each were awarded **Chief of the Army Staff Commendation Card** in 2003.

48A6 Raina

Raina, a Mine Detection Dog of 13 Army Dog Unit, fresh from training, was deployed for the first time with an Infantry Battalion to clear vintage mine field on 22nd July, 1999 along with handler Dfr (ADT) V Venugopal. The dog was successful in detecting two NMM-14 mines and two grenades. The effort was appreciated by one and all. It was during the period 28th July to 10th August, 1999, when the specialized training of the Raina in mine detection was put to real test. ALD (ADT) V Manohar and Raina were deployed with an Infantry Brigade for specific mine clearing operations being conducted by different units. The duo were pressed into action to sanitize vintage mine fields. Manohar deployed young

Raina diligently, applied his professional skills in an exemplary manner and successfully detected and recovered two Non-Metallic Mines (NMM-14). Subsequently, the brave duo cleared the suspected mine field and created safe tracks. Later, between 1st August and 4th August, 1999, Raina and his handler Manohar were deployed for detecting mines and clearing new tracks for reinforcement. Notwithstanding the tall grass, heavy rains and unmindful of his personal safety, the handler and the dog team exhibited extraordinary zeal, dedication and successfully recovered seven NMM-14 mines from one location and additional seven NMM-14 mines from another location. Again in a similar task on 10th August, 1999, the duo recovered mines from vintage mine fields and cleared new safe tracks for reinforcement, thus enhancing the confidence level of the moving troops. The detection of more than twenty mines by Mine Detection Dog Raina and his handler Manohar depicts their bravery and professionalism of very high order. In recognition of the commendable performance ALD (ADT) V Manohar was awarded **GOC-in-C Northern Command Commendation Card.**

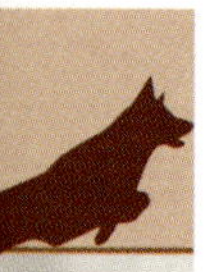

11

Dogs in Disaster Management

A dog is the only thing on earth that loves you more than you love yourself.

... Josh Billings

Animal Rescue Squads have been operating since long in disaster affected areas, either as a result of enemy action or due to natural calamities. During the Second World War, Beauty, a wire-haired Terrier who led one of the PDSA's Animal Rescue Squads with a defined role of searching pet animals that had become trapped with their owners in the rubble following bombing raids in London. She was considered as a pioneer dog for this kind of work and she rescued 63 animals in her wartime service. In recognition of her exemplary services, she received "Dickin Medal" in 1945. Similarly, Jet of Iada aka Jet (21st July, 1942–18th October, 1949) was an Alsatian (German Shepherd), who assisted in the rescue of 150 people trapped under blitzed buildings. He was a pedigree dog, and served with the Civil Defence Services of London. He was awarded both the "Dickin Medal" and the "RSPCA's Medallion of Valor" for his rescue efforts. Jet was born in Liverpool in the Iada kennel of Mrs Babcock Cleaver in July, 1942. He was a black Alsatian, and in the kennel was initially called Jett, with his full pedigree name being Jet of Iada. He was loaned to be trained at the War Dogs School in Gloucester from the age of nine months, where he was trained in antisabotage work. Following eighteen months work on airfields performing antisabotage duties, he was returned to the school for further training in search and rescue duties where he was partnered with Corporal Wardle. They were relocated to London where Jet was known for calling out every night until the end of the air attacks. Corporal Wardle and Jet were the first handler and dog team to be used in an official capacity in Civil Defence rescue duties. He was awarded the "Dickin Medal" on 12th January, 1945 for saving the lives of over fifty people trapped in bombed buildings.

The citation reads: "For being responsible for the rescue of persons trapped under blitzed buildings while serving with the Civil Defence Services of London."

Following the war, he was returned to his owner in Liverpool. On 15th August, 1947, an explosion occurred in the William Pit near Whitehaven, Cumbria. Dogs trained in body recovery work were unavailable, so two dogs were sent from the RAF Police Dog School at Staverton, and Jet was collected from his owner for this assignment. After Jet's efforts helped to save the rescuers he was awarded the "RSPCA's Medallion of Valour".

There is a memorial of Jet in the English flower garden of Calderstones Park, Liverpool, where he is buried.

Some more dogs who became famous while employed in disaster relief operations in recent past are described below:

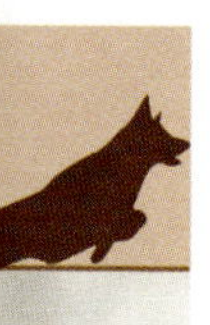

ATTACK ON WORLD TRADE CENTRE SITE IN THE USA

The 11th September attack, also referred to as 9/11, were a series of four coordinated terrorist attacks launched by the Islamic terrorist group Al-Qaeda upon the United States in New York City and the Washington DC metropolitan area on Tuesday, 11th September, 2001. The attack killed almost 3,000 people and caused at least $10 billion in property and infrastructure damage.

Four passenger airliners were hijacked by 19 Al-Qaeda terrorists so they could be flown into buildings in suicide attacks. Two of those planes, American Airlines Flight 11 and United Airlines Flight 175, were crashed into the North and South towers respectively, of the World Trade Centre complex in New York City. Within two hours, both towers collapsed with debris and the resulting fires causing partial or complete collapse of all other buildings in the WTC complex, as well as significant damage to ten other large surrounding structures. A third plane, American Airlines Flight 77, was crashed into the Pentagon (the Headquarters of the United States Department of Defense), leading to a partial collapse in its western side. The fourth plane, United Airlines Flight 93, was targeted at Washington DC, but crashed into a field near Shanksville, Pennsylvania, after its passengers tried to overcome the hijackers. In total, almost 3,000 people died in the attacks, including the 227 civilians and 19 hijackers aboard the four planes. It was the deadliest incident for firefighters and for law enforcement officers in the history of the United States, with 343 and 72 killed respectively.

Suspicion quickly fell on Al-Qaeda. Although the group's leader, Osama Bin Laden, initially denied any involvement but, in 2004, he claimed responsibility for the attacks. Al-Qaeda and Bin Laden cited the US support of Israel, the presence of the US troops in Saudi Arabia, and sanctions against Iraq as motives for the attacks. The United States responded to the attacks by launching the War on Terror and invading Afghanistan to depose the Taliban, which had harboured Al-Qaeda. Many countries strengthened their anti-terrorism legislation and expanded law enforcement powers. Having evaded capture for years, Bin Laden was located and killed by the US Forces in Pakistan in May, 2011.

The destruction of the Twin Towers and other properties caused serious damage to the economy of Lower Manhattan and had a significant effect on global markets, closing Wall Street until 17th September. The civilian airspace in the US and Canada was also closed until 13th September. Many closings, evacuations, and cancellations followed the attack, either out of fear of further attacks or respect for the tragedy. Cleanup of the World Trade Centre site was completed in May, 2002, and the Pentagon was repaired within a year. Numerous memorials have been constructed, including the National September 11 Memorial & Museum in New York, the Pentagon Memorial, and the Flight 93 National Memorial in Pennsylvania.

On November 18th, 2006, construction of one World Trade Centre began at the World Trade Centre site. During the chaos of the 9/11 attacks, nearly 100 loyal Search and Rescue Dogs and their brave owners scoured Ground Zero for survivors. The dogs worked tirelessly to search for anyone trapped alive in the rubble, along with countless emergency service workers and members of the public. Subsequently, more than 300 specially trained Search and Rescue Dogs were deployed at Ground Zero in the days following the 9/11 terrorist attack. They helped in finding survivors in the rubble and later, found trinkets like jewelry that could be returned to victims' families.

One lucky survival was Miss Genelle Guzman-McMillan who was working in her office in the World Trade Centre on that day. She heard a terrible noise outside and as she raced down the stairs, she felt the building collapsing around her. Twenty-seven hours later, she was the final living person rescued from the rubble at Ground Zero. She was not found by a human equipped with special gear, instead, her saviour was a dog.

Still more canines served as Therapy Dogs, helping survivors and first responders to cope up with their emotional trauma. Even though the dogs could not find people still alive, they could provide comfort for the brave firemen and rescue workers of the emergency services. Veterinarian Dr Cynthia Otto, incharge of healthcare for the 9/11 Search and Rescue Dogs, also worked round the clock with other staff to treat dogs who got injured from stepping on debris and also by inhaling smoke.

Appollo, Roselle and Salty

Appollo, a German Shepherd born around 1992, was Search and Rescue Dog of the K9 unit of New York Police Department. In 1994, he graduated from the NYPD Canine Special Operations Division, and was one of the first dogs to learn search and rescue. Appollo passed Type-II training in Florida in 1997, and Type-I in Indianapolis in 1999. He was also part of the first NYPD K9 team for Urban Search and Rescue New York Task Force 1. Appollo and his handler, Peter Davis were called in to assist with the rescue operations after the 11th September terror attack. They arrived at the World Trade Centre site fifteen minutes after the attack, making Appollo the first search and rescue dog to arrive at the site after the collapse of the World Trade Centre. At one point, Appollo was almost killed by flames and falling debris. However, he survived, having been drenched after falling into a pool of water. He started working again as soon as Davis had brushed the debris off him.

Appollo received the "American Kennel Club Ace award" in 2001. He was also honoured for his work at the Westminster Kennel Club Dog Show of 2002, in which he and several other dogs from the New York Police Department's K9 Unit participated.

On 5th March, 2002, Britain honoured America's canine heroes with the PDSA "Dickin Medal" for gallantry. Appollo and his handler, police officer Peter Davis, received the Dickin Medal, equivalent of the Victoria Cross for animals, on behalf of all the search and rescue dogs who participated in the rescue operations at the World Trade Centre site and worked 'the pile' at Ground Zero and through the debris at the Pentagon. Dog and handler representatives from the Port Authority K9 Unit, Task Force 1, Suffolk County Canine Unit, Connecticut State Police K9 Team, FEMA (Federal Emergency Management Agency) were present to receive copies of the PDSA Dickin Medal citation and certificate to take back to their units. Volunteer Search and Rescue teams were represented by Hal Wilson and his German Shepherd "Tsunami" who worked at Ground Zero in those first critical hours after the World Trade Centre towers collapsed. He received the award along with guide dogs Roselle and Salty, who rescued their owners from the World Trade Centre. Guide dog "Salty", owned by Port Authority employee, Omar Rivera, and Guide dog "Roselle" owned by Michael Hingson were also awarded PDSA "Dickin Medal" in recognition of their devotion to duty as they led their owners safely down more than 70 floors of the World Trade Centre and remained devoted to their duty to ensure the safety of their owners. A representative of Guide Dogs for the Blind (California) received the coveted medal on their behalf.

The citation for the award was as follows:

"For tireless courage in the service of humanity during the search and rescue operations in New York and Washington on and after 11th September, 2001. Faithful to words of command and undaunted by the task, the dogs' work and unstinting devotion to duty stand as a testament to those lost or injured".

On presenting the Medals PDSA, Chairman Roy Trustram Eve DL said: "The People of Britain were appalled by the events of 11th September, 2001 and still share in your grief". As a charity devoted to the care of animals, PDSA could not ignore the courageous work undertaken at that time by the many man and dog partnerships. The PDSA Dickin Medal is the highest honour Britain can bestow on any animal in a time of conflict or in the face of danger. In American terms it is the animal equivalent of the Congressional Medal of Honour. The Medals presented at a special ceremony at the Rescue Workers Memorial at Ground Zero, New York on 5th March, were the first PDSA Dickin Medals to be awarded outside the activities of World War II and its aftermath.

Jake

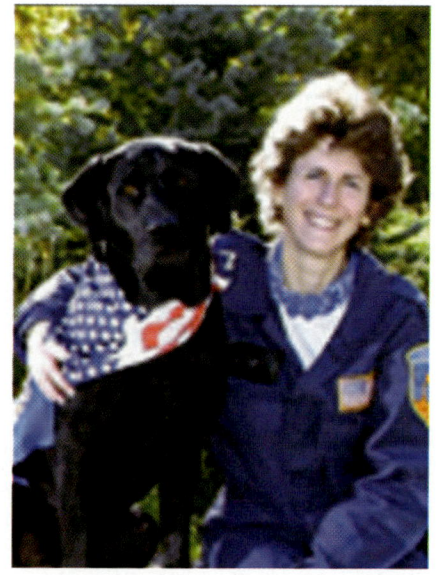

Jake a well-known American black Labrador who served as a Search and Rescue Dog following the September 11 attack and Hurricane Katrina. Jake served as a rescue dog from 1997 until his retirement because of cancer in 2006. Jake was adopted when he was 10 months old by his owner, Mary Flood in 1995, when found abandoned on the streets with several injuries, including a dislocated hip and a broken leg. Jake's owner, Mary Flood, is a member of Utah Task Force 1, a federal search and rescue team, trained to respond to disasters.

Following recovery from injuries, Flood helped to train Jake to become a federal "the US government certified Rescue Dog". There are fewer than 200 of these dogs, who are trained to respond within 24 hours to disasters such as hurricanes, earthquakes, wilderness, water rescue, terrorist attacks, or avalanches. Jake's owner later commented, "Against all odds he became a world-class rescue dog". Jake was most noted for his work following the September 11 attack, where he helped to search for human remains at Ground Zero. Jake, like other rescue workers and dogs, was honoured by New Yorkers as a hero. Jake, wearing his search and rescue vest, was treated to a free steak dinner at an upscale Manhattan restaurant on the evening he arrived to work in New York City. Jake served as a Rescue Dog at the World Trade Centre site for 17 days. Like the humans and other rescue dogs Jake was exposed to the physical hazards of Ground Zero, including sharp debris and suspected unhealthy air.

Jake also served in search and rescue team following Hurricane Katrina in 2005. Jake along with Utah Task Force, drove over 30 hours from Utah to Mississippi to help search for survivors and victims of following the hurricane's landfall. Jake also worked as a Therapy Dog at Utah nursing homes and at a camp for burn victims. He was also deployed to the Gulf Coast in the aftermath of Hurricane Rita.

In his later years, Jake helped to train younger prospective rescue dogs, as well as their handlers. He helped other dogs to learn to track scents in difficult places and terrain, including under the snow and even the trees. Later, Jake was diagnosed with hemangiosarcoma, a blood-borne cancer. He was euthanized on Wednesday, 25th July, 2007, after he was found on his front lawn shaking with high fever. His owner reportedly took him for one last walk through the fields and creeks of Oakley, Utah, before his death at the age of 12 years.

1993 BOMBING IN MUMBAI, INDIA

The 1993, a series of 13 bomb explosions took place in the then Bombay (now Mumbai), Maharashtra, India on Friday, 12th March, 1993. The coordinated attacks were the most destructive bomb explosions in Indian history. The single-day attacks resulted in over 350 fatalities and 1,200 injuries. The attacks were supposedly coordinated by Dawood Ibrahim, don of the Mumbai-based international organized crime syndicate named D-Company. He is believed to have ordered and helped to organize the bombings in Mumbai, through one of his subordinates, Tiger Memon. The bombings are also believed to have been financially assisted by the expatriate Indian smugglers, Hajji Ahmed, Hajji Umar and Taufiq Jaliawala, as well as the Pakistani smugglers, Aslam Bhatti and Dawood Jatt. In the blasts several of the terrorists were recruited from Dubai, UAE and received arms, ammunition and explosives training across the border.

The Supreme Court of India gave its judgement on 21st March, 2013 after over 20 years of judicial proceedings and sentenced the accused. However, the two main suspects in the case, Dawood Ibrahim and Tiger Memon, have not yet been arrested or tried.

One famous dog of Mumbai police, Zanjeer, who also contributed significantly through his sharp senses during this period is described below:

ZANJEER

A Labrador Retriever, served as a detection dog with the Mumbai Police. Zanjeer was trained at the Dog Training Centre of the Criminal Investigation Department at Shivaji Nagar in Pune, India. He joined the Mumbai Police Bomb Detection and Disposal Squad on 29th December, 1992 and was handled by Ganesh Andale and VG Rajput. Zanjeer helped to recover 11 military bombs, 57 country-made bombs, 175 petrol bombs, and 600 detonators. A few months before the 1993 Mumbai bombings, Zanjeer helped to avert at least three more attacks in Mumbai, Mumbra, and Thane. The first incident happened on 15th March, 1993 when Zanjeer alerted his handlers to a scooter bomb on Dhanji Street that contained RDX explosives and gelatin sticks. He was then called to the scene of ten unclaimed suitcases outside the Siddhivinayak Temple where the dog detected three AK-56 rifles, five 9 mm pistols, and 200 grenades marked "Arges 69". Days later, Zanjeer investigated two suitcases at the Zaveri Bazaar that contained nine AK-56 rifles. Further, during the bombing attacks on 12th March, 1993, Zanjeer's contribution was very significant in detection of arms and ammunitions used in serial explosions.

Subsequently, Zanjeer developed swellings in the lungs and paws and died on 16th November, 2000. In recognition of his impeccable service and particularly for detecting explosives and weapons during the 1993 Mumbai bombings, Zanjeer was honoured with a full state funeral.

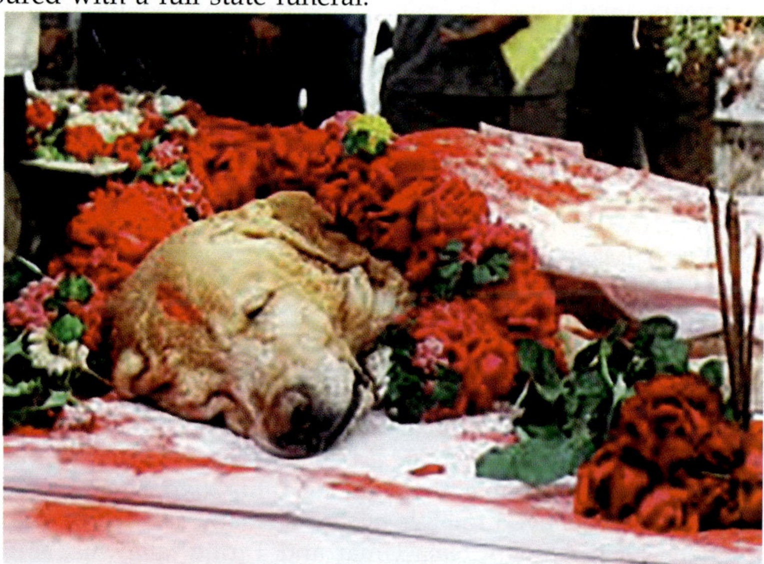

Goodbye Zanjeer

TSUNAMI IN INDIA

060A Bawa, 061A Badi and 5029A Brinda

On 26th December, 2004, Tsunami hit the Andaman and Nicobar group of Islands in India, just minutes after the coastline of Sumatra. After the strike of Tsunami, there was severe fear and chaos not only in the Islands but all over the country. The Tri Services Andaman and Nicobar Command reacted swiftly and declared "OP MADAD" which is one of the biggest peacetime operations undertaken by the Armed forces. Command Headquarters requisitioned for the services of specialized dogs to aid the relief work. Accordingly, three specially trained "Search and Rescue Operation Dogs," 060A Bawa, 061A Badi, 5029A Brinda along with handlers Dfr (ADT) PK Chatri, Dfr (ADT) K Padmanabhan and Dfr (ADT) BJ Chaudhary were immediately sent by RVC Centre and College and they reached Nicobar Island on 31st December, 2004, more than 400 km away from Port Blair. This was the Island where 37 Wing, Air Force Base was damaged extensively and suffered tremendous losses of men and material. The dog teams were placed under the Command of 108 Mountain Brigade (Mtn Bde), the Amphibious Brigade of the Army and the dogs were sheltered in a small portion of Air Force Hanger. Each dog team was assigned to a group of relief workers, which apart from the army personnel also included civilians from different fire brigades of the country. The main task of the group was to search and remove the human bodies from the debris and dispose them *in situ*. More than 450 bodies were recovered from Car-Nicobar alone and the Army dogs and their handlers did put in exceptional efforts in assisting the rescue teams. Army dog teams were also utilized to screen the affected areas from where the relief workers have retrieved the human bodies to the best of their skill. The sharp senses of dogs could again pinpoint the exact location of at least thirteen additional human bodies from the sites which could not be detected earlier by rescue teams. The dog teams also helped the relief workers in retrieving and disposing.

The dog teams took part in relief operations at 37 Wing Air Force Base, Kakana, Mallacca, Lastic, Mus and Chuchukjha. The rescue teams along with Army dog team were required to walk four to five kilometres to reach the site. The main hurdle was, however, the non-availability of drinking water which was grossly insufficient to cater for the individuals and the dogs that were required to perform duty for extended hours. In most of the villages, the ground had become slushy due to the sea water and there were fallen trees, bushes, collapsed buildings and overturned vehicles all over. To negotiate the way, the dogs were often lifted physically and carried across by their handlers. At many places, dogs were put to work on leash as the harness rope used to get entangled in debris. However, the hurdles were overcome by the team efforts and the mission was a grand success. The Army dogs were able to detect many human bodies buried deep under the heaps of rubble and debris.

The relentless working of Search and Rescue dog teams generated immense confidence amongst the rescue teams and rehabilitation workers and their dedicated efforts under such adverse working conditions were lauded by one and all. The search operations were practically completed on 8th January, 2005. **Chief of The Army Staff Commendation Card** was awarded to Dfr (ADT) K Padmanabhan on 15th August, 2005 for the exemplary performance during **'OP MADAD'**.

EARTHQUAKE IN INDIA

068A7 Reeta

On 15th October, 2005, Tracker Dog 68A7 Reeta of 5 Army Dog Unit and Swr (ADT) Chander Shekhar Yadav were deployed for search and rescue operations under OPERATION-IMDAD in earthquake hit area at Goalta near Uri in J&K. The duo depicted great courage, fierce determination and successfully detected mortal remains of two civilians buried deep under rubble. However, after completion of this task, another aftershock tremor hit the region and heavy landslide started. The dog and handler duo while trying to protect them from being washed off under landslide came partially under it and got seriously injured. Notwithstanding their injuries, the duo again started search and rescue operations with indomitable courage, devotion and commitment. Their search covered wide area affected by landslide in highly difficult terrain and they were successful in recovering the mortal remains of another five civilians. For this act of bravery, courage and exemplary sense of devotion to duty displayed by Reeta and Chander Shekhar, the handler Swr (ADT) Chander Shekhar Yadav was awarded **Chief of The Army Staff Commendation Card** on 26th January, 2006.

CLOUD BURST IN LEH, INDIA

B171 Chamkila, B495 Blondy, B437 Hosky and B225 Prince

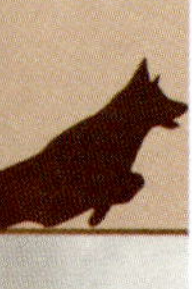

Subsequent to a cloud burst in Leh, J&K, India, in August, 2010 in 102 Brigade Sector located in high altitude area, four teams of Army dogs and their handlers were deployed for search and rescue operations. Army dog B171 Chamkila with handler ALD (ADT) Dharmendra Prasad Yadav and Army dog B495 Blondy with handler ALD (ADT) Satya Rao Kilaparthi of 17 Army Dog Unit were inducted on 6th August, 2010 followed by Army dog B437 Hosky with handler L/Dfr (ADT) Patil Bajirao Yuvaraj of 26 Army dog unit and Army dog B225 Prince with handler Dfr (ADT) Raj Kumar of 17 Army Dog Unit on 10th August, 2010.

Army dogs and their handlers were airlifted from their unit locations to Tyakshi (SSW) Battalion location where many troops and civilians were reported missing/ buried in the rubble of damaged buildings after the severe cloud burst in that area. There were remote chances of survival of buried people. The handlers deployed their dogs very cautiously and with highest degree of professionalism for search of live/mortal remains of individuals buried deep in the heaps of mud, rubble and boulders. The duo of all the teams made untiring efforts displaying exceptional presence of mind, perseverance and utmost dedication to given task in testing circumstances of high altitude area. Search and rescue efforts were continued for 16 to 18 hours every day notwithstanding the severe weather conditions. The untiring efforts and excellent professionalism of the deployed teams led to successful recovery of mortal remains of three JCOs, 39 Other Ranks and 7 Civilians which were buried 10 to 20 feet deep in rubble. Indeed a great feat. In recognition of the excellent work, devotion to duty and professionalism of very high order by the duo of the Army dog teams, ALD (ADT) Dharmendra Prasad Yadav and ALD (ADT) Satya Rao Kilaparthi, both of 17 Army Dog Unit were individually awarded **GOC-in-C Northern Command Commendation Card** on 15th January, 2012. L/Dfr (ADT) Bajirao Yuvaraj Patil of 26 Army Dog Unit and Dfr (ADT) Raj Kumar of 17 Army Dog Unit were individually awarded **Chief of The Army Staff Commendation Card** on 26th January, 2012. Further, Army dog B225 Prince, a Labrador, trained as Avalanche Rescue Operation Dog of 17 Army Dog Unit, who depicted extraordinary efficiency, endurance and excellent ground scent work indicating exact spots leading to recovery of mortal remains of 6 soldiers buried under and up to 20 feet of slush, debris and boulders at Tyakshi was honoured with **Chief of The Army Staff Commendation Card** on 26th January, 2012.

12

Dogs in the UN Peacekeeping Missions

"It's not the size of the dog in the fight;
It's the size of the fight in the dog."

... Mark Twain

The United Nations peacekeeping mission is one of the most effective tools presently available to assist host countries in their difficult path from conflict to peace. It has unique strengths, including legitimacy, burden sharing, and an ability to deploy and sustain troops and police from around the globe, integrating them with civilian peacekeepers to advance multidimensional mandates. The UN Peacekeepers provide security and the political and peace building support to help countries make the early transition from conflict to peace. Multidimensional peacekeeping operations are also to facilitate the political process, protect civilians, assist in the disarmament, demobilization and reintegration of former combatants, support the organization of elections, protect and promote human rights and assist in restoring the rule of law. The UN peacekeeping is guided by three basic principles, consent of the parties, impartiality and no use of force except in self-defence and defence of the mandate.

Peacekeeping is flexible and over the past two decades has been practiced in many configurations. As on today, 17 UN Peacekeeping Operations are ongoing in four continents and one special political mission, the United Nations Assistance Mission in Afghanistan (UNAMA), led by the Department of Peacekeeping Operations.

The UN peacekeepers, soldiers and military officers, civilian police officers and civilian personnel from many countries, monitor and observe peace processes that emerge in post-conflict situations and assist ex-combatants in implementing the peace agreements they have signed. Such assistance comes in many forms, including confidence-building measures, power-sharing arrangements, electoral support, strengthening the rule of law, and economic and social developments. All operations must include the resolution of conflicts through the use of force to be considered valid under the charter of the United Nations which gives the Security Council the power and responsibility to take collective action to maintain international peace and security. For this reason, the international community usually looks to the Security Council to authorize peacekeeping operations. Most of these operations are established and implemented by the United Nations itself with troops serving under the UN Operational Command. In other cases, where the direct UN involvement is not considered appropriate or feasible, the Council authorizes regional organizations such as the North Atlantic Treaty Organization, the Economic Community the West African States or coalitions of willing countries to implement certain peacekeeping or peace enforcement functions.

Armies of various countries, including India, take part in various UN peace missions, deploy their Military Working Dogs in their peacekeeping efforts. These dog contingents play their significant role in enhancing the Battalion's operational efficiency. Battalion Dog Unit, as they are commonly called, generally form an integral part of the troops in the United Nations peacekeeping force. The Army Dog teams in the UN Missions usually consist of War Dogs which are trained to carry out specific tasks in support of the troops. The dogs give advance warning of ambushes and help in maintaining security of areas/installations of vital military significance. They are also tasked to detect and confirm the presence of explosives/ mines, Improvised Explosive Devices (IEDs), suspicious objects, plastic explosives, etc. and thereby render invaluable assistance in confirming known/unknown explosives in marked/unmarked areas leading to confidence building in their own troops as well as civilians in the vicinity. Various duties being entrusted to Army Dogs in these missions are as follows:

Patrolling: An Infantry Patrol (IP) Dog is trained to indicate the presence of any group or individual in a patrolled area, thus preventing any danger of ambush to own troops. Further, while ensuring security of own area, it is important that no infiltration of armed elements takes place inside the Blue Line within Infantry Battalion area of operations. Patrol dogs, by leading the foot patrols, heighten the confidence of troops to detect any infiltration in adverse weather conditions, poor visibility and during night. The dogs adds to the security measures and act as deterrent to infiltrators by their presence.

Explosive Search: Explosive Sniffer Dogs are extremely useful in detecting and confirming presence of explosives, IEDs, human bombs, human-carrying explosives, hidden weapons and for road clearance duties. The Sniffer Dogs in these missions were gainfully tasked for sanitization of vehicles, helipads and other areas, buildings, aircrafts and baggage.

Guarding: When troops are committed for various tasks round the clock, there is a need to guard the camps and various UN installations. Guard/Attack dogs are extremely efficient in guarding premises and are a vital deterrence at night. These dogs also give early alert to their own troops about likely intruders up to a distance of 250–300 yards.

Riot control: Whenever there is a situation involving a civilian unruly crowd, which gets out of control and the UN help is sought, the task of peacekeepers become challenging. During such testing time, deployment of trained dogs acts as a deterrent and greatly helps in pacifying and dispersing the crowd.

In addition to the Military Working Dogs being deployed by the UN peacekeeping forces, the UN Mission Headquarters deploy dogs as security and safety measure. Recently dogs have been deployed in Sudan (UNMISS), for the protection of civilian sites and also at the main gates both at the UN house and Tomping compound to search and indicate if people are bringing in weapons or explosives or other contraband. The dogs may also be flown to other areas like Bentiu and Malakal when needed since the dogs are good visual deterrent. On 12th February 2014, eight Sniffer Dogs arrived from the UN Mission in Afghanistan (UNAMA) to help with random searches in and around the UN Bases and some displacement camps in strife-torn South Sudan. Most of these dogs are Labradors and Cocker Spaniels originally from South Africa. These dogs had undergone specialized training for three months before their deployment. They were stationed at main gates of the UNMISS and protect sites in the capital, Juba alongside the UN Department of Security and Safety and the UN Police to carry out daily searches.

The UN Mine Action Service (UNMAS) demonstrated the work of Sniffer Dogs in the Protection of Civilians (POC) camp at the Tomping site of the UN Mission in South Sudan, in Juba and also used to screen internally displaced people (IDPs) arriving at the entrance gate, as well as to conduct random searches throughout the camp. The dogs successfully detected unexploded cluster bomblets along the Juba-Bor Road in Malek and proved their mettle.

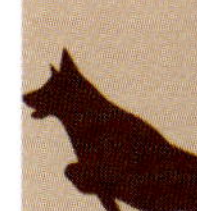

Such dog teams might have been deployed in the UN missions in other countries also as on required basis.

13

New Horizons

"No animal I know of can consistently be more of a friend and companion than a dog."

... Stanley Leinwoll

The use of dogs in new fields is being continuously explored. In some of these new fields, dogs have already demonstrated their potential which in times to come may be widely utilized for betterment of mankind. A few of these fields are mentioned below:

POLYCARBONATE DETECTION

Polycarbonates are the chemicals which are used in the DVDs manufacturing process and detection of this chemical by the sharp smelling power of dog has opened a new avenue for training and employment of dogs so as to check illegal smuggling of CDs and DVDs. Two dogs trained in this job have already proven their mettle and the details are as under:

Lucky and FLO

They are a pair of black Labrador Retrievers notable for being the first animals trained to detect optical discs by scent. It took around nine months to train these dogs to detect polycarbonates, chemicals used in the disc manufacturing process. Although the dogs cannot tell the difference between the real and pirated disc, they can detect if DVDs are hidden among shipments signed off as a consignment of something else. They are sponsored by the Motion Picture Association of America (MPAA) and Federation Against Copyright Theft (FACT) as part of an initiative to combat copyright infringement of film DVDs. The dogs' abilities were first demonstrated in May, 2006 at the FedEx shipping hub at London Stansted Airport. Inspectors found all the discs the dogs detected that day to be legitimate. Another successful demonstration was held at the MPAA's Washington DC office on 26th September, 2006.

In March, 2007, the two dogs were sent to Malaysia to sniff out DVDs and on 13th March, 2007, Malaysia's Domestic Trade and Consumer Affair Ministry used

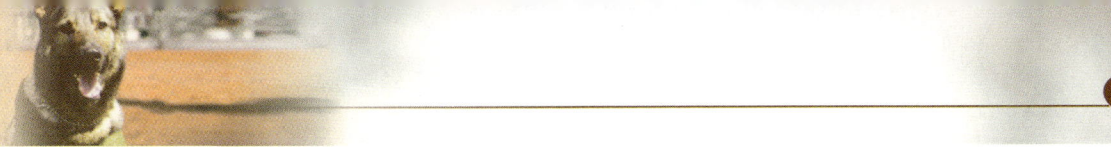

these two sniffer dogs, to detect huge stashes of pirated pornographic DVDs hidden among more than 50 boxes scattered around the cargo complex at the country's biggest international airport Sepang, Kuala Lumpur.

After a raid on a pirated DVD ring in Johor Bahru on 20th March, 2007, it came to light that the dogs were now targeted by the DVD pirates and that a bounty had been put on their heads. Notwithstanding this fear, the twin black Labrador counterfeit detection dogs were successful in sniffing out nearly 2 million pirated counterfeit DVDs on a six-month secondment to Malaysia in 2007. Following the multimillion dollar detection, they became the first dogs to be awarded Malaysia's "Outstanding Service Award."

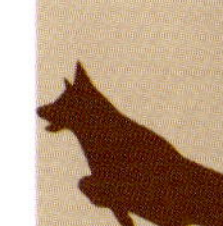

In March, 2008, the MPAA along with children's magazine the Weekly Reader, released a curriculum for grades 5 to 7, featuring Lucky and Flo to be distributed to nearly 60,000 classrooms in 20,000 schools across the 10 US states and designed to "educate children about the importance of respecting copyrights while presenting it in a fun and exciting way." MPAA chairman and CEO Dan Glickman lavished praise on the canines, saying that the dogs "are some of the smartest employees we have here at the MPAA".

THERAPY DOGS

A Therapy dog is trained to provide affection and comfort to people in hospitals, retirement homes, nursing homes, hospices, disaster areas and to people with hearing difficulties. It is believed that interaction with therapy dogs can temporarily affect the release of various neurotransmitters in the brain, levels of oxytocin which is linked with bonding and levels of dopamine, involved in the reward-motivation system are increased, while levels of cortisol, an immunosuppressant associated with stress are decreased.

During World War II, Smoky worked as a Therapy Dog when Wynne was hospitalized for a jungle disease. As Wynne recovered, his friends brought Smoky to the hospital to cheer the soldier up. Smoky immediately became popular with the other wounded soldiers. The Commanding Officer, Dr Charles Mayo of the Mayo Clinic, allowed Smoky to go on ward rounds and also to sleep with Wynne on his hospital bed. Smoky's use as a Therapy Dog continued for 12 years, during and after World War II.

The systematic use of therapy dogs is attributed to Elaine Smith, who worked as a registered nurse. Smith noticed how well patients responded to visits by a chaplain and his Golden Retriever. In 1976, Smith started a programme for training dogs to visit institutions. Other healthcare professionals noticed the therapeutic effect of animal companionship such as relieving stress, lowering blood pressure, and raising mood. As such, the demand for therapy dogs continued to grow. In recent years, therapy dogs have been enlisted to help children overcome speech and emotional disorders.

In 1982, Nancy Stanley founded Tender Loving Zoo (TLZ), a non-profit organization that introduced animal therapy to severely disabled children and convalescent hospitals for the elderly. She got the idea while working at the Los Angeles Zoo, where she noticed how disabled visitors responded eagerly to animals. She researched the beneficial effects that animals can have on patients and then

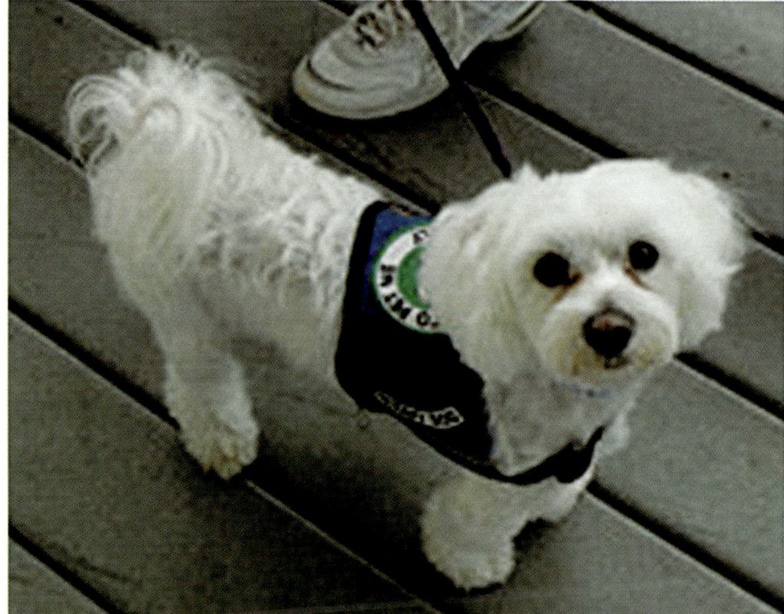

A Therapy Dog

began taking her pet miniature poodle, Freeway, to the Revere Developmental Center for the severely disabled. Inspired by the response of the patients and the encouragement of the staff, she bought a van, recruited helpers and persuaded a pet store to lend baby animals. Soon requests for TLZ visits were coming from schools, hospitals and convalescent homes throughout the country.

There are three different types of therapy dogs:

Therapeutic Visitation Dogs

These dogs are household pets whose owners take time to visit hospitals, nursing homes, detention facilities, and rehabilitation facilities. Visitation dogs help people who have to be away from home due to mental or physical illness or court order. These people miss their pets, and a visit from a visitation dog can brighten the day, lift spirits, and help to motivate them in their therapy or treatment with the goal of going home to see their own pets.

Animal Assisted Therapy Dog

These dogs assist physical and occupational therapists in meeting goals important to a person's recovery. Tasks that a dog can help achieve include gaining motion in limbs, fine motor control, or regaining pet care skills for caring for pets at home. Animal Assisted Therapy dogs usually work in rehabilitation facilities.

Facility Therapy Dog

These dogs primarily work in nursing homes and are often trained to help keep patients with Alzheimer's disease or other mental illness from getting into trouble. They are handled by a trained member of the staff and live at the facility.

Therapy Dogs must be well-tempered, should not shed excessively, should be well-socialized (exposed to many environments) and love to cheer up others. These dogs must be certified as the certification provides liability insurance and temperament testing for all certified dogs. Many organizations provide evaluation and registration for therapy dogs. In the United States, some organizations require that a dog pass the equivalent of the American Kennel Club's Canine Good Citizen test and then add further requirements specific to the environments in which the dogs will be working. Other organizations have their own testing requirements. Typical tests might ensure that a dog can handle sudden loud or strange noises, can walk on assorted unfamiliar surfaces comfortably, not frightened by people with canes, wheelchairs, or unusual styles of walking or moving, get along well with children and with the elderly, and so on.

THERAPY DOGS IN IRAQ AND AFGHANISTAN

Iraq

Therapy Dogs were inducted into Iraq which took the dogs to the next level on the battlefield. In June, 2010, two black Labrador Retrievers, Budge and Boe, were deployed to Iraq to help relieve combat stress of soldiers in the field. They provide emotional comfort through physical interactions such as playing fetch or simple petting.

Afghanistan

Therapy Dogs were used in Afghanistan to provide emotional support and to relieve the combat stress of soldiers.

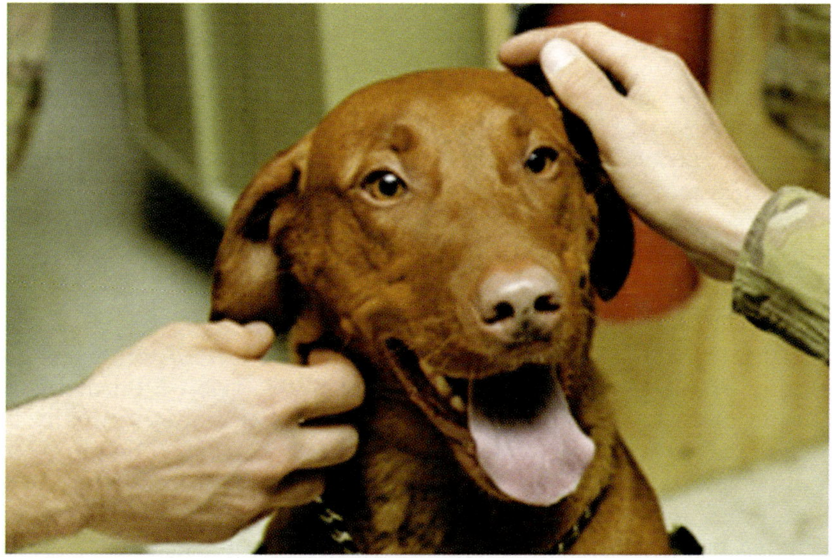

Service members pet the Combat Stress Dog of 98th Medical Detachment Combat Stress Control at Bagram Air Field on 21st January, 2014.

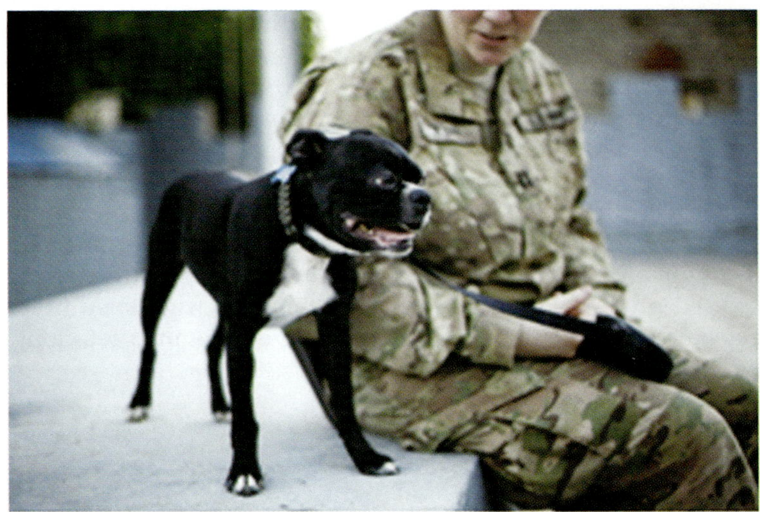

Captain Katie Kopp from 2nd Battalion, 12th Infantry Regiment of the 4th Brigade Combat Team, talks to Therapy Dog Hank during Hank's visit to Combat Outpost Nangalam in the Pech River Valley of Afghanistan's Kunar Province on 3rd July, 2012. Hank is the Boston Terrier therapy dog deployed in this region to interact with soldiers as a stress relief.

CANINE MEDICAL SCENT DETECTION

Dogs have been successfully trained to identify urine containing *E. coli*, the bacteria that causes a certain type of urinary tract infection, and to distinguish these samples from healthy urine samples. This will change the lives of disabled people, who often become hospitalized and even die from urinary tract infections.

Published studies have also shown that dogs can detect early stage cancer with 88% specificity, and 99% sensitivity. As such, dogs could help to provide an extremely accurate, low-cost, non-invasive, early detection screening for cancer. Early detection is the greatest cure, as of now. The next mission is to study the diagnostic accuracy of canine scent detection on early stage stomach and pancreatic cancer. These cancers have no screening methods, and are almost always found too late. The dogs may be widely utilized for canine scent detection so as to provide a diagnostic screening method for the early detection of cancer in large number of humans in times to come.

PENETRATION OF FORTIFIED BARRIERS

On 2nd May, 2011, Cairo, a Malinois, became, the USA's newest four-pawed superhero. The hero dog that accompanied SEAL Team 6 on their raid into the compound of Osama Bin Laden in Abbottabad, Pakistan, eventually killing him. Cairo was tasked with tracking down anyone who tried to flee from Bin Laden's compound in Pakistan. The Canine SEAL fitted with a high-tech kit was able to take high definition videos. Like all superheroes Cairo had a "cape", technically customized body armour. Cairo's specialized working gear is designed to make him bulletproof and enable him to hear through concrete and record missions in high-definition, even on the darkest nights. Cairo was amongst the growing number

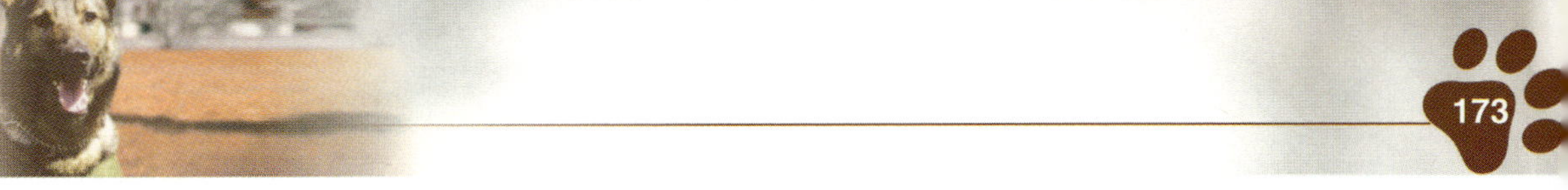

of dogs deployed in the battlefields and are also trained to jump from choppers and parachute at great heights or sniff out drugs and even roadside bombs.

The canine tactical assault vests for these wonder dogs weigh just three to five pounds. Since, communication is a key for the relationship with the dog and his master (warrior), these "Dogs of War" are trained one-on-one that is one dog:one warrior. The bond with the duo is closer than that of Batman and Robin with an aim to make working dogs more efficient and safe while deployed for specific operations in hostile circumstances. The patented load-bearing harness enable handler to rappel from the helicopter with his dog strapped to his body. Once on ground, the dog could run ahead to scout as the handler issue commands through an integrated microphone and speaker in the armour. The proprietary speaker system enables handlers to relay commands at low levels to the dog. However, the handlers need to see and hear how their dogs are responding. In a tactical situation, every second counts. Hence, the encrypted signal from dog to handler penetrates fortified barriers like concrete, steel-fortified ships, and tunnels. These gears translate to standard operating ranges up to four football fields.

The appearance of the ancient warrior with his war dog has not altered greatly over time. The ancient soldier was lightly armed and clad for speed of movement on the battlefield. The War Dog wore a light protective jacket made up of leather with spikes and matching collar for throat protection at most. Today, both dog and man are more valued in society and greater protection is afforded to both. Today's War Dogs have bulletproof vests and rubber booties for protection. Communication devices and video systems can be attached to the dogs, so handlers cannot only see and command dogs in the heat of battle, but also allow them to be recalled to safety if required.

New areas of innovative training and dog safety measures are being explored. These require visionary approach and creativity in training and equipping the dogs suitably for the task to be performed. While the deeds of these four-legged heroes are worth a look, so is the high-tech gear that helps them to do their job. Tactical body armour for dogs, is available with a price of $20,000 to $30,000 a piece, depending on the version. The tactical body armour is wired with a collapsible video arm, two-way audio, and other attachable supersecret gadgets that one can only speculate about. Customized bulletproof body armour has also been designed exclusively for working dogs. The high-tech equipment fitted on the armour can enable the dog to hear through concrete, and can record high-definition video of missions, even in the dead of night. To operate efficiently in a tactical situation, they need to be connected and a high-definition camera mounted on the dog's back makes it possible for handlers to see whatever the dog sees, using handheld monitors. The footage is stable because the entire module is sewn into the vest. With unpredictable light conditions, like middle-of-the-night missions, the camera adjusts automatically to night vision. The lens is protected by impact-resistant shielding and the system is waterproof.

The armour itself protects against shots from 9 mm and 0.45 magnum handguns. The weave technology catches bullets, knives and sharpened screwdrivers. Keeping the armour strong, but light, is a priority. Entire communication module weighs only 20 ounces and the average armour weighs between three to seven pounds, depending on the size of the dog and the level of protection. Of course, these systems don't come cheap but it's the dogs themselves that are the real investment. However,

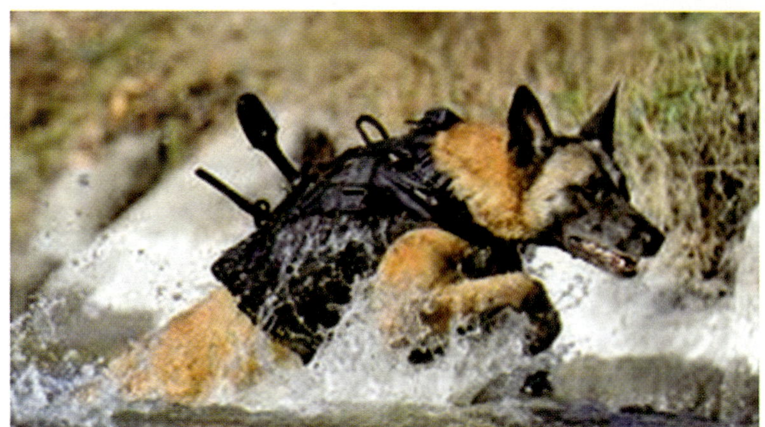

Bulletproof vest attached to a camera

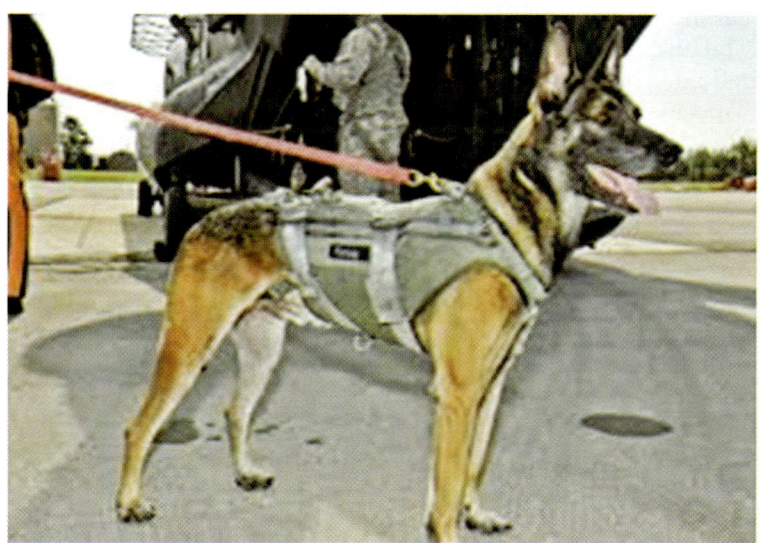

Tactical body armour vest

no amount of money can replace the life of a canine that saves the precious lives of troops. The new technology and the equipment is the buzz but the fit has to be perfect otherwise it will flop around and will hinder mobility and can also cause injury. The military dogs are now being equipped with special equipment which includes doggles (goggles designed to fit a dog) to provide protection from bright sunlight and dust and fine sand often found blowing into the desert. More recent vest designs come with many special features besides cameras. Some vests have compartments on the inside for the insertion of cold packs (soft, flat plastic bags containing a chemical that, when activated, becomes very cool and prevents heat stroke). There are also attachments on the vest to enable the dog to be dropped by parachute, or hauled up via a rope. Vests now allow identifying badges to be easily added and more of them have various grips for the handlers to pick up an injured dog. One vest design even has straps so that a handler can carry the dog on his back like a pack. While vests hinder dogs' mobility a bit, especially when they are jumping, however, the dogs quickly adjust. Some handlers still prefer unarmoured vests, because they are lighter and less constrictive but vests protect the dogs from stab wounds, shell fragments, and some bullets. The expense on the vests is justified because of the value of the dogs. The dogs take over a year, and some $60,000 (in the West) to train. So spending some money on life-saving equipment and efficient functioning of the dogs is a good investment.

AIRBORNE CAMERA DOGS

The dogs are being trained for the United Kingdom's Special Air Service Regiment, to be used in a highly skilled technique called 'high altitude high opening', jumping as much as 32 kilometres from their targets and gliding towards them for up to 30 minutes. Fearless MWDs will jump from aircraft at 7,000 metres (25,000 feet) wearing their own oxygen masks and strapped to special forces assault team members. Once down in hostile terrain such as in Iraq or Afghanistan, the dogs will be sent first to seek out insurgents' hideouts, with tiny cameras fixed to their heads. The cameras beam live TV pictures back to the troops, warning of ambushes or showing enemy leaders' locations. Two such dogs have been issued to each of the Regiment's four squadrons and paratroopers have been specially selected to be their handlers. This amazing tactic has been devised to cut down the soaring SAS Regiment's casualty rates.

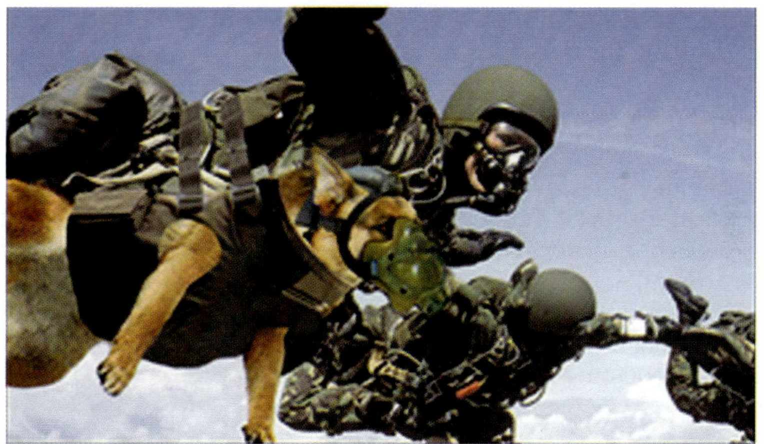

Aerial insertion vests

ANTI-NUCLEAR DEVICE

Just as the Russians previously trained anti-tank dogs in the World War II for suicide missions, the Soviet doctrine in any modern European war called on the use of dogs to carry out similar missions and destroy the enemy's nuclear weapons sites. It is a great deal easier to teach a dog to get up to a missile or an aircraft unnoticed than it is to get it to go under a roaring, thundering tank. As before, the dog may carry a charge weighing about 4 kilograms, but much more powerful as they were in World War II and the detonators, incomparably more sophisticated and fool-proof. Detonators have been developed that detonate only on contact with metal but do not go off on accidental contact with long grass, branches or other objects. The intelligent dog, with proper training, quickly becomes capable of seeking out, correctly identifying and attacking important targets. Such targets include complicated electronic equipment, aerials, missiles, aircraft, etc. All of this makes the "Spetsnaz" (Russian Special forces) dog a frightening and dangerous enemy. Apart from everything else, the presence of dogs with a Spetsnaz group appreciably raises the morale of the officers and the men. Some especially powerful and vicious dogs are trained for one purpose alone to guard the group and to destroy the enemy's dogs if they appear. No electronic devices and no enemy firepower has such an effect on his morale as the appearance of dogs. The enemy's dogs always appear at the most awkward moment, when a group exhausted by a long trek is enjoying a brief uneasy sleep, when their legs are totally worn out and their ammunition is used up. Surveys conducted among Soldiers, Sergeants and Officers in Spetsnaz produce the same answer again and again that the last thing they want to come up against, is the enemy's dogs. The heads of the GRU (Russian foreign military intelligence) have conducted far-reaching studies into this question and come to the conclusion that the best way to deal with dogs is to use dogs as well.

SUBMARINE SEARCH

American Military successfully used a Jack Russel terrier dog named Lara (J2740) for sniffing out bombs in submarines in Cameron Frost, into the USS Norfolk. It is now widely accepted that the nose of a good bomb sniffer dog far surpasses any technology available for detecting makeshift bombs.

NEW AREAS OF TRAINING AND EMPLOYBILITY

The next phase of development could be plans for remote-delivery systems and enhanced accessory functionality. They describe a system that would help dogs transport medical supplies, walkie-talkies, or water into constricted areas like rubble. New appendages like air-level quality meters for mines are also being planned and experimented. Small dogs weighing only 15 pounds such as West Highland Terriers, who look like playful white puffballs may in future help in drug raids in confined spaces like air ducts. Hence, new horizons have to be explored for employability of working dogs for boosting the war efforts as well as for the counter insurgency and anti-terrorism.

14

Breeds of Modern War Dogs

"To a dog the whole world is smell."

... Unknown

By the time World War II started, two breeds had become synonymous with war dog. The first was the German Shepherd, a breed developed in the late 1800s in Karlsruhe, Germany, by Capt Max Von Stephanitz and others. Shepherds descended from herding and farm dogs, but selective breeding accentuated the traits such as high trainability, extreme loyalty and commitment that make them such fine military animals. The other iconic war dog was the Doberman Pinscher, a breed that originated in Germany around 1900 and possesses great endurance and speed. More importantly, they are highly intelligent and could absorb and retain training better than other dogs.

Many countries trying to establish the fledgling War Dog programme were perfectly willing to learn from European success stories and both, German Shepherds and Doberman Pinschers, became the choicest Military Working Dogs. The US Marine Corps adopted the Doberman as its official dog, and the breed saw action throughout the Pacific Theatre. The US Military used German Shepherds extensively, both as scout and sentry dogs. Today, German Shepherds remain one of the most popular breeds in armies around the world. Defense officials also rely heavily on Labrador Retrievers and Malinois dogs. Labs earned their reputation as diligent workers on docks and wharves in Newfoundland, where they worked alongside fishermen to pull in nets and catch escaped fish, but their even temperament and trainability made them ideal Military Working Dogs. The Malinois, a breed developed in the Belgian city of Mechelen (Malines in French), looks like a German Shepherd, but has a slighter build. Its smaller size makes it no less valuable, however, it is a strong, agile dog with an impeccable work ethic and an obedient disposition. Of course, having a trainable breed is just the beginning, it still takes a great deal of effort to transform a raw canine recruit into a war-ready soldier.

The use of various breeds of dogs in armed forces are based on the fundamental principle that each dog should be able to effectively perform the assigned task for which the dog has been trained, suitable for performing in all types of terrain and climatic conditions and breed extensively enough to meet demands. German Shepherd Dog (GSD), Labrador Retriever (Labs) and Malinois (Belgian Shepherd) are mostly used due to the convenience in training, adaptability and field requirements. Other breeds such as Doberman Pinscher, Boxer and Rottweiler are also used in some countries.

GERMAN SHEPHERD

The breed was established in Germany in the 1880s, although there is still some debate about its ancestry. It is also believed that the German Shepherd Dog, or Alsatian may be a descendant of the Bronze age wolf. Around 7th century, there existed in Germany a Shepherd dog of similar type but with a lighter coat. By the 16th century, the coat is said to have darkened appreciably. It is one of the most versatile working dogs ever developed. Throughout the world, armies and police forces use them as a guard dog and farmers use as a sheep herding dog. It is also a popular pet and a very good companion. The German Army used these dogs during World War I and noticing their success, these dogs were soon introduced into the US and the British Commonwealth Armies by returning allied soldiers. Since then, German Shepherds have rapidly achieved widespread popularity. This dog is extremely intelligent, dependable and eminently trainable.

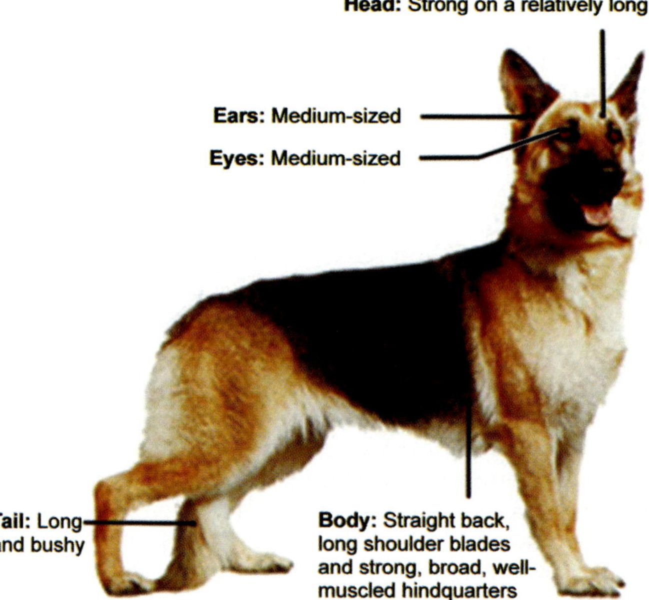

Breed Characteristics

The German Shepherd Dog (GSD) is well-proportioned and strong having a sturdy, muscular, slightly elongated body with a light, solid bone structure. The head should be in proportion to its body, and the forehead a little rounded. Male dogs are 60–65 cm and female dogs 55–60 cm in height. The body weight of male dog is 35–40 kg and of female dog is 30–32 kg. Length of the body is greater than height with deep broad chest, straight back and sloping hindquarters. The eyes are almond-shaped and usually dark brown in colour. Nose is most often black and the ears are wide at base, pointed, upright and turned forward. The teeth meet in a strong scissors bite and lips are firm, close tightly over the teeth. The front legs and shoulders are muscular and thighs are thick and sturdy. The feet have very hard sole and are compact with rounded, arched toes with well-developed pads and dark nails.

There are three varieties of German Shepherd, i.e. double coat, plush coat and long-haired coat. Body coat should be of medium length, straight, hard and close with a dense thick undercoat. Colours are solid black or grey, black saddle with tan or gold to light grey markings, grey with lighter or brown markings which are also referred to as sables. The tail is of medium length, bushy and set low and reaches below the hock, hangs down with a sabre-like curve when the dog is at rest and slightly raised when moving.

LABRADOR RETRIEVER

This breed is thought to have originated in Devon, England, and taken to North America by fishermen. On the coast of Newfoundland, these dogs were trained to bring in fishing nets through icy waters. In the nineteenth century Newfoundland's fisherman came to the English West Country to sell fish and some were persuaded to sell their dogs too. The breed was immediately successful as a gun dog. It was the Earl of Malmesbury, who first called them Labrador, based on location, in 1887. Subsequently, this breed was recognized by the English Kennel Club in 1903. The Labrador is most popular Retriever, loyal, even-tempered intelligent dog and is exceptionally reliable. It is renowned for its versatility and is widely used as police dog, guide dogs for the blind and excellent gun dog. Labrador is a fine swimmer, good tracker and ideally combine the role of pet, sporting companion and working dog. Always eager to please the master, but guards against intruders boldly.

Breed Characteristics

This breed has broad skull, with pronounced top. Body coat is short, straight dense and hard to touch. Colours are solid black, yellow or liver/chocolate. Body coat is short and dense, without wave or feathering and a water-resistant under coat. Eyes

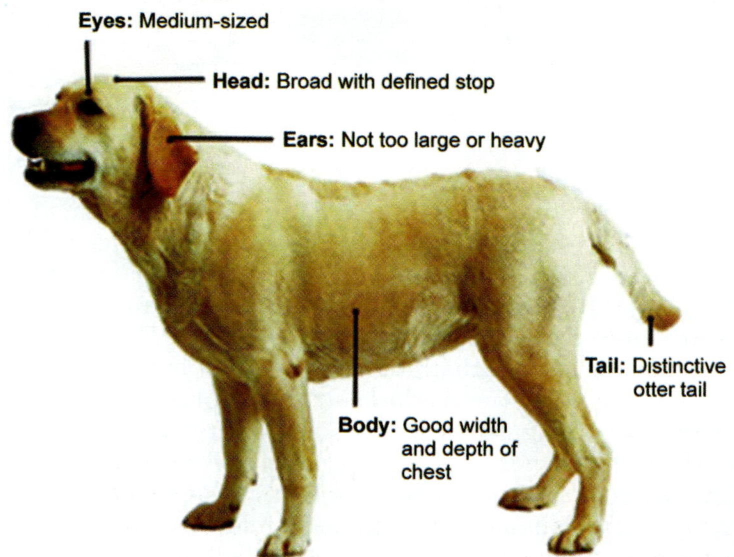

are medium-sized, brown or hazel, with intelligent expression. Nose is large and well-developed. Jaws are powerful with upper teeth closely overlapping lower teeth. Well built body, with deep, broad chest, level back and wide loins. Forelegs are straight from elbow and hindquarters are powerful. Male dogs are 56–61 cm and female dogs 53–58 cm in height with body weight 27–34 kg and 25–32 kg respectively. Feet are compact, round with well-arched toes and generous pads.

MALINOIS (BELGIAN SHEPHERD)

The Belgian Malinois was named after the Belgian city of Malines. It is one of the four varieties of Belgian sheep dogs, the Belgian Malinois (soft-coated), Belgian Tervuren (long-coated, other than black), Belgian Groenendael (long-coated black) and the less popular Belgian Laekenois (wire-coated) which all share a common foundation. In most countries and breed clubs all four dogs are considered the same breed with different varieties in coat types.

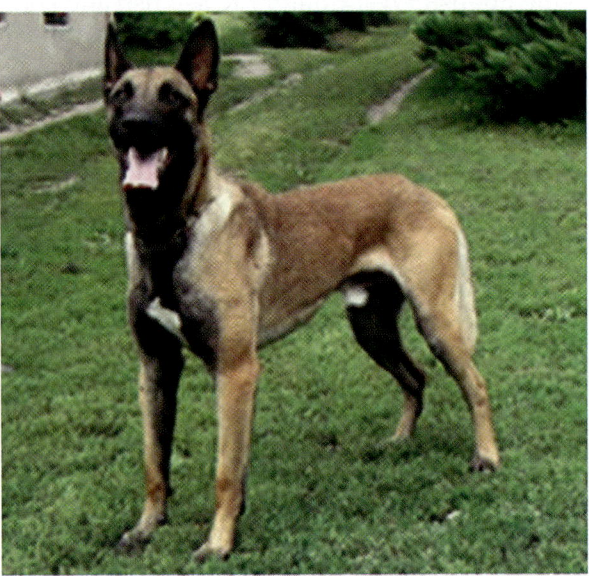

Belgian Malinois

Breed Characteristics

The body often described as square, as that is the shape it appears to have when the legs and top line are viewed from the side. The overall size of the head is in proportion to the body. The skull is flat with the width and length being of the same distance. The body is moderately long with a firm straight back, which shows a slight slope downwards towards the croup. The chest is deep and capacious. The muzzle is somewhat pointed and equal in length to the top of the skull with a moderate stop. The medium-sized, almond-shaped eyes are brown and the erect ears are triangular in shape. The legs are of good bone with round compact feet. The coat is short and wiry in texture. The coat colours are mainly ash grey, rich fawn to mahogany to black, with black tips on the hairs. The masks and ears are black. The tail and back end and underneath the body are a lighter fawn. The hairs around the neck look like a collar as these are slightly longer. The

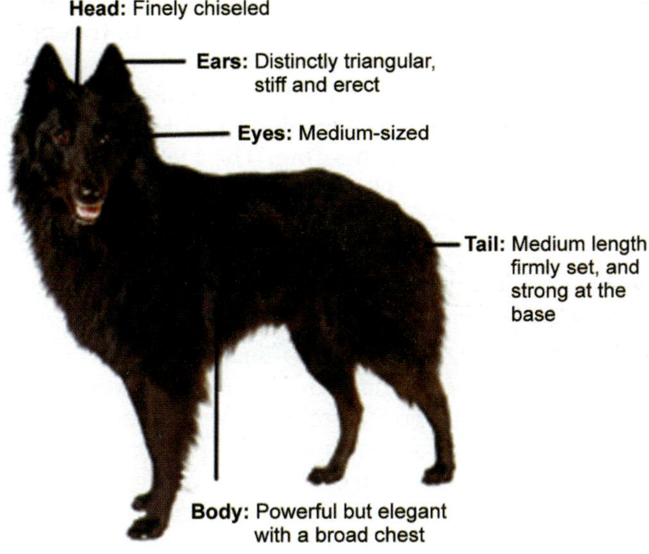

Belgian Tervuren

height of male dog is 61–66 cm and that of female is 56–61 cm with weight ranging from 24–29 kg. This breed is known for vigour, intelligence and versatility.

DOBERMAN PINSCHER

The Doberman was developed in the 1880s by Louis Doberman of Apolda in Germany. He wanted a ferocious, short-coated, medium to large dog with courage

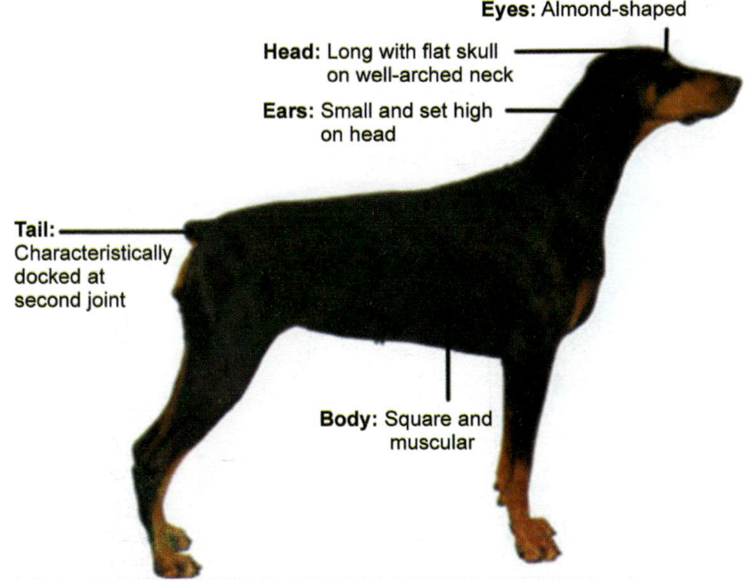

Doberman Pinscher

and stamina. As such, he developed his stock around the German Pinscher, which was both alert and aggressive. To this he introduced the Rottweiler with its stamina and tracking ability, and Manchester Terrier from which the Doberman inherited its marking. The Doberman was given official recognition as a breed standard in Germany in 1900. An exceptionally powerful dog that can be trained for guarding, tracking, retrieving and even sheep herding. The Doberman is intelligent, strong and aggressive when necessary. This dog needs knowledgeable handling and training, being wary of strangers and constantly on guard.

Breed Characteristics

Squarely built body with well-developed muscular chest and tucked up belly. Head is long with blunt, wedge-shaped profile. Top of skull is flat and parallel to muzzle. Tail continues the line of the spine, usually docked at the first or second joint. The height of male dog is 66–72 cm and female dog is 61–66 cm with body weight ranging from 30–40 kg. Back is short and straight. Eyes are almond-shaped, dark brown in black dogs or tones with coat colours and gives keen, alert expression to the dog. Lips are set tightly over jaws. Forelegs are straight. Hind legs are powerful and the feet are cat like and compact, with well-arched toes. Body coat is, smooth and hard, lying close to the body. Colours are black, blue, brown or fawn with rusty marking above eyes, on muzzle, throat, chest, legs and below tail. Colour of the nose varies according to the coat colours.

BOXER

The Boxer's main ancestors were German dogs of the Mastiff type, the Bullenbeiszer and the Barenbeiszer that were used in the middle ages for bull baiting and hunting boar. It was bred with the Bulldog to create the Boxer. Despite its German origin,

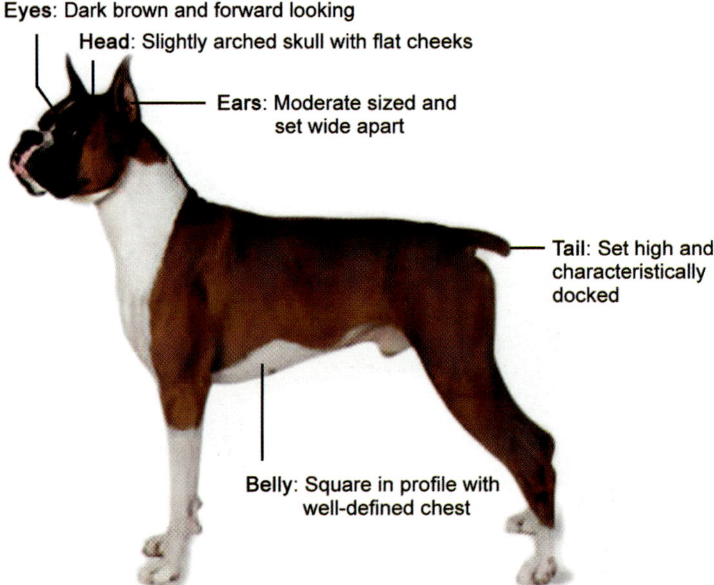

Boxer

'Boxer' is an English name that aptly describes the dog's punchy fighting style. Boxer is well-known for its courage and makes an excellent guard dog due to its natural guarding instincts. It has ferocious looks that further contribute to its deterrence. It makes a good family dog, very affectionate and playful. The Boxer is always keen to work and play, but can be rather boisterous and extremely athletic even in old age. This breed is known for courage as well as discipline.

Breed Characteristics

Head is square, with deep broad muzzle and upturned nose. Lower jaw projects beyond the upper and curves slightly upwards. Deep chest with well-arched ribs and short Loins. The back is broad, short and well-muscled. Eyes are medium-sized, dark brown with dark eye rims. Nose is broad and black with a line between wide nostrils. Neither the teeth nor the tongue should be visible when the mouth is closed. Tail is set high, carried erect and usually docked short to 5 cm. Feet are small, with ample pads and well-arched toes. Forelegs are long, straight and parallel and hind legs are longer than fore feet, well-muscled with broad curved thighs. Body coat is short, smooth, shiny and lying flat to the body. Colours are fawn or bindle and any white marking should not take up more than one-third of the coat colour. When the Boxer is pleased, happy or excited, it tends to wag its whole body instead of the docked short tail. Height of male dog is 56–63 cm and female dog is 53–61 cm with body weight ranging from 27–30 kg and 24–29 kg respectively.

ROTTWEILER

The Rottweiler has probably descended from the Italian Mastiff, which accompanied the herds that the Romans brought with them when they invaded Europe. During the middle ages, it was used as a herder, as a guard, messenger dog, draught dog and for police work. It was bred in German town of Rottweiler in Wurttemberg.

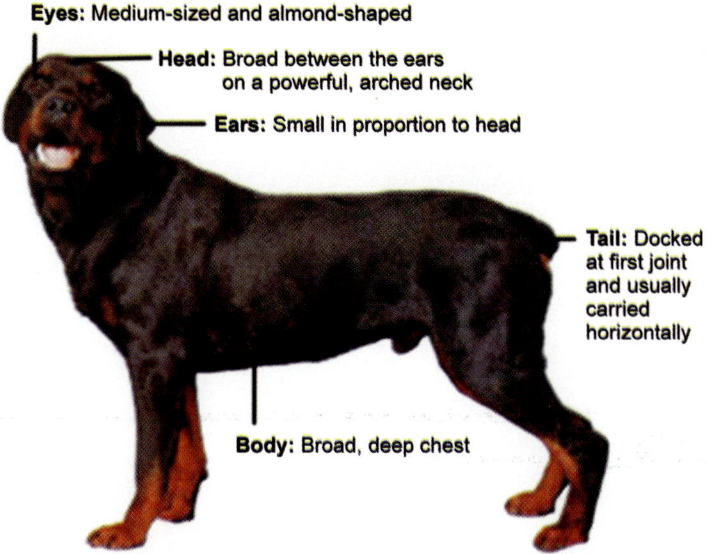

Rottweiler

The breed became practically extinct in the 1800s but made a come back in the early twentieth century due to the efforts of enthusiastic breeders centered in Stuttgurt and the breed was first recognized by American Kennel Club (AKC) in 1931.

Breed Characteristics

The Rottweiler has a heavily built, muscular, massive and powerful body. The head is broad with a rounded forehead and it has a well-defined top. The muzzle is well-developed and the teeth meet in a scissors bite. The wide nose is black. The lips are black and the inside of the mouth is dark. Eyes are medium-sized and almond-shaped and the ears are triangular and carried forward. The tail is customarily docked. The chest is broad and deep. The coat is short, hard and thick and is black in colour with well-defined tan or mahogany brown markings on the cheeks, muzzle, paws and legs. A red colour with brown markings also exists. The height of male dog is 61 to 69 cm and that of female dog is 56–63 cm with weight ranging from 43–59 kg and 38–52 kg respectively. This breed is intelligent, naturally obedient and courageous. Rottweiler's talents includes tracking, herding, guarding, search and rescue, guide dog for the blinds and police work.

There is, of course, no perfect war dog breed. Many a Mongrel (meaning a dog or bitch whose sire and dam are likely to owe their make up to any number of different breeds) has served the colours with heroic distinction. Recently in Australia, several crossbreed dogs that had been given a second chance from a dog pound have served in Afghanistan searching for explosives. Many have made the ultimate sacrifice. How true is the adage:

"It's the fight in the dog, not the dog in the fight that counts".

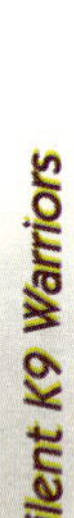

15

Canine Olfaction, Character and Personality

"He is your friend, your partner, your defender, your dog. You are his life, his love, his leader. He will be yours, faithful and true, to the last beat of his heart. You owe it to him to be worthy of such devotion."

... Unknown

BASIC SENSES

The dogs prior to their domestication used their hunting skills to kill the prey. In their quest for food, they were assisted by their natural gifts of highly developed senses of smell, hearing and vision. The dog must use his basic senses to carry out this role effectively. These basic senses, in their order of importance in the training and employment of dogs, are considered in details in the succeeding paragraphs.

Smell (Olfaction)

Undoubtedly, the dog's sense of smell is more developed than his other senses. The 'Organum olfactorium' of dogs is better developed than that of man. By virtue of extensively large number of receptor cells (225 million in the nasal mucosa of dogs as compared to only 5 million in human beings), the dog's sense of smell is 40–45 times better than that of human beings. Under favourable conditions, the dog is able to track on a many hours or even many days old trail. The dog's nose is capable of detecting the faintest odour at great distances from the source of origin of such odour. Studies have shown that a dog responds to traces of odour in very high dilutions as compared to human beings and he can distinguish between many odours, which to human beings, seems identical. The dog's sense of smell is invaluable to the trainer because a great part of the dog's role as a working dog depends upon his ability to pick up a scent.

Hearing

A dog has much more acute sense of hearing than man, which means that a dog can detect sounds that would completely escape the notice of his trainer or any other human being. It is an invaluable trait for special role of working dogs in peace and hostile circumstances. Dogs can detect most sounds from four times the distance than a man. The dog's sense of hearing is greatly utilized while training them for

the role of Infantry Patrol. More so, hearing is also one of the main media through which the handler/trainer communicates with the dog.

Vision

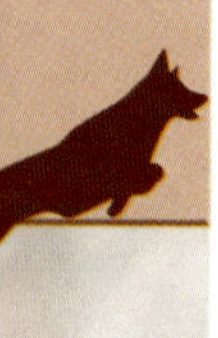

Due to predominance of rod receptors in the retina, dogs can see much better than humans in poor light conditions. Their ability to see at night is further enhanced by the presence of a special reflective layer (tapetum) at the back of their eyes. It is the reflection from this, which causes a dog's eyes to shine green or yellow green when reflected against headlights of automobile/torch at night. The dogs can perceive moving objects better than human beings extremely sensitive to anything that takes a sudden or unusual movement. This unique asset is most gainfully used by retrievers, pointers and hunting dogs during their work.

Touch

Dogs show considerable degree of variation amongst themselves in their response to the sense of touch. Certain dogs are very susceptible to a caress for physical corrections whereas others appear to be rather insensitive to it. As such, a dog's sense of touch can be determined when he is patted or corrected. Some dogs seem to understand physical praise or correction better than oral praise or correction.

Sixth Sense

The important question that has intrigued human since time immemorial is, whether dogs have sixth sense? There is a strong belief amongst people particularly in tribal areas that early warning of fire, prediction of earthquakes and tsunamis and other natural calamities are generally indicated by unusual behaviour of dogs. Such instances when seen in conjunction with subsequent reporting of such natural calamity make us believe that dogs do have sixth sense. In case of earthquake prediction, it is believed that dogs can smell seepage from the ground. Another view is that they detect low frequency warning vibrations. However, the exact mechanism by which the dogs sense the natural calamities is still not clear but human being do have a strong belief on their unusual capabilities.

It is the power of their highly developed natural senses, coupled with speed, stamina, ferocity, faithfulness as well as their ever-readiness to do anything to please the master that has been exploited by human beings to their best advantage. Anyone who has been fortunate to own a dog, is bound to be impressed with the extraordinary relationship because of which the dog is considered a part of human society.

Dogs like the rest of the animal kingdom, are subject to outside influences, which have a direct bearing on their behaviour. Accordingly, a dog, no matter how highly trained, cannot be expected to work with the same precision under all adverse circumstances. The dog is a special ancillary weapon and should be used judiciously only after a careful appreciation of the tactical situation, climatic condition and the terrain.

CHARACTER AND PERSONALITY OF DOGS

Knowledge of dog's character and personality help to specify the duties to which a particular dog may be best suited. Some of the facets considered are:

Courage: It is the ability of the dog to react in the given circumstances. It must confront the danger situation. A good guard dog must be courageous and aggressive. A courageous dog will attack the intruder even if his own life is in danger.

Virtual Curiosity: When a dog is being trained, this is an important indicator of willingness to learn. Keen expressions certainly point to good training potential. This trait is most evident in puppies and young dogs.

Defense: The defensive impulse will make a dog rush to the aid of his master in the face of a threat without caring even for his own safety.

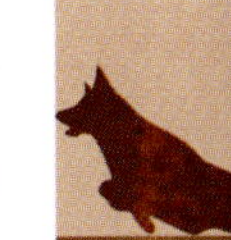

Docility: This feature enables a dog to become part of a human group. Docility should not to be confused with weak character. Some dogs are strong willed and docile, while others are weak willed and not docile at all.

Tendency to bite: A dog's hostile as well as defensive reaction is depicted by tendency to bite when faced with unpleasant stimuli. Many breeds like Dachshunds, Mastiffs are known to have tendency to bite. However, some dogs act cowardly but tend to bite, while others may be brave but will not bite.

Endurance: This enables the dog to summon up energy both mental and physical as required to perform various duties. A well-fed and nicely cared dog has tremendous stamina and staying power which makes him fit for all physical activities.

Self-Control

Man and his best friend dog have something in common as both behave aggressively when they run out of control. Researchers at the University of Lile Nord de France found that dogs that "run out" of self-control make more impulsive decisions very similar to human beings.

Accordingly, selecting the best dog for training is dependent on the character suited to the task it will be asked to carry out. A dog with very strong or very weak character cannot be trained well.

16

Specialities and Training of Working Dogs

"A dog has the soul of a philosopher."

... Marcus Tullius Cicero

SPECIALITIES OF WORKING DOGS

Working dogs are required to perform various tasks as confronted by their masters. Accordingly, after perfecting the use of dogs in one specialty successfully, their use in new fields becomes the vision and this cycle goes on. Hence, spectrum of specialty of working dogs keeps ever increasing as per the functional needs, success rate in training and subsequent utility to mankind.

Tracker (TR) Dogs

These dogs pick up human scent from human telltale marks, dropped clothing/ items of kit or articles touched by the individual. It can track down its quarry to a distance of 15–20 km even on 72 hours old tracks under ideal conditions. Notwithstanding this, a tracker dog should be deployed on the site at the earliest possible time. In addition to the German Shepherds and Labradors, Malinois has also proved to be excellent trackers.

Guard Dogs

These dogs provide security of very high order by utilization of inherent powers of sight, smell and ferocity that humans do not possess to the same degree. By rendering the sentries more effective they are invaluable in the security needs of battlefield areas as well as for guarding of vital installations of strategic importance. At night, human sentries are seriously handicapped due to darkness, the fear of the unknown and the sense of isolation which at times erodes their morale. On the contrary, guard dogs are extremely alert to the slightest sound/movement and generate confidence in the environment. Training makes them very bold and extremely ferocious. These dogs are employed to augment, strengthen and supplement the security arrangements at high risk installations, and premises such as ammunition dumps, air force stations, missiles sites, satellite stations, rocket launching batteries, ordnance and fuel depot, etc. They can also be employed as escorts and for riot and mob control. The bold, aggressive and versatile German Shepherds make ideal guard dogs.

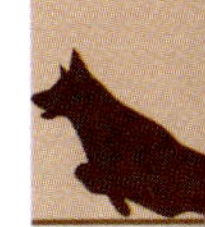

Mine Detection (MD) Dogs

These dogs detect anti-personnel and anti-tank mines buried in the ground. They are much lighter in weight and smaller in size in comparison to human beings and can move in minefield with comparative immunity. After spotting the mine, the dog sits down within 60 cm of actual mine location, pointing its nose towards the mine. Subsequently, the engineer's representative confirms, defuses and lifts the mine. These dogs are the only answer to the detection of plastic mines where costly electronic gadgets also fail to detect. Labradors, Malinois and German Shepherds have proved to be successful MD dogs.

Explosive Detection (ED) Dogs

The Labradors, because of their cool temperament and better intelligent expression have proved to be most successful and dependable ED dogs. However, German Shepherds and Malinois are also often used. These dogs detect various types of explosives and Improvised Explosive Devices used by terrorist outfits for their criminal and anti-national activities. ED Dogs are employed for security, anti-sabotage checks and checks of crowded public places including terrorist hideouts, road opening patrols and sanitization of specific vulnerable areas. The excellent performance of these dogs has led to their extensive use for anti-militancy and anti-terrorism operations.

Infantry Patrol (IP) Dogs

The Labradors, German Shepherds and Malinois bestowed with naturally gifted senses of smell, hearing, aggression and suspicion have been successfully utilized as IP dogs. These dogs pick up unfamiliar scent while on patrol and indicate it by giving an alert from a distance of 300 to 500 metres. They have proven ability to detect ambush sites and enemy caches of weapons and ammunition in the area being patrolled. IP dogs may also detect the enemy hiding under water, if using need to breathe through, which makes it possible for the dog to pick up the scent. Such dogs are deployed to lead patrols and render valuable service to own troops by fore-warning them about the likely presence of concealed enemy. This act also saves the patrol from surprise ambush. These dogs can be deployed at any time irrespective of weather and terrain conditions and are important means of preventing loss of life.

Avalanche Rescue Operation (ARO) Dogs

These dogs detect casualties/trapped victims buried in fresh/wet snow under 6–8 feet or even more. They also can indicate personal articles such as items of kit, books, equipment and can also pick up the sounds of radio sets buried along with casualties. It is obvious that many lives can be saved by timely detection and prompt treatment. The Labradors naturally gifted with retrieving qualities and cool temperaments have proved to be very successful ARO Dogs.

Search and Rescue (SAR) Dogs

SAR dogs are an effective instrument to save human lives as they have proved their mettle in the past in a number of disaster management missions undertaken by multifarious relief agencies across the world. SAR dog is of immense help in conjunction with the main rescue team by utilizing its exemplary sniffing power. A pair of fully trained SAR dogs can sanitize 5 acres of area in an hour depending on the degree of inclement conditions whereas 20 men are required to search the same area in two hours and may still fail to locate the victim if buried deeper. A well-trained SAR dog is able to locate the victim or his articles buried under 6–8 feet of debris and at times under 20 feet debris also. SAR dog with his agility and compact body is able to maneuver difficult slopes, turns, narrow passages, heaps of rubble/debris and unstable structures, thus being able to search every inch of the area. A strong, light to medium built Labrador dog who is staunch, active, willing and intelligent prove to be a good candidate to become a SAR dog, though German Shepherds and Malinois are also used.

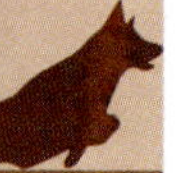

TRAINING OF WORKING DOGS

The basis of all training and performance is the relationship between the dog and his trained handler. The dog has been gifted by nature with characteristics like acuteness of his senses, ferocity, speed, watchfulness and above all faithfulness to his master. These extraordinary characteristics enable him to be of immense value. To exploit full potential of the natural gifts to canines, the dogs should be trained scientifically and trainers have to be selected carefully and discretely. Prior to initiating pups into training, it is necessary to assess their suitability by subjecting them to certain tests such as cool chamber, spin maze, step ladder, alertness rag play and chambers test. They are graded as per their behaviour and performance. Pups meeting the standards are selected for training.

Principles of Dog Training

Dog training is an art. It establishes a working relationship between the dog and the handler. Obedience is the first essential element to be taught. It serves to develop in dog, the behaviour that is essential for efficient and effective training. Basic obedience training is based on practical knowledge of how a dog's mind works, constant repetition of training exercise, suitable recognition of a dog's progress and patience, firmness and kindness. The effectiveness and success of a dog training programme depend on certain basic principles, which are discussed in detail in the succeeding paragraphs.

Know–How

The trainer must know as to how a dog's mind works and should understand its limitations. In the beginning, a dog may be uncertain of what is expected of him, however, in due course of time with proper handling, the trainer is able to establish himself as the master and win over the confidence and faithfulness of his dog. He only should pat, praise, feed and handle the dog assigned to him and should not permit anyone else to make friends with his dog.

The trainer must know-how each maneuver, act, technique, method and position is perfect before he can properly train his dog. The degree of proficiency prescribed for each exercise should be carefully studied. The trainer, then, should adhere to the proper methods and techniques so that high standards are achieved. In doing so, he must conscientiously apply all these principles with keen interest, enthusiasm and a desire to achieve perfection. He must demand complete obedience from his dog at all times. It is very essential that the trainer himself practice personal discipline so as to achieve success. The trainer should understand that next to voice, gestures and hand signals are the chief means of influencing dogs. Often, vocal commands and gestures are to be combined. To start with, gestures may have to be exaggerated to help convey the desired commands to the dog. As the training progresses, exaggeration in gestures is reduced.

Repetition

Repetition is one of the most important factors in implanting the requirement of a command on a dog's memory. It is essential to make the dog carry out the same command over and over until it learns to respond without hesitation. However, both the trainer and his dog can lose efficiency by practicing anyone command too much during one period. After practicing a command for 4 to 5 minutes, the trainer should move on to another command or give an interval of 10 minutes before resuming practice of the original command.

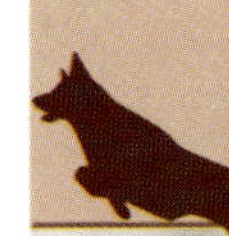

Patience

One of the most important requirements of a dog trainer is patience. To train a dog to perform the same exercise repeatedly until the task is properly executed calls for the ultimate in self-control. The trainer must never lose patience or become irritated. If he does, his dog will become hard to handle because the dog takes his clue from the trainer's attitude. Patience should always be judiciously combined with firmness.

Reward

To enable a dog to understand that he has carried out its trainer's wishes, it should immediately be rewarded when an order has been correctly obeyed. It is the natural desire of a dog to please his master and full advantage should be taken of this admirable trait during his training. Several effective methods are used to reward a dog. Kind words often do the trick. Patting, praising, offering tidbits such as a small piece of meat or biscuit, etc., a few minutes romp and play, can all bring in good results. Each dog might require a special method and the trainer must determine during his early association with the dog, which method of reward best suits his dog.

Correction

A dog does not understand right or wrong. Reward and correction are the means by which a dog is taught. If the dog does an exercise incorrectly, he should be immediately checked and corrected. Correction can be done either orally or manually. Withholding praise, or a simple admonition, 'No' spoken re-approvingly, or a jerk on the leash, may all be resorted to. Correction, in whatever form, should be administered immediately. The time factor is very important in administering any form of correction, since the dog connects a reprimand with an incorrect performance. Proper correction demands correct observation, patience, self-control, discretion and proper thinking on the part of the trainer.

End all exercises on a successful note. If the trainer is to maintain his dog's enthusiasm for work, each training period must be concluded with patting, praise and encouragement. Whatever the type of training, the lesson must always finish on a successful note. When the exercise is difficult, and the trainer realizes that the dog is unable to grasp it in that particular lesson, he should be allowed to perform some other exercises in which he is proficient before returning him to the kennel.

Punishment

The purpose of punishment should be aimed at improvement, not reprisal. The trainer should never slap a dog with his hand or strike him with the leash. The dog looks upon his trainer's hand as an instrument of praise and pleasure and he must never be allowed to fear it. Beating him with the leash will make him shy of it and lessen the effectiveness of its legitimate use. In short, physical violence, even for willful disobedience must never be resorted to, as the dog may become sullen, stubborn or cowed. Withholding praise, using a rebuking tone, or a sharp tap on the hindquarters may be enough in most cases. Timing in punishment is most important and the punishment, whatever form it takes, must be administered immediately after the dog misbehaves.

Length of Lessons

Training periods should not be too long otherwise the dog becomes bored and loses interest. It is definitely better to have two training periods of half an hour than one period of one hour. In specialized dog training the following additional points should be kept in mind:

Only one Job: A dog can be successfully trained for only one job because of its natural limitations. Any effort to train it for more than one job will, therefore, diminish the contribution the dog can make.

Trainer–dog relationship: The dog and his trainer should work as one team and once the team has been established, the relationship must be maintained. Frequent changes of trainers or dogs should not be resorted to.

Motivation: The dog should be motivated by praise, patting and reward as well as by the goal of accomplishing a mission. The dog can and should be trained to complete a task as an end in itself, not simply for the sake of reward from its trainer.

Training over different terrain and conditions: The trainer should conduct training over varying terrain and in the face of other distractions, to develop the dog's responsibility for given tasks and to ensure the accomplishment of its mission.

Review: Review of previous training lessons maintains and raises each dog's level of performance. The trainer is the best judge.

Welfare of the dog: Successful training of dogs depends to a great extent on the care taken by the trainer for their welfare. Unless the dogs are kept in good health, properly groomed, fed and kenneled, the effectiveness of the training programme will be considerably reduced.

Basic Obedience Training

Before any special form of training is attempted, the foundation of basic obedience training must be well-established in each dog. It is during this initial training that the trainer masters his dog and the latter is conditioned to become a reliable, obedient and well-trained. The dogs are generally initiated into the basic obedience training at 6 months of age and the training lasts 12 weeks. The dog learns to "Heel" while marching, a lesson which becomes the basis for orderly movement of dogs and their handlers. To heel properly, the dog must walk at the handler's left side with his head even at the handler's knee level. This lesson is followed by other words of command on and off leash which train the dog to sit, lie down, stand, stay, move out and recall. Later the dog learns to crawl under and jump over obstacles. Simultaneously the dog is taught to obey hand gestures also. Perfection in each lesson is gained through repetition of each exercise until the dog can be depended upon to obey under all circumstances.

Obedience Course Training

The obedience course exposes the dogs to various obstacles that simulate walls, open windows, tunnels, ramps, or steps. The dog's exposure to these obstacles reduces the amount of time required to adapt dogs to different environments. The dog learns to negotiate each of the obstacles. When confronted with a similar obstacle in the working environment, the dog is not deterred from completing his mission. The obedience course also develops the handler's ability to control the dog's behaviour both on and off leash. However, the obedience course is not a substitute for exercise and the dog should never be required to negotiate the obedience course until he has been warmed up by proper exercise. The specification of various obstacles may be as under:

Hurdles: The hurdles consist of four obstacles measuring 3 ft × 3 ft and standing in a straight line 16 feet apart. There may be a picket fence, a chain link fence, a simulated brick wall, a 30″ × 30″ open window the dog must jump through, a wall or board jump and a shrub jump. The dog must jump over or through all four of these hurdles following only voice commands before returning to his handler.

Catwalk: The catwalk portion of the course evaluates the dog's ability to climb a ladder and stay at a mid-point of a raised platform on command before dismounting. The ladder consists of five steps placed 12 inches apart, with the first 12 inches off the ground. The ladder sits at a 25 to 30 degree angle leading up to a 24-inch wide platform 6 feet off the ground. A 10-foot long dismount ramp on the opposite end of the raised platform completes the obstacle.

Broad Jump: The broad jump obstacle tests the dog's ability to leap a distance of 6 feet over a set of progressively taller boards. The four boards that make up this stage of a dog agility course are 6 inches wide and 5 feet long. The lowest of the boards is 6 inches off the ground, with height gradually increasing to a final height of 12 inches off the ground. To succeed in this portion of the course, the dog must jump over the boards on a single voice command without stepping on or knocking over any of the boards.

A-Frame: A-frame is another obstacle designed to challenge the dog's agility and enables him to confidently handle circumstances in the field. It consists of two boards measuring 4 feet × 6 feet which spread 4 feet apart at the base and their top edges come together at a 6-foot high peak. On a single voice command, the dog jumps to the top of the obstacle, then dismounts and returns to his handler's side. The dismount side includes a platform 3 feet off the ground to prevent the dog from being injured as he leaps from the top of the A-frame.

Crawl: The final piece of the agility course evaluates the dog's ability to crawl through a tight tunnel on command. The obstacle consists of pipes wrapped with chain-link fencing that leaves an opening 4 feet wide and 16 inches high at the base. The tunnel is covered with a sheet of plywood measuring 4 feet × 8 feet. Upon a single voice command, the dog must lower to the ground and crawl into the tunnel for a distance of 8 feet, exit and return to his handler's side.

The layout of the obstacle course may be planned as under:

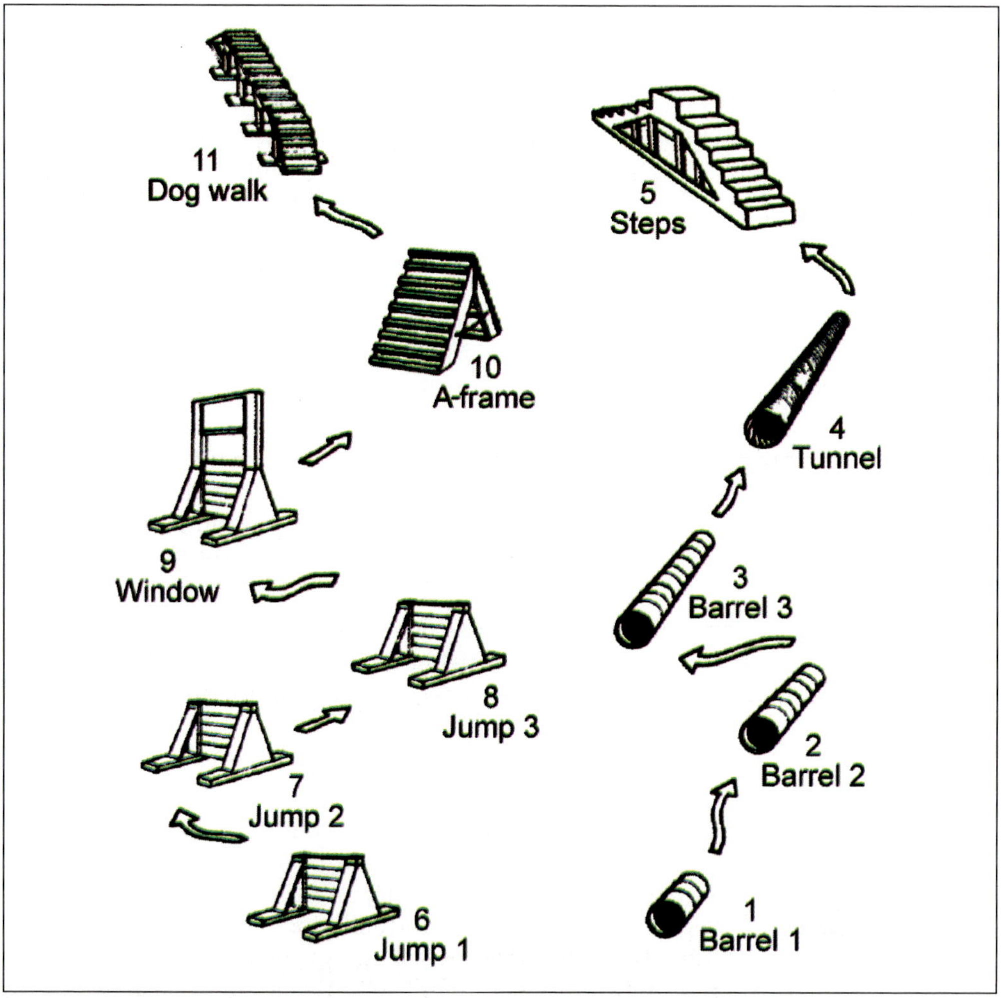

Weapon Fire Training

Training on weapon firing ranges is essential for the war dogs to become proficient and not be deterred from attacking agitators during gunfire. The dog must not attack the handler during gunfire. The firing of the weapon assigned to the handler should be done in the presence of war dog, whenever possible. The dogs can also be desensitized with the firing of many different types of weapons. This can often be accomplished by arranging for the handlers to take the dogs to weapon ranges of different units. Determine the dog's reaction to the sound of gunfire. It may be necessary for the handler to use counterconditioning techniques until the desired proficiency is achieved. These include starting the fire at distances of 300 metres and slowly bringing the gunfire closer to the dog (or as safety allows, bringing the dog closer to the weapon). The goal is for the dog not to bark or show any signs of aggression when the handler fires all assigned weapons. This can be a slow process over the course of several days.

On completion of basic training course with his handler, the dog should be selected for the specialty for which he is best suited. Extremely aggressive dogs are ideal to become Guard Dogs, whereas dogs with above average alertness and sense of smell are usually suitable for Infantry Patrol and dogs proven to be highly intelligent coupled with power of endurance and willing aptitude for track work are considered for Tracker Dogs, Mine Detection Dogs, Explosive Detection Dogs and Search and Rescue Operation Dogs. Obstacle course training and weapon training should be inclusive in all specialized training programmes.

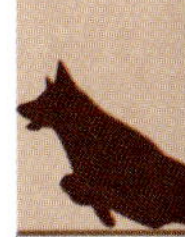

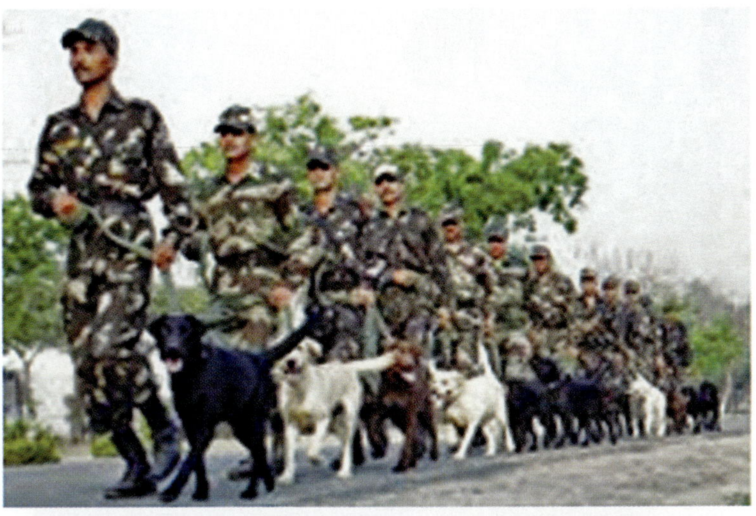

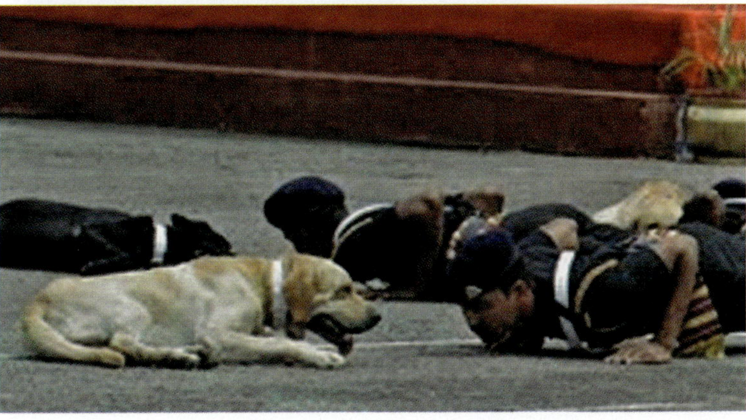

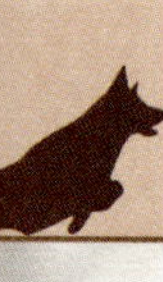

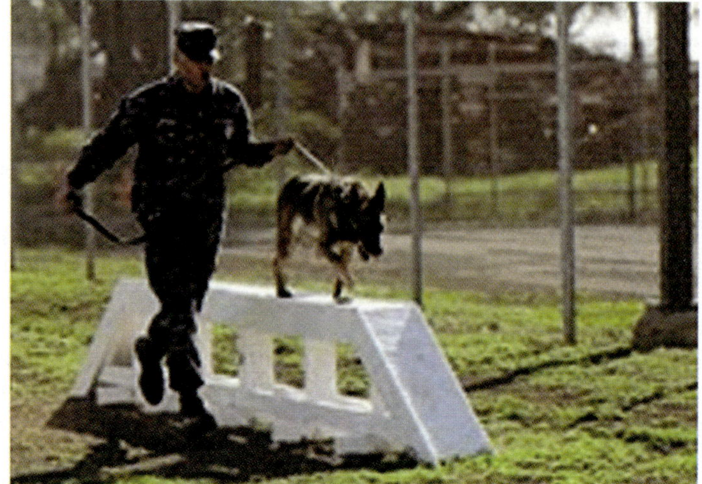

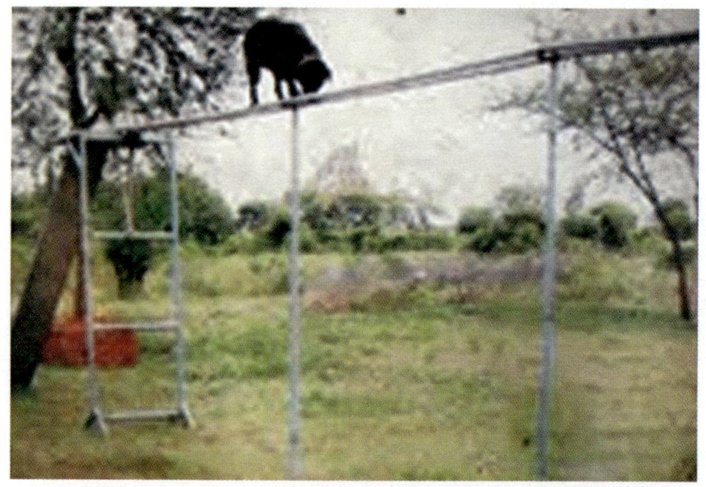

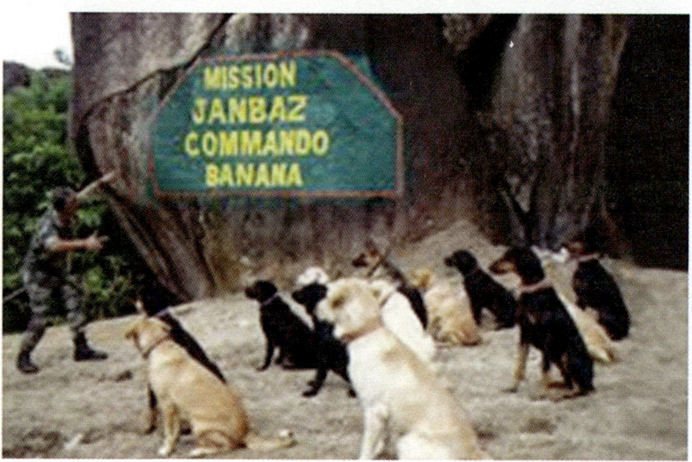
MISSION
JANBAZ
COMMANDO
BANANA

SPECIALIZED TRAINING OF DOGS

Guard Dog

Guard Dogs are trained to warn their handlers about the approach or presence of strangers inside the guarded premise by giving a silent indication about the same. These dogs are also trained to pursue attack and delay the intruder on command of the handler. The dogs are trained for this discipline over a period of 12 weeks after completion of the basic training. The four stages of guard dog training are sack batting, sleeve batting, suit attack and muzzle attack.

Training

The dog is taken to the training area on a chock chain, and when the handler attaches the leather collar it means that the dog is now on duty. In sack bating stage, another man called an agitator approaches with a small stick and a sack. He begins to tease the dog by sack batting so as to arouse the dog's natural aggressiveness. The handler, keeping the dog on leash, commands "Dekho" ("watch him") and as soon as the dog makes an aggressive move, the agitator retreats while the dog is encouraged to chase him. After each successful attempt, the dog receives praise from his handler. The psychology of the dog to always win over the agitator and his natural desire to please the master makes the learning perfect. The dog is now taught to attack a padded arm guard, also called as sleeve batting, which the agitator drops whenever the dog seizes it. The agitator later dons a long padded garment called "attack suit" and runs while the dog is encouraged to chase him. Subsequently, the dog is permitted to attack the suit while on leash. Finally, the dog is unleashed and taught to attack and release his hold on command from the handle, and thus leaving his handler free to use his weapon.

Trained guard dogs are utilized for patrolling around vital installations and places of strategic importance. They are always alert for smells which no human could detect and are of immense value where security against intruders must be maintained. The guard dog may be employed, as a patrolling sentry, static sentry, attached by a running chain to a long wire within a specified area and confined loose in a building or fenced area, etc., depending upon the requirement of deployment in various situations. The ever present human fear of a vicious dog coupled with the dog's alertness in detecting intruders makes the guard dogs invaluable in all types of security work.

Specially selected guard dogs may also be suitably trained as ambush dogs where 'non-barker' characteristic of dog along with the training to 'stay still till further command' is essential. Accordingly, additional training on this aspect is given before employing on such duties. Such dog should be able to give silent warning of any one approaching by tensing its body and or pricking its ears. Further, once the ambush has been sprung, the dog should be able to attack and hold the intruder who has escaped. Similarly, with slight variation in training schedule, guard dogs may also be trained as a security dogs that is not required to attack and bite. Such dogs should be medium to large in size with ferocious looks. They should have bold but non-aggressive temperament in complement with a natural aptitude to quarter and search.

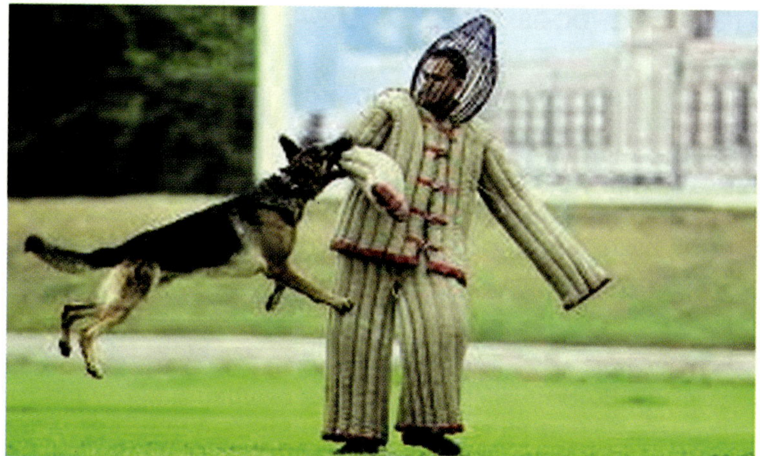

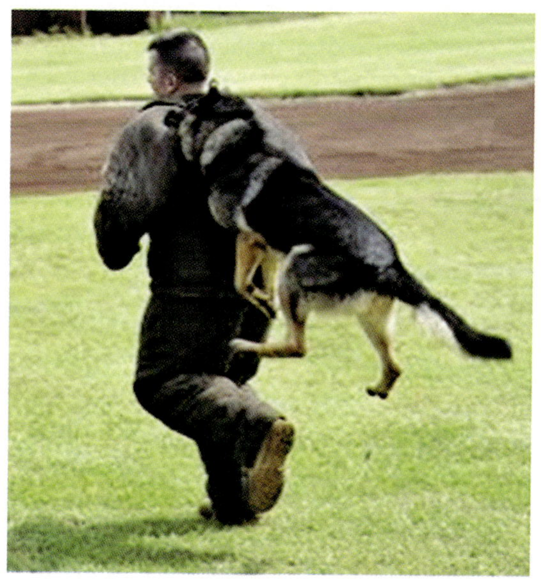

Tracker Dog

Training of a tracker dog requires basic knowledge of scent, and the track. Dog has a highly developed sense of smell and is able to track a man even over a trail which is many hours old. A dog becomes conscious of the scent through the air he breathes and comes in contact with the olfactory nerve ending in the delicate mucous membrane lining of nostrils. The degree of discernment is, therefore, proportional to the concentration of the scent in the air.

There are many factors which affect the track and the tracking procedure. Wind is an important factor to be considered in tracking as the tracker dog takes human scent from ground and follows the variations as per the pattern of the wind. If a dog is following a track across a strong wind, then the dog is required to move down the wind of the original track because in this scenario the scent get diffused and spread in the direction of the wind. Similarly, a strong wind will obliterate the scent completely or may spread it very thinly over the entire area and the dog will have difficulty in detecting the scent owing to low or negligible concentration in the air. As such, in the nascent stages of tracker dog training, the dog is taught to keep its head down at ground level and initiated to track the ground scent.

Another important factor is terrain and surface. The ideal surface to hold the tracks of scent well is one which is damp and covered with grass or short vegetation. Such surface tends to preserve the scent even after the subsequent drying up of the surface. Further, evaporation of scent is faster at higher temperature and to avoid this, early morning hours as well as the late afternoon are the most favourable time for the track work. Heavy rains over a fresh track tend to wash away the scent whereas light rain may be advantageous as it will lead to dampness which is considered good to hold the scent.

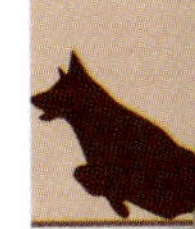

Age of the track is another factor, although a dog can follow a track laid several hours earlier yet during training, the dog should not be made to follow a track laid for more than two hours so as to have good concentration of scent. Dogs selected for tracker dog training should have a well-developed nose which is essential for scenting capabilities. A medium to large size Labrador showing willingness for track work, intelligent and with power of endurance is considered most suitable. However, German Shepherds, and Doberman Pinschers are also suitable based on requirement and availability.

Training

Initial condition for tracker dog training is done by inducing the dog to use his nose on the track laid of soup scent, tracking, and master's scent for a distance of 20 metres down wind and then tracking a quarry for a distance of 50 metres down wind. It is followed by tracking scent from articles and following ten minutes old scent as well as tracking articles dropped at a distance of 40 metres along the track and tracking 15 minutes old scent. Tracking length is gradually increased up to 400 metres and age of the scent is increased to 25 minutes. The dog is exposed to fresh scent across less frequented streets and on 20 minutes old scent along much frequented street ending in a house. It is followed by tracking on 30 minutes old scent intercepted with one right angle turn and then on obstacles like ditches, fences, etc. The age of scent is gradually increased to 40 minutes and then to 60 minutes over obstacles/interceptors with a turn. Subsequently, the length of the track is further increased to 500 metres intercepted with a turn. It is gradually increased to 1 km with two turns and then 2 km with more than two turns. The dog is now trained for identification of quarry amongst a group of 3 to 4 people at the end of the track and catching of the right forearm of the quarry.

After adequate practice and perfection on above-mentioned track work, the dog is conditioned to distinguish the diversionary tracks and conditioned to work under different types of climatic conditions as well as on all types of tracks so as to track up to 2 to 6 km on scent up to 24 hours old.

Identification Parades: The dog, after taking scent from the belongings, identifies the correct man from close line up or from a crowd immediately followed by identification of the correct man from well-spaced line-up of assorted people after following 50 metres track or the wanted person.

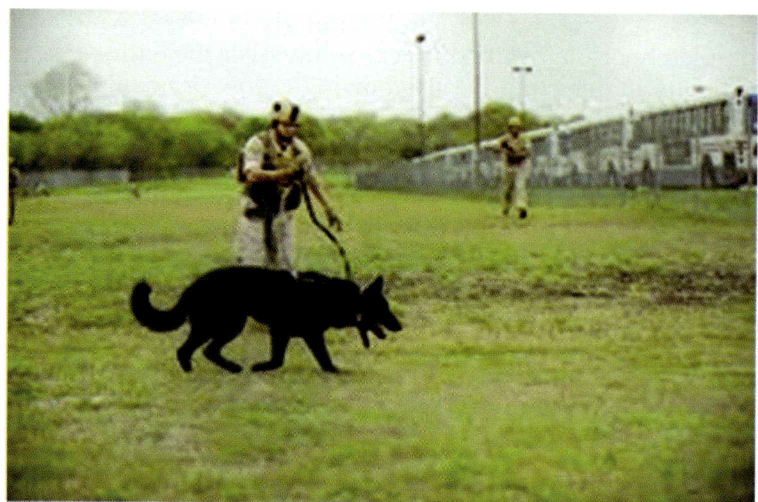

Distinguishing a quarry's article by scent: The dog is first trained to pick up the trainer's article from a pile after taking scent from the hand of trainer. Subsequently, the dog learns to pick out articles of strangers from pile after taking their scent.

Infantry Patrol (IP) Dog

The infantry patrol dog should be of medium to large size, intelligent, bold and possessing highly developed olfactory and acoustic capabilities which are respectively 40 and 20 times more developed than human beings. These traits are essential for an infantry patrol dog to learn detection of a human decoy by smell.

Training

With friendly encouragement from his handler and moving up wind, he is motivated to sniff air scent and he quickly learns as to what is expected of him on the word of command "move out." Immediately he starts sniffing the wind as well as the ground for scent of a human decoy and learns to give alert by some signs such as straining on leash or raising the ears. Each dog has his own way of alerting his handler who must watch carefully for the signals. While reading the dog, the handler must prevent his barking, growling, whining or making a noise otherwise which would be audible to the hidden enemy and may prove fatal in combat for both the dog and the handler.

Subsequently, the dog is encouraged to move towards the decoy, which runs away. The dog is now allowed to chase while being held on leash and after each successful performance, the dog is praised lavishly. After learning the basic rules the dog is then trained to detect decoys planted further and further away. To develop confidence, lessons are repeated under varied conditions, at different times of the day and night until the dog becomes expert enough to detect a decoy at distance up to five hundred yards or more. By quartering the area, the handler is able to determine the location of the strange sounds or smell detected by the dog. Trained to work silently, these dogs are used to accompany the patrols and give silent warning of a concealed enemy in a patrolled area so as to reduce the chances of fatal surprise or ambush. German Shepherds are more suitable for this specialty. However, Labradors, Collies and Malinois may also be used. Such dogs should not be easily excitable and not in the habit of barking, growling and whining. When the dog gives an alert and indicates the presence of strange scent, the handler is required to take a lying position, recall the dog with the help of a silent whistle and inform the patrol commander about the direction and location of the enemy depending upon the wind conditions.

The infantry patrol dog is also trained to pick up the scent of any cache of arms and ammunition along the route of deployment. Initially, haversacks, water bottles or some bundles of used clothing should be placed about 5 metres off the lane in upwind direction, and should be left uncovered so that the dog gets a strong scent and can give an observable alert. After interpreting the alert, the handler should recall the dog with the help of a silent whistle and take a lying position. The handler and the dog should behave in the same manner as in case of finding a decoy. The follow-up party then retrieves the arms, ammunition and equipment/stores slowly and suspiciously. The dog is now allowed to smell, sniff and investigate his find and the handler build up the dog's curiosity by whispering "good boy", etc. in his ears. Listening to his praise by his handler, the dog realizes that what has been found is as important as an alert on detecting the presence of decoy. The attentive handler must watch carefully for any weak alert to indicate the presence of cache in comparison to a strong alert to indicate an ambush since many a times the human scent of cache may not be as strong as it is of human decoy. The handler should concentrate on the modes of alert being given by a dog as this may vary slightly with each dog. At the word "move out", the infantry patrol dog carrying its head high should be able to move ahead of his handler and start scenting by sniffing into the air while maintaining visual contact with the handler for any change in the direction. Any tendency to bark whine or scowl should be discouraged, and if necessary, the dog may be muzzled.

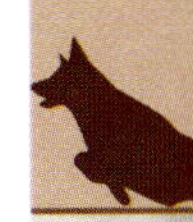

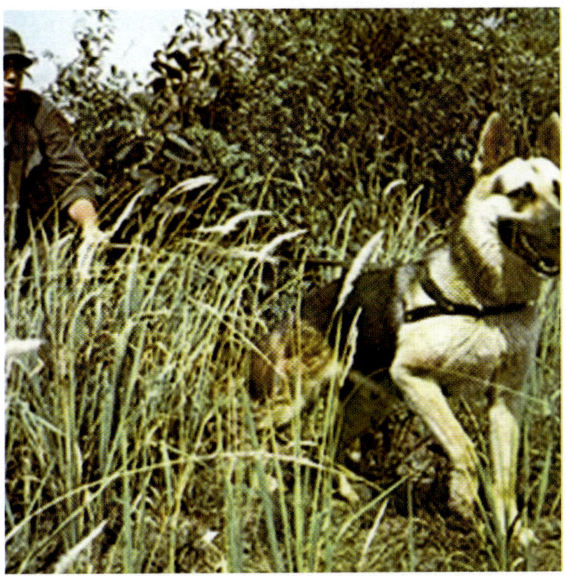

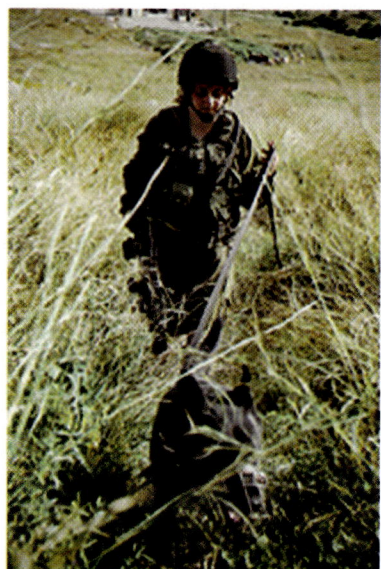

The infantry patrol dogs should be conditioned to work by day or night in all types of terrain and weather conditions up to 2 hours at a time and may again be re-employed after some rest. Properly trained dogs should not be disturbed by various kinds of noises. An infantry patrol dog is able to give an alert up to 300 metres or even more in most suitable conditions and up to 30 metres under adverse conditions.

Mine Detection (MD) Dog

The mine detection dog is non-aggressive and capable of giving response to indicate various types of mines and trip wires by smelling the scent given off by the buried object and its contents inclusive of the scent of the person who planted it. The mine detection dog also observes the physical changes in soil at the site and can indicate the presence of mine by sitting with in 60 cm of the target. For mine detection work, smaller to medium size Labradors, German Shepherds and Malinois, who are intelligent, willing and show inquisitiveness for ground scent, are considered suitable.

Training

Before starting the actual training, initial conditioning is a must which includes pen work to sniff training cans in a straight line having a piece of meat or a dog biscuit on top followed by making the dog to sit with in 60 cm of the sniffed cans. Subsequently, the track is widened to 1 metre and the cans are replaced by unprimed mines placed in a zigzag manner. After achieving the initial conditioning, width of the track is gradually increased and partially concealed mines are placed in a zigzag fashion. Later, concealment of mine is increased to 50% by using twigs or grass followed by fully concealed mines and the dog is initiated to use its nose more than its sight to locate the mine. Afterwards, the mines are partially buried leaving the edges of the holes unsealed followed by the mines fully concealed and camouflaged.

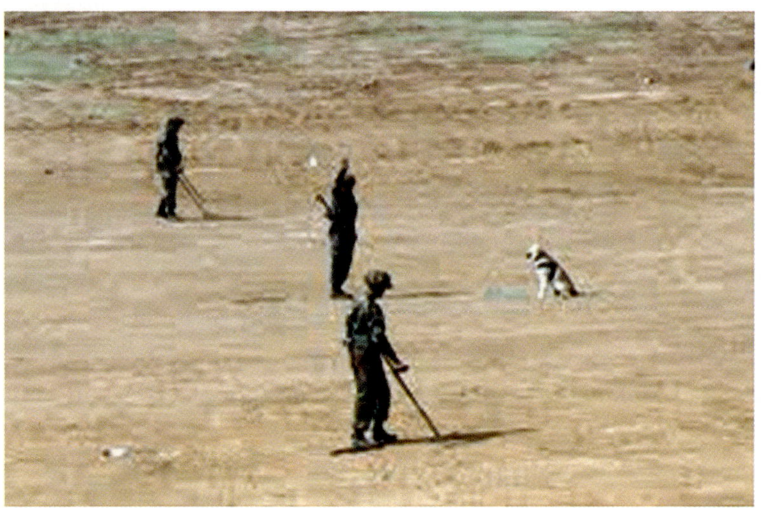

Trip Wire Detection

Trip wire detection training starts after the dog has completed the mine detection training and has learnt how to use his nose to detect the fully concealed mine complementing the teaching of sitting within 60 cm of the trip wire. To simulate the trip wire, initially white-coloured thick twine is stalked about 30 cm above the ground level across the trail followed by gradual reduction in the thickness of the twine. Dark-coloured twines are subsequently used along with some obviously visible colours. Later, all the dark-coloured threads are used to simulate trip wires and the height of threads, simulating as trip wire, is reduced or actual trip wire may also be used to replace threads. It is followed by placing the trip wires at varying height and different angles to the trail. After the dog has developed sufficient confidence in detecting the trip wire at various heights and various angles,the trip wire detection training is integrated with mine detection training. During the training, mine detection dogs should be taught how to work at appropriate pace of 30 metres per minute for a two metres lane. The trainer should take corrective measures for dogs having tendency either to run fast or move very slowly. Dogs should not be allowed to sit more than 60 cm on either side of the trail and tendency of some dogs to dig at the site of mine before or after giving indication must be curbed.

Explosive Detection (ED) Dog

The training of explosive detection dog involves olfactory sensitization to a primary explosive odour so as to make the dog capable of discrete odour discrimination for qualitative detection of various explosives. It is possible owing to the fact that dogs have a highly developed olfactory apparatus. The olfactory epithelium of dog is 30 times larger, olfactory receptors are 20 to 40 times more and cilia in the cells are double in the dogs as compared to the human being. Similarly, dogs have 150 sq. cm of surface area of nasal mucous membrane and possess about 225 million receptor cells and each of the receptor cells has 125 cilia whereas man has 5 sq. cm surface areas of nasal mucosa and possess 5 million receptor cells only.

An explosive detection dog should be of less aggressive temperament and friendlier appearance with good retrieving potential. He should be bold, inquisitive and willing to go to small places without shying from noises of traffic, etc. It is a known fact that a majority of explosive combinations are composed of a relatively small number of chemical ingredients that produce the primary odour for which the dog has to be conditioned and training of ED dogs on these common ingredients is considered adequate to detect all types of combinations. The explosive compounds commonly used in various types of explosives are categorized into following chemical families for the training purposes.

Nitro compounds: This group includes TNT and picric acid.

Nitrate esters: These compounds include nitro glycerin, ethylene glycol dinitrate, commonly called EGDN or dynamite, PETN, also called cordex, and nitrocellulose also called Gun cotton.

Nitramines: Tetryl also called PEK, RDX and HMX are the various compounds in this group.

Acid salts: These include ammonium nitrate, potassium chlorate and ammonium perchlorate.

Training

During the training, main emphasis is on the habit of sniffing to which the dog is initiated by sniffing of soup scent. Repeated learning and practice makes the dog to develop the habit of sniffing. It is followed by teaching the dog to sniff on word of command with and without leash. Later, pattern sniffing by spiral method and strip/ zigzag method and then article sniffing is taught and practiced. On satisfactory performance the dog is praised by saying "good boy" and is offered a tidbit so as to shape the dog's behaviour to the limit that the sniffing response becomes nearly habitual.

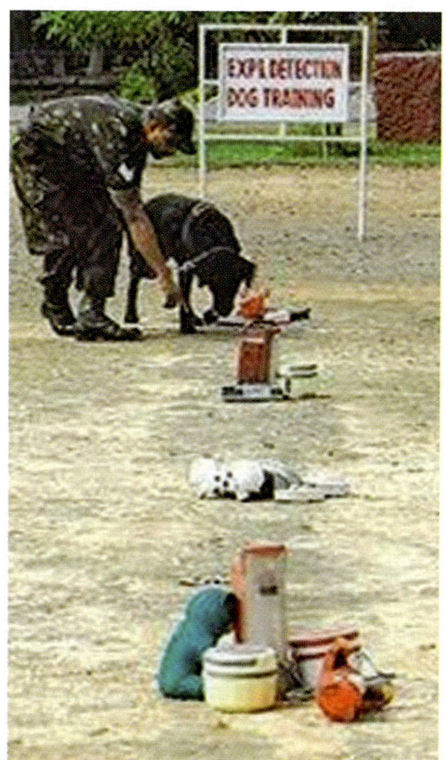

Further training includes sniffing packed explosives and gradually forming the habit to sniff explosives. To start with, high vapour pressure explosives are used for conditioning the dog. A small quantity of such explosive like gun powder is placed in a tin box/plastic jar, perforated with holes, and the dog is trained to sniff. The conditioning proceeds with the dog obtaining a reward upon inhaling/exhaling at the command "Sniff" and taught to respond by sitting on a positive target odour while ignoring negative and distracting odours. Gradually, the low vapour pressure explosives are used in descending order and the least volatile being the last. Soon the dog learns to respond by sitting for all primary explosive odour detection. It is followed by sniffing and conditioning on wrapped explosives followed by response to explosive vapours at various depths under the ground, in luggage/toys/airtight plastic containers/improvised explosive devices/landmines, etc. in different environment and climatic conditions. After this the dog is trained on odour signatures with captured explosives and conditioned to discriminate explosive vapours from distracting/masking vapours.

Finally, the dog is trained on various scenarios which include training for systemic sterilization (also called sanitization) of buildings, vehicles, aircrafts, ships, ground search and open area search which includes scenario based on environmental task training, etc.

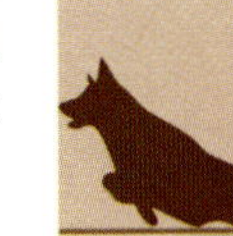

Performance Evaluation

The dog should be advanced from one stage to another only when he is constantly scoring at least eight out of ten positive indications on two consecutive evaluations and those failing to come up to the desired standard should be relegated. A fully trained ED Dog should be able to sterilize approximately 330 sq. ft area in 20 minutes and 2–4 km stretch of narrow lane depending upon environmental conditions. Normally a dog may do sniffing at the rate of 200 times per minute and gets tired after 20–30 minutes of continuous sniffing. As such, a rest of 10–15 minutes should be given to dog after each work session of 20–30 minutes.

Avalanche Rescue Operation (ARO) Dog

The dogs selected for this specialty should be of average size, strong, active, intelligent and possessing a good nose. Normally Labradors are preferred but German Shepherds and Malinois are also trainable. ARO Dogs are trained to trace the human scent under the snow and a fully trained dog should be able to locate the victim or his belongings 6–8 feet or even more deep in the snow. Before commencing the training, the dog and his handler are required to be acclimatized for ten days at an altitude of 9,000 feet. During this period, the handler should walk and play with dog on the snow for hardening the footpads of the dog and proper acclimatization.

Training

Initially, the dog is trained on the smell of a bone wrapped in a cloth or gunny bag which is buried 6 inches deep in the snow followed by other articles of the trainer buried up to 2 feet deep in the snow with the help of the trainer himself. The depth of the trainer's articles buried in snow is now increased up to 4 feet and the dog is given full freedom to search the area without any help of the trainer. Gradually, the trainer's articles are replaced by other articles of different types and the dog is trained and practiced to develop confidence in smelling all types of articles in fresh and wet snow. To avoid telltale marks, article should be buried before the fresh snow. Later, more than one article is buried six feet deep and the dog is trained to search these articles without distraction as well as with distraction.

Subsequently, a man, adequately clothed, is placed in a trench measuring 7 ft × 6 ft × 2 ft which is covered by snow up to one feet height and no telltale marks are left; followed by increasing the depth of the trench up to 6 feet. After the dog has developed confidence in detecting a human being and his belongings up to 6 to 7 feet

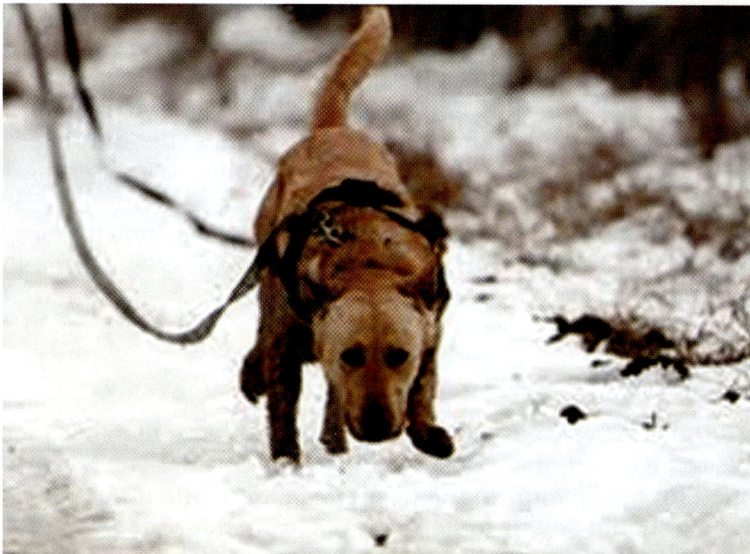

deep in the fresh and wet snow, more number of dummy victims are buried in zigzag fashion and distractions like food items, radio sets, weapons and equipment, etc. are added and the dog is practiced till perfection is achieved.

Finally, the subjects buried in a defined area are concealed from the sight of the dog as well as his handler and the dog along with his handler is left to search the area to detect the buried subjects. A well-trained team of ARO dog and his handler should be able to locate any one buried up to 6–7 feet deep in the snow in an area of around 5 acres in one hour. It must be kept in mind that a live man will survive if he can be recovered within 40 minutes of his burial in avalanche. It is a known fact that earliest employment and fast recovery save lives.

Search and Rescue Operation (SAR) Dog

A medium size, staunch, active, willing, intelligent and under aggressive dog is suitable for being trained as the SAR dog. Labradors, less aggressive German Shepherds, Malinois and Collies are commonly used for this purpose. These dogs are trained for unfamiliar scent of human beings in damaged buildings, heaps of rubble and debris, razed and fallen structures and natural environmental disaster and other calamities like earthquake, tsunami, etc.

Training

For training of SAR dogs, different types of damaging, devastating and natural calamities scenarios are simulated in the training area, for detection of scent of unfamiliar human beings, clothes and other belongings. Putting on the harness on dog is the sign of work, as such, it should only be used when the dog is employed. During training and practice dummy victims should avoid leaving ground scent as it will assist the dog to quarter at the appropriate site. The handler should follow closely behind the dog and when successful in search, the dog is encouraged to scratch the site or tuned to any other indication.

Environmental Effects on Training and Performance

Just as the environment affects soldiers performing their duties, the dog is also affected by his surroundings. It is important to become aware of the many different conditions that can affect their performance. However, all dogs are not affected in the same manner. Special consideration is given to the following factors:

Wind: Always consider the direction and velocity of the wind when using a war dog for any detection operations. This consideration holds true even indoors. There may be a slight breeze that will move a scent away from the location of its source. Fans, air conditioning units, and objects in motion can create winds that will affect the performance of a detector dog. In addition to these operational concerns, wind may create medical issues (such as blowing sand) that are negative. Wind also creates increased cooling, which is positive in hot weather but negative in cold weather.

Inclement weather: Precipitation can degrade the dog's performance of detection operations but do not assume that a dog will not be able to perform satisfactorily. The amount of moisture accumulated and the amount of time elapsed since the scent was left are variables. Dogs have been proven to be effective even in inclement weather.

Heat: When operating in locations of extreme heat, the dogs should be allowed sufficient time to acclimate. Care should be given to ensure that the dog does not sustain injuries to the pads of his paws due to excessive walking on concrete or pavement in extreme heat conditions. Always ensure that the dog has a fresh and constant source of drinking water.

Cold: Extreme cold temperatures should not deter war dog operations but special care should be taken to enable the dog to perform optimally in cold locations. The accumulation of moisture on the dog's paw pads can freeze and injure him. Using paw pad protectors to aid in the prevention of injury due to cold weather may be helpful, but the dog must be trained to wear them.

Terrain: The safety of the handler and the dog must be given the highest consideration when operating in hazardous terrain. Care should be taken when employment will take place in rocky or mountainous areas. Unfamiliar locations can pose threats in the form of caves, holes, loose footing, and other hazards.

Distraction: There are numerous distractions that can affect dog's performance. These are conditions that can cause the dog to focus his attention away from the desired task at hand. Planning and consideration should be given to eliminate or reduce distractions that hinder operations. Distractions are natural and also man-made such as the presence of other animals, a large number of people activities in the area of deployment, and various types of noise and smell.

Evaluation of Trained Dog's Performance

The evaluation authority should witness a demonstration of the dog's capabilities. All substances, the dog has been taught to respond on, should be used. Additionally, the dog's capability to detect past/present odour should be demonstrated by the dog and the handler. At the completion of the demonstration, the dog must obtain a 90–95 percent accuracy rate for the number of trials conducted. After clearing the evaluation test, the dog is considered fit to undertake task pertaining to its assigned role. Such evaluation of dog's performance should be carried out by the appropriate authority periodically so as to ensure the dog's reliability on a continuing basis. All the trained dogs in various disciplines must always maintain high standards of accuracy to provide the desired level of confidence in their tasks.

Training the Trainers

Continuous professional development of the dog trainers is the key to success of dogs. With the change in methods of employment over the ages, use of dogs has also undergone a sea change. Dogs are presently being used in various specialized jobs and being trained for many new tasks. However, it may be remembered that performances of dogs, no matter how highly trained, are not constant and they cannot be expected to work with same efficiency under all conditions. In order to ensure consistency in their performance, regular training and practice is of utmost important. The aim of training the trainers is to ensure professional competence of handlers and supervisory staff in employment of working dogs at all times and in every mission. Competency of dog handlers may be ensured by the following:

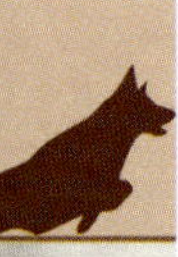

Refresher Training

Periodic refresher training is essential to enhance professional efficiency of dog handlers at appropriate time intervals. They should learn latest trends in dog psychology, training methodology, employment and retraining of specialized dogs. They should also update themselves about dog foods, feeding practices, care and management of dogs including first aid, kennel care and the management and transportation of dogs, etc.

Professional Update

Dog handler has to undergo various upgradation courses/training programmes and attain necessary qualification to become more and more proficient in his field. Higher standards should constantly be aimed for and in the process, he should be honed to achieve perfection. The most important factors in ensuring positive and result-oriented performance is on the job training, regular training and practice, special courses and monitored development along with the ability to demonstrate their proficiency, when subjected to simulated conditions.

Motivation

Only a motivated person, with dedication and commitment to team building, knowledge sharing and interaction can deliver the desired results. It is pertinent to mention that laid down methodology will impart the knowledge on the subject along with its effects, impact and uses but how perfectly the particular job is done depends upon the individual who has to be motivated to become a competent and a dedicated dog handler.

Assessment

The personnel are regularly assessed to ensure their proficiency for the assigned job. They should have a friendly attitude towards dogs along with patience and perseverance. All dog handlers should be good in physical endurance and must be able to exercise common sense. The handlers and the dogs must demonstrate their ability to work as perfect team.

Part 2

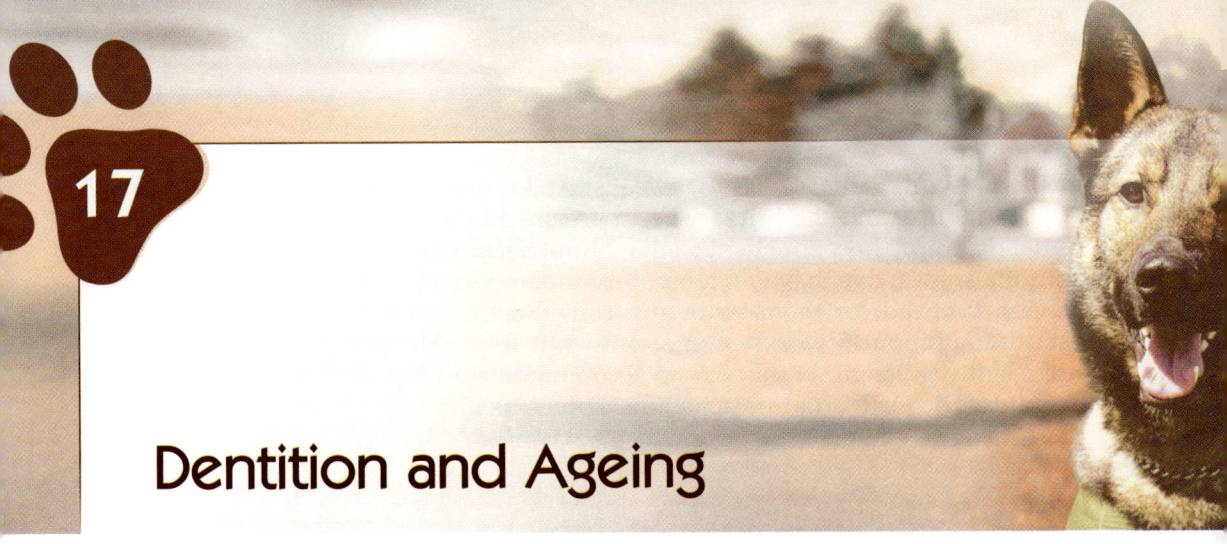

Dentition and Ageing

"Dogs have given us their absolute all. We are the center of their universe. We are the focus of their love and faith and trust. They serve us in return for scraps. It is without a doubt the best deal man has ever made."

... Roger A Caras

Dogs are carnivores and have teeth that reflect their meat-eating evolutionary history. Pet dogs, of course, have been turned into omnivores, as most dry dog foods contain substantial amounts of plant material. There are four types of teeth and they are designed to perform a specific function.

Symbol	*Teeth*	*Description*
I or i	Incisors	These are small teeth with a sharp cutting surface and are used for scraping meat remnants from bones, nibbling during grooming and to grasp food.
C or c	Canines	These teeth are ideal for piercing food and killing prey as they have pointed crowns.
P or p	Premolars	These teeth are used for crushing and cutting food.
M or m	Molars	These are larger than premolars and used for crushing and grinding food.

The layout of the teeth in the mouth can be described by a standard formula. As the structure of a normal skull is symmetrical (the left hand side being mirrored by the right hand side), the formula along the top line, describes only one side of the mouth with the maxillary teeth (those in the upper jaw) whereas the bottom line describes the mandibular (lower jaw) teeth. Capital letters are used to indicate permanent teeth, and lowercase for deciduous. Puppies have a total of 28 deciduous teeth consisting of: 3 upper and 3 lower incisors, 1 upper and 1 lower canine, 3 upper and 3 lower premolars on each side.

The dental formula of puppies is: $\mathbf{i^3/_3\ c^1/_1\ p^3/_3\ m^0/_0}$

Puppies initially develop a set of teeth collectively referred to as the primary, or deciduous, dentition. These primary teeth generally erupt or emerge into the oral cavity between the ages of 3 to 6 weeks. At 3 months of age, the permanent teeth begin to erupt, and the primary teeth are shed or exfoliated. The first premolars and molars erupt as permanent teeth without deciduous predecessors. As the dental formula shows, they have no temporary molars. At such an early age the puppies have little need for them—moving from their mothers milk through weaning (starting at about 3 weeks of age) onto soft food. The jaw bone has not grown sufficiently in length at that age to accommodate all the teeth types an adult dog requires. The teeth eruption schedule is given as under:

	Deciduous	*Permanent*
Incisors	4–6 weeks	3–5 months
Canines	5–6 weeks	4–6 months
Premolars	6 weeks	4–5 months
Molars		5–7 months

Adult dogs have a total of 42 permanent teeth consisting of: 3 upper and 3 lower incisors, 1 upper and 1 lower canines, 4 upper and 4 lower premolars and 2 upper and 3 lower molars on each side.

The dental formula of adult dog is: $\mathbf{I^3/_3\ C^1/_1\ P^4/_4\ M^2/_3}$

As permanent teeth develop within the jaws, resorption causes the roots of the deciduous teeth to be absorbed by the surrounding tissues. This process of exfoliation of primary teeth and eruption of permanent teeth is usually complete by 6 months of age. The time when the mouth contains both primary and permanent teeth in functional positions is called the period of mixed dentition. Tooth eruption is facilitated by osteoclasts that resorb alveolar bone, forming an eruption pathway for the tooth to exit its bony crypt. Eruption is controlled by genetic, environmental, infectious and traumatic factors. As noted, in most dogs, the deciduous teeth are fully erupted by 2 months of age, and usually by 6 months they are replaced by permanent (secondary or adult teeth). The canines erupt first, followed by the incisors, then the fourth, third and second premolars, for a total of 28 primary teeth.

Each tooth is divided into three parts:

Crown: It is the free part of tooth, which is seen above the gum.

Neck: The constricted part which is encircled by the gum, and divides the crown from the root.

Root: This is that part of tooth which is inserted in a cavity in the jaw bone.

The structure of the crown is different in each jaw, in the upper jaw it is composed of one main lobe and two lateral lobes whereas in the lower jaw it has one main and one lateral lobe. It is by noting the number and type of teeth erupted and the wear of the main lobes that an estimation of the age is made. Unfortunately, the wear, depending on factors such as the set of the jaws, the inherent hardness of the teeth and the habits of individual dogs, exhibit considerable individual variations. The lobe of a dog which habitually gnaws stones and bones will wear much more rapidly. Ageing process in relation to eruption of teeth and their wearing off can be correlated to the actual age of dogs when in dispute. Although proper documentation of dogs

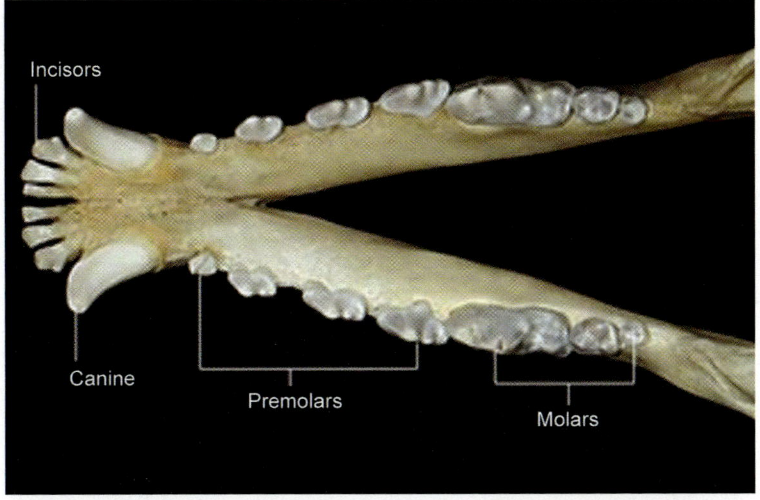

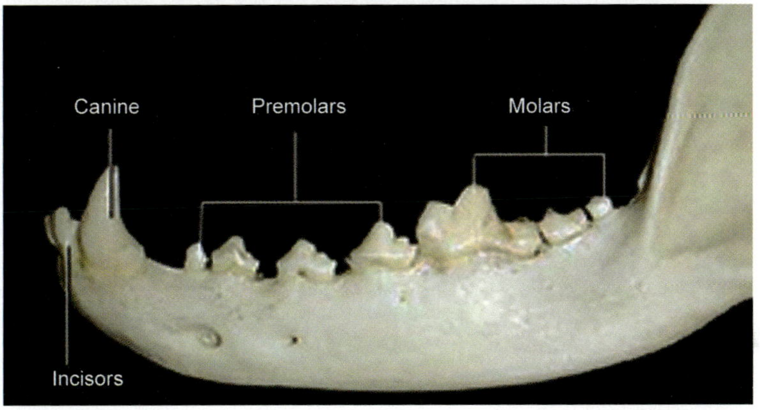

contain all details including correct age, however, in case of ambiguity, teeth of the dog are of utmost value in determination of the dog's age besides other factors such as the general appearance of the animal and the graying of the muzzle.

The following table shows the changes which occur in the teeth of the average dog:

At birth	*No teeth*
1 to 2 months	Milk teeth erupt.
3½ to 5 months	Milk incisor teeth are shed and the permanent incisors appear.
5 to 6 months	Milk canines (fangs) are shed and the permanent canines erupt.

(Contd.)

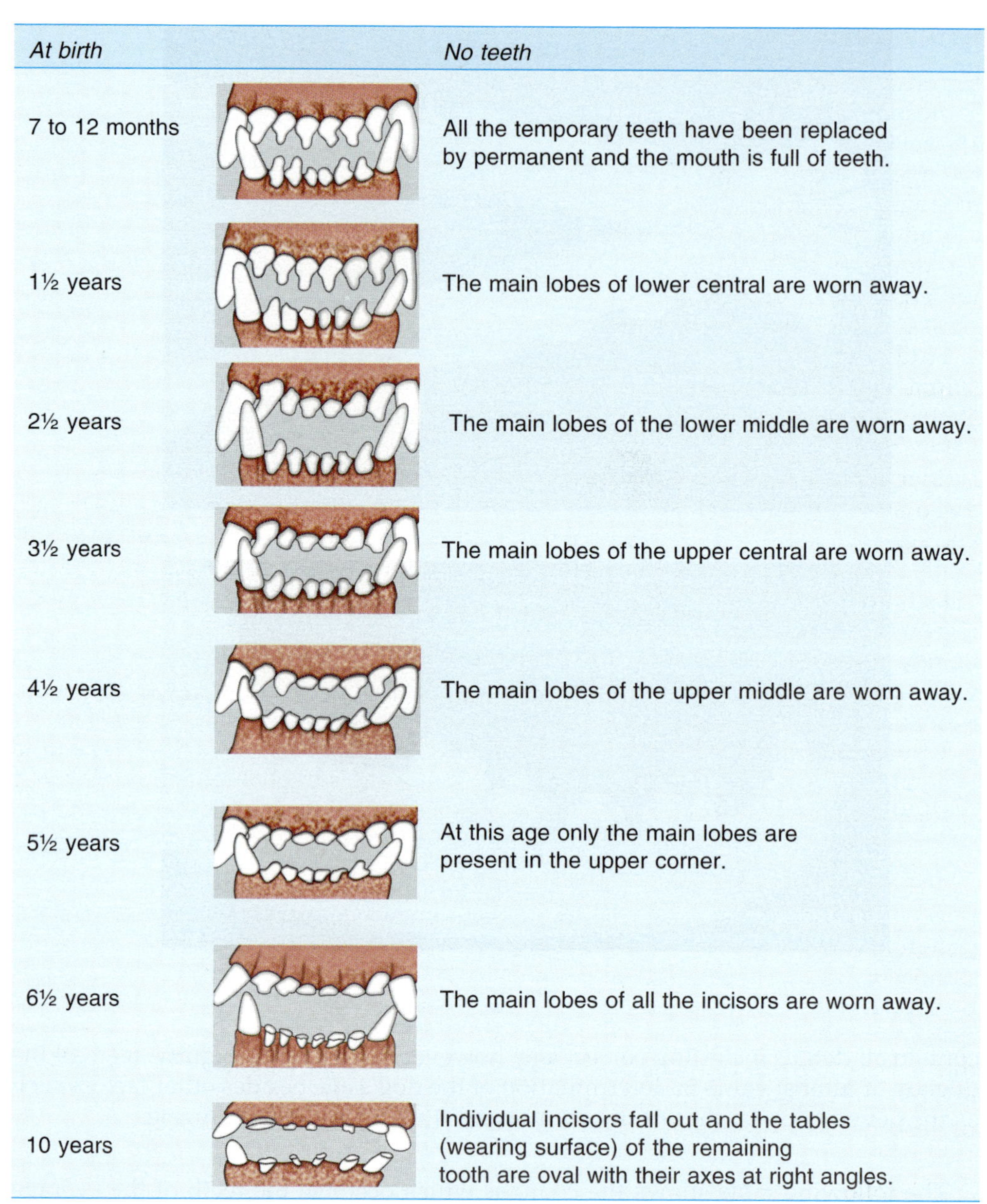

At birth	*No teeth*
7 to 12 months	All the temporary teeth have been replaced by permanent and the mouth is full of teeth.
1½ years	The main lobes of lower central are worn away.
2½ years	The main lobes of the lower middle are worn away.
3½ years	The main lobes of the upper central are worn away.
4½ years	The main lobes of the upper middle are worn away.
5½ years	At this age only the main lobes are present in the upper corner.
6½ years	The main lobes of all the incisors are worn away.
10 years	Individual incisors fall out and the tables (wearing surface) of the remaining tooth are oval with their axes at right angles.

Other changes that help in assessing the age are:

- At 4–5 years, in the majority of dogs, grey hairs appear on the muzzle.
- At 6–7 years, there is very often cataract formation which causes blurring of vision.
- At 10 years, hollows appear above the eyes and there is dishing of the face below the eyes due to sinking of the bones of the cheeks as a result of teeth falling out.

TEETH AND BITE GENETICS

Heredity of teeth and bite is mostly unknown and presents a confusing pattern. It is mostly unknown if it is dominant, recessive or polygenic for each abnormality. However, these teeth and bite faults can be seen with a simple visual inspection by the age of 1 year, which means that affected dogs can easily be kept away from breeding. The most commonly seen issues in dogs are missing teeth, fused teeth, oligodontia (absence of most if not all teeth), overbite/overshot bite, retained deciduous teeth (baby teeth do not fall out by themselves), extra teeth, underbite/ undershot bite and wry mouth (or wry nose or jaw). Dogs with brachycephalic skull type (Bulldog, Boxer) may frequently have imperfect dentition.

Studies of dentition done with German Shepherds, were not indicative of any simple mode of inheritance. The difficulty of identifying the heredity of missing teeth is compounded by the fact that apparently missing teeth are sometimes present below the gum rather than totally absent. Such dog is considered unsuitable for further breeding and should be discarded from a breeding programme, even if the dog otherwise possess outstanding qualities. Abnormal bites vary in levels of severity and some breeds and lines within breeds appear to have a higher incidence of bite faults than others. It is seen that some lines or individuals do produce more incorrect bites than breed averages, leading to a general familial inheritance pattern. Some researchers have suggested that the shortening of the lower jaw and muzzle might be responsible for incorrect bites and missing teeth. It has been observed that dogs with undershot bites usually have parents with scissors bites, suggesting that the trait is recessive.

Upper and lower jaw structures appear to be independently inherited traits and even the size of the incisors may play a role in occlusion. Abnormal size and overly vertical incisors can also create incorrect bite.

Puppy Bite Information

In general, a puppy's bottom jaw will continue to grow until they are approximately 9 months old, which means the bite is in transition until 9–11 months of age. It should be noted that the upper jaw is also in transition and growing during this period. The bite can go either way, from scissors to underbite or from scissors to overbite, or from scissors to level bite. It is a general observation in some breeds that a puppy which starts off with an overbite, even if it corrects later on, can have a higher incidence of producing more puppies with overbites. Puppies with underbites almost never correct themselves.

18

Foods and Feeding

"The dog in life, the finest friend, first to welcome, foremost to defend, Whose heart is still his master's own, Who labours, fights, breathes for him alone."

... Lord Byron

Food is necessary to the dog to build up the tissues and organs during growth, make good the wastage due to wear and tear, keep up the body temperature, supply the necessary energy for internal and external work. After ingestion the food is broken down into the main nutrients, which are then utilized by the dog for various body functions. Working dogs require a balanced diet to grow and to maintain health once they are mature. Nutrients are components in the diet that have specific functions within the body and that contribute growth, reproduction, body tissue maintenance and optimal health performance. Essential nutrients are those components that cannot be synthesized by the body at a rate that is required to meet the body's needs. Therefore, essential nutrients must be supplied in diet whereas non-essential nutrients can be synthesized in body hence not required in diet. The dogs require six major categories of nutrients, i.e. water, carbohydrates, proteins, fats, minerals and vitamins.

Water

All foods, even those that have been naturally air-dried, contain a certain amount of water. Most of the water a dog requires is consumed as drinking water but a small amount is derived from the food. Dogs can live for long periods without taking solid food but very quickly suffer dehydration if given no water. This is illustrated by the fact that a dog can lose practically all its fat and over half its flesh but still lives whereas a loss of one tenth of its water content will result in death. Without water the dry matter of the food can neither be digested nor absorbed. The total water needs of the animal vary with its environment and the quantity of food it consumes.

Carbohydrates

These are energy producing substances and are contained mainly in cereals and vegetables. Foods of animal origin contain very little carbohydrates.

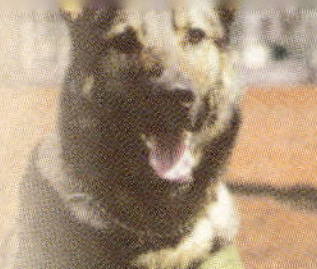

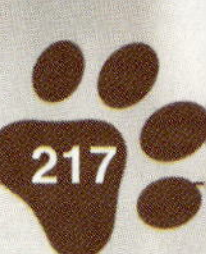

Fats

These are found mainly in the fat portion of meat. After being absorbed they are then oxidized to provide energy or are deposited in the tissues as reserve fat for future use.

Proteins

These substances are required for flesh making and tissue building. A young growing dog needs a higher proportion of proteins than the mature animal in which they are mainly utilized to make good, general wear and tear. They are mostly contained in meat, fish, milk and eggs.

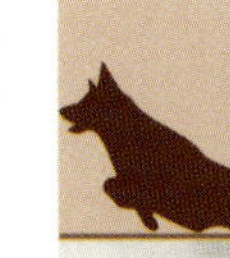

Minerals

They form about 3 per cent of the dog's weight, the presence of mineral salts in the diet is most essential especially in young animals. In the body they are found in the bones, hair, muscles, sweat and some fats. They are required mostly as compound of calcium and phosphorus and are contained in vegetables, cereals and bones.

Vitamins

These accessory food factors are essential to the health and growth of the animal. They exercise an influence in the nutrition in proportion to the required quantity consumed. Their absence from diet leads to definite symptoms of disease. They are of special importance during the period of growth of young animals and are present in milk, fresh vegetables, meat and liver.

TOTAL ENERGY REQUIREMENT OF DIFFERENT CATEGORIES OF DOGS

For this purpose working dogs can be classified as growing, moderately working and hardworking dogs. Dogs which have not yet attained adulthood, i.e. till 1 year of age are termed as growing. Dogs performing job involving less than 6 km of walk/run per day are classified as moderately working whereas dogs running more than 6 km per day are termed as hardworking dogs.

When it comes to nutrition, dogs are a lot like humans. They are omnivores, meaning they can live healthy lives while eating a variety of food. Meats, vegetables, and grains, all can be a part of a dog's diet. But also like us, dogs need balanced, moderately-sized meals that fuel their activities. An over indulgent diet will expand their waistlines and put them at risk of diseases. It is simply true saying that for a perfect food for dogs, return them to their environmental roots. They need daily interesting activity, fresh air, clean water, romps in nature, lots of love and food as close to the form they would find in the nature. Fresh whole natural foods when fed in variety are good, if health is the goal. However, to get a natural or packaged food as close as possible to that goal, requires the expertise to design and manufacture such foods.

Working dogs are provided nutritious ration which is based on job requirement. The total energy requirement of such dogs can be met by 680 gm meat, 480 gm atta/rice, 230 gm fresh seasonal vegetables and 30 gm dog biscuits. In addition, vitamins and minerals should be given as on required basis. Dogs are able to digest a variety of foods and this remarkable adaptability of the dog has led to the successful use of commercial diets that differ widely in their ingredient composition. The pet food industry has well-established markets in developed countries but it plays minor role in developing countries. Good quality ready to eat pellet feed are available in market which is convenient to carry and easier to feed at any location. The quantity of feed to be given to dogs is determined based on the size, weight and work being performed by the dog. Each brand of such feed gives guidelines to calculate the daily quantity of feed required by various categories of working dogs.

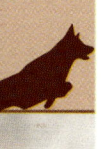

The dogs are normally fed twice daily by the handler himself, the evening meal being heavier. There should not be frequent changes in feeding time and the food should be properly made before giving to the dog. Dogs should not be fed immediately before or after work and those employed at night should be given light meal early in the evening and heavy meal in the morning. The dog should not be disturbed when having food, otherwise he tends to become aggressive. Fresh, clean drinking water should always be available near the dog for drinking as on required basis.

Requirement of feed

Requirement of feed components	*Proteins* (%)	*Carbohydrates* (%)	*Fat* (%)
Growing dogs	27	32	41
Moderately working dogs	26	36	38
Hardworking dogs	32	36	38

19

Care and Management of Working Dogs

"All knowledge, the totality of all questions and answers, is contained in the dog."

...Franz Kafka—Investigations of the dog

Working dogs should be kept physically fit at all times so as to make optimal use of their work potential for which they have been trained. It is, therefore, imperative for the users to remain acquainted with the general information pertaining to kenneling, feeding, health and daily routine which keeps them in excellent working state.

KENNELS

The kennel whether permanent or temporary must be comfortable for the dog, watertight and windproof, adequately ventilated without being draughty. Selection of site for kennels should be done keeping in view the important requirement such as quietness of the surroundings, drainage facilities, adequate area availability for training and support utilities and other functional considerations.

Permanent Kennel

A permanent kennel complex for the required number of dogs should consist of individual dog kennels, a support building, an obedience course, an exercise area, a dog break area, a exterior storage and a training area, etc. The entire complex should be enclosed, with a heavy-duty, 8-feet-high chain-link fence with three strands of straight wire (no barbed) at the top to prevent a war dog from climbing or jumping out. Ideally, there should be one kennel for each dog, comprising a room with floor area of 3.50 square metres, 1 metre wide veranda in front of room and a 3 metres deep courtyard. Normal height of room should be 3 metres and that of veranda and courtyard may be 2 metres. Central covered passage with doors at either side should be 1.50 metres wide and 3 metres high. Hence each kennel inclusive of sleeping accommodation and run should not be less than 11 square metres.

Ventilation system in kennel should ensure a proper circulation of fresh air and avoid draughts. The lighting system should ensure maximum benefit from the sunlight. In addition, artificial light system with electricity and heating/cooling arrangements must also be provisioned. All electrical wires should be encased in metal tubes so as to avoid accidental shock through damaged wires. The kennels may be grouped into blocks depending upon the number of kennels required. These may be single or double and when double blocks are built they may be erected back to back or separated by a central passage. The plinths should be raised 6 to 10 inches from the ground with proper drainage facilities. The floor and passages should be made up of concrete and cement and the slope of the floor be such that it drains out all water in the drainage pipe/channel outside the block. A tick channel may be provisioned around the kennels so as to avoid crawling of ticks inside. Kennels should be kept clean at all times and routinely disinfected using diluted antiseptic solutions or by using blow lamp/flame gun. **However, use of carbolic group disinfectants are not recommended since dogs are highly susceptible to carbolic poisoning**. Warning signs should be posted on the exterior fencing and buildings of the kennel and exercise area. Signs should contain the following words: **"DANGER—WAR/MILITARY/ARMY DOG AREA."** Personnel approaching the kennel area should be able to see and read the warning signs under normal daylight conditions from a distance of 50 m.

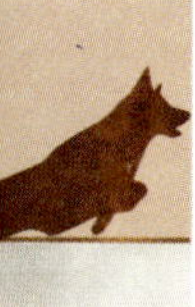

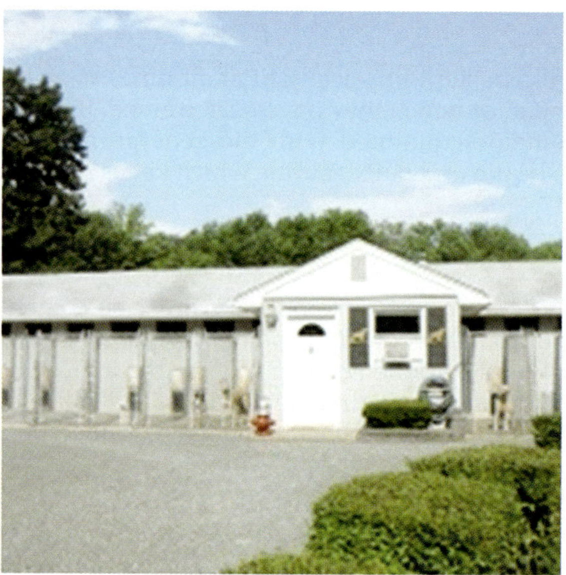

Permanent kennel

Obedience Course

The obedience course measuring 150 feet × 150 feet should be provisioned near the permanent kennel complex. It plays an important role in maintaining the dog's agility and stamina as well as in reinforcing obedience and proficiency training. The course should be grassed and free of hazards, e.g. trees, large rocks, holes, and burrs, etc. that may be harmful to dogs and handlers. The site should be graded for drainage but minimally sloped to provide a level field for training. The area should be enclosed with an 8-feet-high chain-link fence.

Dog break area: A dog break area measuring 10 feet × 20 feet should be located near the kennels. A break area allows the handler to release the dog immediately after exiting the kennels or before entering the kennels so that the dog can relieve himself. The area should be enclosed with an 8-feet-high chain-link fence. The ground can be a sandy area for cleaning ease and should have a water source.

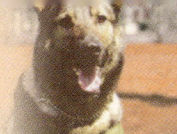

Exercise area: The exercise area measuring 20 feet × 40 feet is a space where the dog can be released without the handler being present. The exercise area should not be a shared area with the obedience course, as it would conflict with training objectives. The exercise area should be visually separated from the obedience course to prevent dog from being distracted during training and should preferably be grassed, hazard free, and graded slightly for drainage purposes.

Temporary Kennel

The temporary kennels often, as a result of the location, various facilities are limited at the site but it does not imply that the kennel itself should give any less comfort or protection to the dog. The structure should be sufficiently durable to withstand the

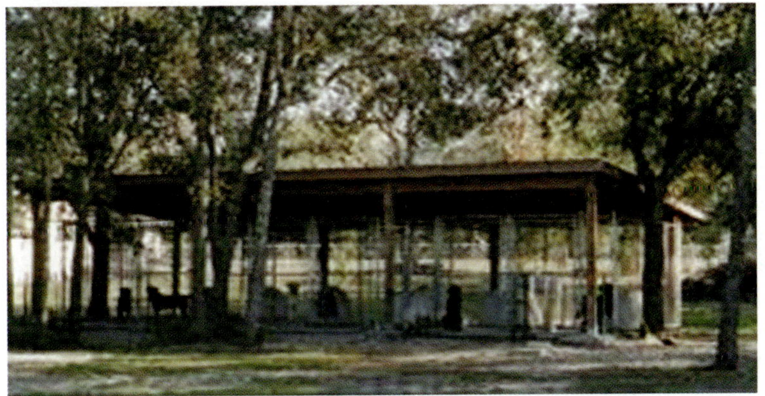

Temporary kennels

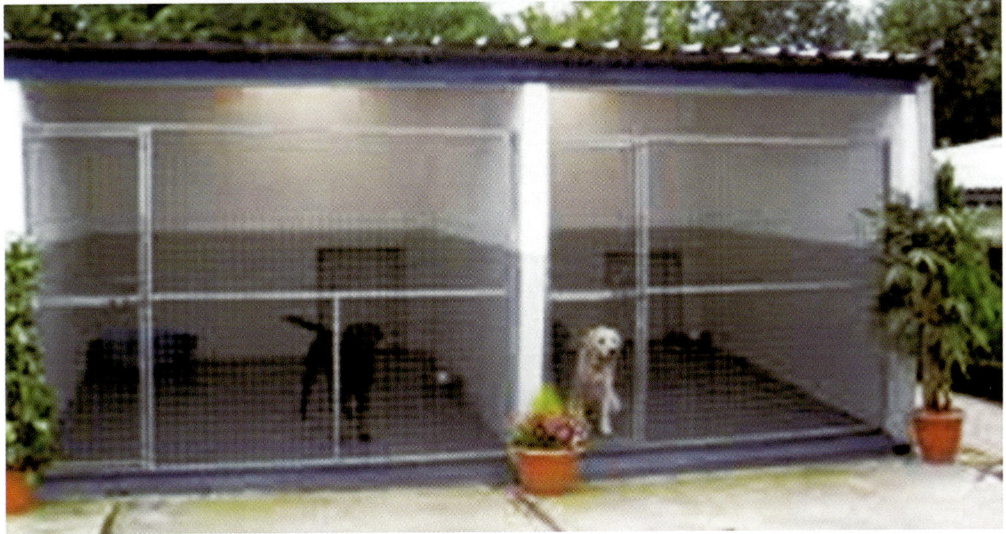

Temporary kennel

vagaries of harsh weather conditions. In addition, potable water, sanitary measures, electric and telephone facilities are considered bare essential. At times, it may be possible to obtain the use of an existing building or other structures for temporary kennels. In this case it should be ensured that the building is well-ventilated, safe, and structurally sound and without hazards (such as chemicals, bare wires, holes, or debris) that can cause injury to the dogs. Improvised kennel may be constructed for a limited period, out of any available resource locally. The design is not standard and varies from site to site depending on the location, mission, and duration of operations. Using a concept similar to constructing fighting positions, the temporary kennels will be improved continuously as needed or until a permanent facility is completed. Using tents may be a quick method of setting up temporary kennels. Although this method is not optimal for sustained operations, it may be useful until other accommodations can be coordinated. Erect the tents at a location that allows the dogs a safe place to rest away from other troop activities after operations. Whenever possible, place a barrier between troop activities area and the temporary kennel. Temporary kennel site should never be selected near motor pools, dining facilities, or high noise areas. In these kennels, space availability for each dog should be adequate. The structure should have proper ventilation facility and properly cleanable with drainage facility as per the requirement.

Portable Kennel

Portable kennels are also available in various designs for use in field conditions and also for transporting dogs. These kennels house a dog comfortably and can be easily shifted from one place to another. These kennels should preferably have a length of 1.43 metres, width 1.13 metres, height 1.05 metres in front and minimum 90 centimetres in rear. Use of these kennels should be for a limited period only and not as an alternative to permanent kennel.

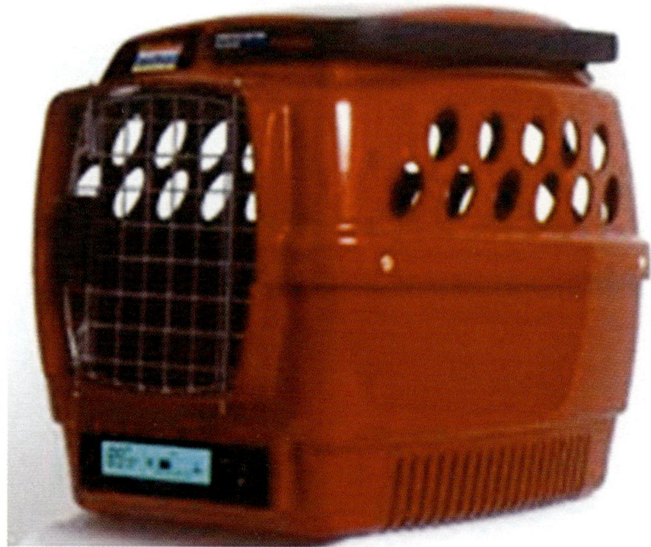

Portable kennel

It is a common practice that wherever possible, a dog be provided with its own shelter, however, there are occasions especially in the jungles where sharing of its handler's bivouac might be necessary to stop restlessness or whining. It will also ensure that any silent warning, the dog might give, will be immediately transmitted to its handler. High altitudes and extra cold climates do not pose great problem since the dogs withstand the cold quite well. However, physical strain on body and likelihood of respiratory disorders should always be taken care off. When the dogs work in high altitude for prolonged time, they should be protected against breathlessness, loss of appetite and photosensitization. Accordingly, as far as possible, kennel should be sited near the hill cliff to avoid winds and draught. Temperature inside kennel needs to be regulated, alternatively, the dog should be provided with appropriate cold extreme cold clothing. Flooring in kennel may be of wooden or concrete and cement and should always be kept dry. Further, before kenneling, dogs should be properly dried after work and adequately groomed along with necessary care of footpads. Food and water should be given at body temperature and older dogs should be constantly monitored for disorders of urinary system and respiratory system.

Hygiene and Sanitation

Removal of all excreta from the kennel and its cleanliness as well as that of surrounding area is the most essential routine every day. It is not necessary to wash the kennel, especially in cold weather, however, if washing of kennel is required then it should be ensured that it is dry before the dog is put back into it. Mild disinfectants, other than those belonging to carbolic group, may be used, though they are not necessary unless there is prevalence of some infectious diseases.

Exercise and Daily Routine

The daily routine of working dogs consists of kennel out for stool site and recording of temperature before sunrise, walk and run exercise for 3–5 kilometres in 45 minutes and occasionally getting the dog to negotiate small obstacles. Practice/training session as per the requirement of working dog, for about 2 hours with a break in the middle of session, is considered necessary to ensure the optimal work efficiency of the dog. This is followed by grooming for 30 minutes, feeding and kennel out for stool site and midday rest. The afternoon routine is repetition of light exercise and job specific training/practices with special reference to any weakness in performance earlier observed.

To maintain a dog in a healthy, well-muscled and physically fit condition, he must be given exercise every day even if the dog is regularly working. A dog which is not under the complete control of his trainer/handler should be exercised individually on leash. Similarly, in the initial stages, while employed for working on snow, occasional bleeding from the footpads may be observed, accordingly, the dog should be carefully observed for such condition during first two weeks till the footpads are suitably hardened. During acclimatization, training and work, making snow balls/heaps at regular intervals should be a part of the practice to easily find out the starting point. However, working in bright sunshine, rains and snowing weather conditions should only be when absolutely essential.

Rest and Sleep

The working dog should be provided with a wooden sleeping board (5 feet × 3 feet), a dog blanket and a dog coat besides other items. In case the sleeping board is not available, improvised bedding should be arranged to give adequate comfort to the dog.

Dog Equipment

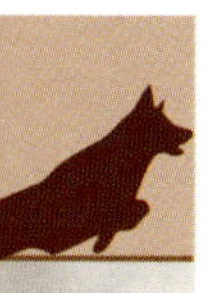

The equipment that is required for care of a working dog includes brushes, tweezers, blankets, towel, durries, putties, water bottle, rubber ball, stainless steel feeding basin, chain tether, waterproof dog coat, dog collar, steel comb, wooden dumbbell, dog harness, leash rope, dog muzzle, pilot rope and any other item which may be required as per training and employment needs.

Grooming

A dog is groomed twice daily for 30 minutes throughout the year as well as when he returns from any outdoor assignment. The grooming offers the handler an opportunity to become friendly with his dog and to find out any wounds, injuries, external parasites or any skin infections, etc. troubling the dog. While grooming, firstly, the dog is checked for the presence of ticks to prevent tick-borne infections. Ticks also cause irritation to dogs resulting in loss of condition. Particular attention is paid to the favourite sites of ticks like between the paws, behind the ears and in the folds of neck. The ticks are manually picked up with the help of forceps/tweezers and put in kerosene oil and later destroyed by burning. Next, the hair and skin are attended to. The hairy coat of the dog provides protection against the vagaries of climate and also acts as a safeguard against injuries. The coat grows thick in winter and thin in summer. The German Shepherds have two coats, soft woolly under coat, which lies close to the body, and an outer coat composed of longer and coarser hair. This outer layer also serves the purpose of water repellent. The other breed of dogs, i.e. Labradors and Malinois have short coat. The actual cleaning of the coat and skin is done with the help of brush and steel comb. To start with, the dog is given a vigorous massage with the tips of the fingers which brings out the hidden dust, loosens the broken hair and stimulates the blood circulation of the skin. Then the hair coat is brushed with a body brush in circular manner followed by brushing in the direction of the hair. After this, a steel comb is used to untangle the mated hairs and to remove the dead and tangled hair. Finally, the dog is massaged vigorously with the flat of the palm to give a shiny and glossy appearance. During the grooming process following organs are specially attended to:

Eyes: Any discharge, when present, should be removed with clean cotton soaked in warm water. If any symptoms of infection or injury are noted, for example, lacrimation, congestion, injury and opacity, the dog must be taken for veterinary examination and appropriate treatment.

Teeth: The teeth of the dog require regular attention. Discoloured or stained teeth may be cleaned with a weak solution of hydrogen peroxide once a month. Should the accumulation of tartar be excessive, it may be necessary to scale them from time to time. This should be carried out under supervision of expert/veterinarian.

Ears: The daily inspection and cleaning of the ears is most important. The accumulation of wax and dirt can, especially in long-eared dogs, cause severe inflammation and irritation. Wax and dirt are best removed with the aid of either dry/wet cotton wool.

Nails: With regular exercise nails remain in proper shape. However, they must be watched for overgrowth. Overgrown nails should be trimmed so as to avoid splitting leading to lameness. Excessive cutting of nails should not be practiced as it may also cause lameness.

Anus: Regular inspection of the anal sphincter is required to see if any segments of tapeworms are sticking or protruding. Regular watch is also kept to see if anal glands are impacted. The anal sphincter and anal glands lubricate the passage of stools and are normally prevented from getting impacted by the process of defecation. However, if they are impacted, a piece of cotton wool is placed over the anus and firm pressure is applied with the forefinger and thumb which relieves the impaction.

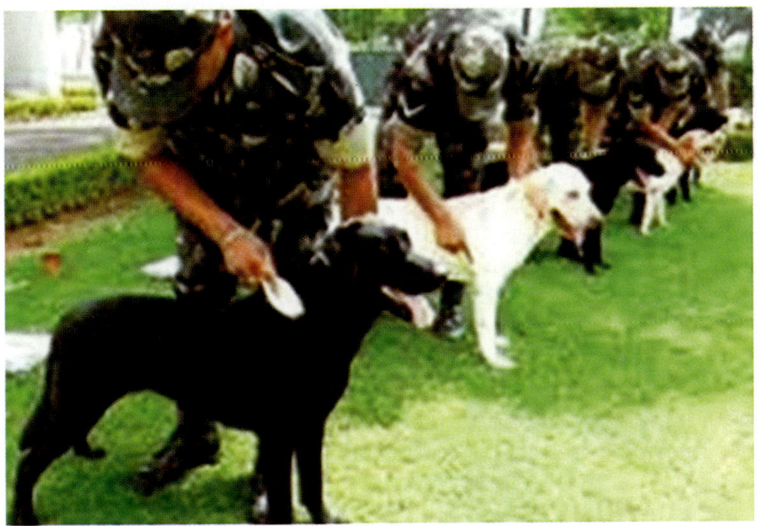

Grooming of dogs

The sequence of grooming which should be followed is as under:

Examination of the dog	1 minute
De ticking	5 minutes
Massage with tips of the fingers	6 minutes
Brushing	10 minutes
Combing	2 minutes
Cleaning of eyes, ears, teeth and anus	3 minutes
Setting the hair	2 minutes
Final touch	1 minute
Total	**30 minutes**

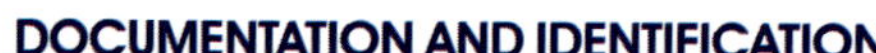

DOCUMENTATION AND IDENTIFICATION

The individual details of working dogs should be documented appropriately so that they may be readily identified at the time of birth. It is also the time to get the pup registered with the national/regional kennel club as per the local requirement. Furthermore, a complete record of their details should always be maintained. The individual details are its number, name, breed, sex, age and description. All this information should be on a working dog history sheet/card and a separate sheet/card should be made and maintained for each dog.

Numbering

Each dog should be given a number which is tattooed on the inside of the left ear. The following system known as Preston system of numbering may be followed to number 4,000 animals with each letter selected. If the letter "A" is to be used the first number in the series will be "A000", the second "A001", the third "A002" and so on up to "A999" which completes the first thousand. The second thousand will be numbered "0A00", "0A01", "0A02" up to "9A99". The third thousand will commence "00A0" and finish "99A9" and the fourth thousand will commence "000A" and finish with "999A".

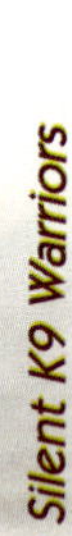

Tattooing

For tattooing, the dog is required to be securely muzzled and firmly held by its handler. The most suitable method of restraint requires handler to straddle the dog, which has been put in the sitting position, and to grasp the collar and a fold of skin on either side of the neck. The operator then thoroughly clips the hair on the inside of the left ear, and after cleaning with methylated spirit, infiltrates the area with a local anaesthetic. A liberal coating of tattooing ink is then applied and the operator standing in front of the dog, opens the jaws of the tattooing instrument and slips the ear flap between them. By pressing firmly on the handles, the jaws of the instruments are brought together and the needles forced into the body of the ear. They are kept in this position for about 3 seconds and then the ear is released. To ensure that sufficient ink penetrates the punctured site, a further application is smeared with cotton wool.

Naming

The name of dog should be short, not more than two syllables, easy to remember and, when possible, describe some outstanding characteristics of the dog. It may also be ensured that in one group of dog population, names are not repeated so as to avoid confusion at a later date.

Description

For description purposes, the general colour of the dog is noted first. It is followed by description of each body regions, i.e. head, neck, body, legs and tail. The general colours of the dog usually consist of one or two primary colours, the dominant colour being recorded, e.g. black and tan, sable and fawn. However, frequently seen colours also include black, brindle, fawn, sable, tan and yellow (golden). When describing the individual regions, variations of colour and any unusual markings are noted, e.g. tail fawn, light fawn underneath, etc. Besides the colour, any distinguishing feature such as crop, prick or lop ears, curled or docked tail and scars which are considered to be permanent are recorded.

PROTECTIVE VACCINATION

To ensure good health, working dogs are regularly vaccinated against contagious and infectious diseases, e.g. canine parvovirus, canine coronavirus, canine distemper, infectious canine hepatitis, canine parainfluenza, rabies, leptospirosis and tetanus, etc. so as to develop immunity against these diseases and to keep the dogs in physically fit state. Vaccinating a dog has long been considered one of the easiest ways to help him to live a long, healthy life. There are different vaccines for different diseases and also different types and combinations of vaccines.

A veterinarian can determine a vaccination regime that will provide the safest and best protection for the dog. Vaccines help to prepare the body's immune system to fight the invasion of disease-causing organisms. Vaccines contain antigens, which look like the disease-causing organism to the immune system but don't actually cause disease. When the vaccine is introduced to the body, the immune system is mildly stimulated. If a dog is ever exposed to the real disease, his immune system is now prepared to recognize and fight it off entirely or reduce the severity of the illness.

Bottom line vaccines are very important in managing the health of the dog and every dog needs to be vaccinated against the diseases. It is very important to discuss with the veterinarian a vaccination protocol that's right for the dog in a particular geographical area. Factors that should be examined include age, medical history, environment, travel habits and lifestyle. Most veterinarians highly recommend administering core vaccines to healthy dogs.

In 2006, the American Animal Hospital Association's Canine Task Force published a revised version of guidelines regarding canine vaccinations. The guidelines divide vaccines into three categories, i.e. core vaccines, non-core vaccines and vaccines which are not recommended. Core vaccines are considered vital to all dogs based on risk of exposure, severity of disease or transmissibility to humans. Canine parvovirus, canine distemper, canine hepatitis and rabies are considered core vaccines. Non-core vaccines are given depending on the dog's exposure risk and the geographical areas and country, where the dog is located and a veterinarian must take decision in this regard keeping in view the ibid aspects.

PARASITE CONTROL

Dogs are at risk of becoming infested with internal parasites (intestinal worms and heartworms), and external parasites (fleas, ticks, and mange mites). Some of these parasites may also transmit infectious diseases to the dogs. In order to prevent infestation and disease transmission, all dogs must be on a routine parasite control programme supervised by the responsible veterinarian. When deployed to areas with high parasitic risk, additional preventive measures will be prescribed by the veterinarian. The handler must ensure that flea and tick collars will only be used when prescribed by the veterinarian and must be removed when the dog is not under direct physical control (when off the choke chain and leash) of the handler to prevent accidental ingestion.

SIGNS OF GOOD HEALTH

An understanding of the signs of health is necessary before sickness can be recognized. A healthy dog is active, alert, lively and keen to work or play and does not tire easily. The eyes are bright and shining; nose cold and moist; the mouth, tongue and teeth are clean; the breath is wholesome, the coat is glossy

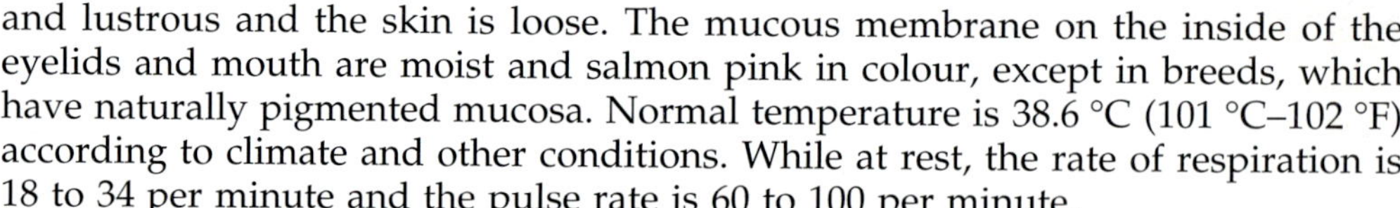

and lustrous and the skin is loose. The mucous membrane on the inside of the eyelids and mouth are moist and salmon pink in colour, except in breeds, which have naturally pigmented mucosa. Normal temperature is 38.6 °C (101 °C–102 °F) according to climate and other conditions. While at rest, the rate of respiration is 18 to 34 per minute and the pulse rate is 60 to 100 per minute.

A healthy dog has a ready appetite for food, relishes its meals and consumes it quickly. The bowels are emptied regularly and the stools, which may vary in colour from dark greenish black to a light orange brown, are well-formed and passed without difficulty. The urine is clear, usually light orange brown in colour and is passed in small quantities at frequent intervals. The inner surface of the ears is clean, and in prick-eared dogs, the ears are carried erect. A healthy dog has a happy appearance generally but disposition varies and alteration of disposition is usually one of the first signs of the dog being off colour.

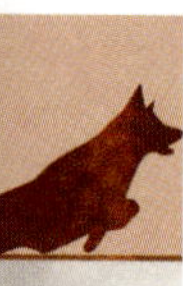

CARE AND MANAGEMENT OF SICK AND INJURED DOGS

An ailing or injured dog is apt to bite anyone handling it, because either he is in pain and afraid, or not fully aware of his actions. For this reason care must be taken while handling and the animal must be restrained to prevent him biting. The dog should be approached and handled calmly, confidently, quietly, firmly and deliberately, but with sympathy and understanding. It is usually preferable to allow the dog to see one approaching and to let it realize that it is about to be handled. The dog should be muzzled, or its mouth should be taped, while the head is held by an assistant. If the dog is inclined to snap, a loop made up of bandage or other such material may be slipped over the muzzle for holding so that the hands are too far away to be bitten. If the injuries are extensive and severe, it may be necessary to improvise some forms of stretcher on which it can lie down comfortably. Ordinarily an injured animal can be lifted after muzzling, by kneeling behind its shoulders, slipping one hand under its neck and the other hand under the body in front of the hips and raising the animal on the forearms. If the dog is not muzzled, one hand should grasp the scruff of the dog's neck instead of being slipped underneath it. A dog may be carried satisfactorily for a short distance by placing one arm around the breast and the other around the quarters and raising the dog breast high. To carry a longer distance, the handler should place his head under the dog's chest and so carry the animal on his neck and shoulders while holding its legs in his hands.

HOSPITALIZATION

Veterinary hospital should be provisioned to provide advanced treatment to canines hurt in combat or while training and also to cater for all emergencies. Like soldiers, Military Working Dogs suffer from war injuries and routine health issues that need to be treated to ensure they can continue working. The dogs deployed on various tasks get emergency medical treatment on the spot or in near vicinity where such facilities are provisioned. However, for advanced treatment the dogs are evacuated to the nearest veterinary hospital designed for the purpose. The hospital should have proper operating room, digital radiography, scanning equipment, an intensive care unit, behavioural specialist and rehabilitation rooms with an underwater treadmill and exercise balls among other features.

20

Breeding and Reproduction of Working Dogs

"No animal I know of can consistently be more of a friend and companion than a dog."

... Stanley Leinwoll

Dog breeding should always be aimed to breed good quality breeding stock so as to obtain high quality pups to meet the functional requirement. Genetic makeup and environment are the two important factors, which determine how a puppy will develop later on. The breed characteristics express themselves in the offsprings and are known to get influenced by environmental factors like temperature, nutrition and exercise. An organized, systematic and scientific approach has to be followed for attaining desired results in breeding programme. Factors to be considered before breeding: the bitch and the male dog should be in breeding fit condition, free of diseases and physical abnormalities. Dogs selected for breeding should be free from hereditary disorders that are common to the dog breed (canine hip dysplasia, oligodontia, etc.). Both the bitch and the male dog must be of sound temperament. Both dogs should preferably be registered with national kennel club so as to facilitate puppies registration subsequently.

FEMALE REPRODUCTIVE TRACT

The reproductive tract of breeding bitches should be of sound health which comprises following organs:

Ovaries: These are two in number, i.e. left ovary and right ovary. Both produce ova (eggs) and certain reproductive hormones. The eggs in the ovaries develop within fluid filled sacs called follicles.

Oviducts: These tubes move the ovulated and released eggs from the ovaries to the uterus in approximately two days. Also, the oviducts are the sites of egg maturation and fertilization.

Uterus: This consists of two long horns and a short body. The uterus is the site of implantation and placental and fetal development.

Cervix: This structure is a constricted orifice that serves as a channel from the uterus to the vagina. During pregnancy, the cervix closes the birth canal and serves as a barrier against the entry of microorganisms into the uterus.

Vagina: It is a hollow organ which extends from the cervix to the vulva. The inner lining of the vagina is made up of cells that undergo particular changes during the estrous cycle.

Vulva: This structure is composed of the external genitalia, which includes the clitoris (sexual organ) and two vertical lips.

MALE REPRODUCTIVE TRACT

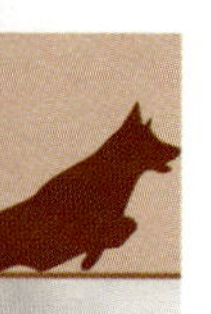

The reproductive tract of male dogs should be of sound health and comprises:

Testicles: These masses of seminiferous tubules are responsible for the production of sperm cells and the male sex hormone, testosterone. Cells lining the seminiferous tubules produce sperm, while cells found between the seminiferous tubules produce testosterone.

Epididymis: These ductules are the sites of sperm maturation.

Vas Deferens: This is the ejaculatory sperm duct that is also called ductus deferens.

Prostate: This accessory sex gland is responsible for the production of the fluid portion of the semen.

Urethra: This hollow tube originates at the neck of the bladder and runs through the penis to transport urine. During mating, it transports semen.

Penis: The dog's penis contains two rather unique characteristics:

Os-Penis: The objective of this small bone within the free extremity of the penis (glans penis) is to direct the male non-erect penis into the bitch's vulva and vagina during the early stages of mating.

Bulbus Glandis: This swelling of the penis is locateds toward the rear end of the os-penis. As soon as the male dog inserts his penis into the bitch's vagina and begins to thrust, the bulbus glandis enlarges to a firm spherical shape, resulting in the so-called "coital tie." This tie prevents the male dog and the bitch from separating immediately after ejaculation and may last from 5 to 60 minutes.

Prepuce: This foreskin or outer covering is where the external opening of the penis usually lies.

Scrotum: This is a sac of skin where the testicles are suspended outside the peritoneal cavity.

ESTROUS CYCLE OF FEMALE DOG

Bitches become sexually mature when they exhibit their first heat period, usually between 6 and 16 months of age, depending on the size and breed. Most bitches come into heat twice a year. The estrous or heat cycle of an intact (unspayed) and non-pregnant bitch is divided into four separate phases:

Proestrous: The most reliable indicator of the beginning of this phase is the bloody vaginal discharge which is due to the leaking of red blood cells from capillary vessels lining the uterus into the lumen of the uterus. Other indicators include swelling of the vulva and frequent licking of the external genitalia. During proestrous the bitch will attract male dogs but will not allow mounting or mating. Proestrous usually ranges between 6–11 days, but on an average lasts for nine days. During this phase the Follicle-Stimulating Hormone (FSH) and the Luteinizing Hormone (LH), both secreted by the pituitary gland, stimulate growth and development of follicles within the ovaries. Furthermore, the levels of the hormone estrogen rise gradually in the bloodstream causing behavioural estrous in the bitch.

Estrous: This phase begins when the bitch allows mounting or mating. To indicate sexual receptivity, the bitch crouches, elevates the rear quarters towards the male and moves the tail to side. The vaginal discharge becomes straw or light pink colour. The average duration of estrous phase is about 9 days, but it can last from 2–21 days. During this phase oestrogen levels decrease and progesterone levels increase. It is during estrous that ovulation (release of eggs from ovarian follicles) takes place. A surge in LH from the pituitary gland triggers ovulation, which occurs 1–3 days after LH levels peak in the bitch's bloodstream. All mature ovarian follicles rupture and release their eggs into the oviducts within 24–48 hours. Generally, larger dog breeds, ovulate more eggs than smaller breeds. Released eggs undergo maturation in 2–3 days and then remain viable for a period of 12–72 hours. Following ovulation, each ruptured follicle changes to corpus luteum, a yellow body responsible for increasing progesterone levels during estrous. Extreme care must be taken during the estrous phase in order to prevent unwanted pregnancies. The bitch must be supervised when she is allowed to go out into the yard or taken out for walks.

Diestrous: This phase, which lasts about two months, begins with the bitch becoming unattractive to the male dog and lasts until the corpora lutea (plural of corpus luteum) regress. Hence, diestrous is under the influence of the hormone, progesterone. If the bitch has been bred, this phase is the beginning of pregnancy. However, the corpora lutea are maintained and remain functional, secreting progesterone, which is otherwise important for the maintenance of pregnancy.

Anestrous: This phase is considered to be a quiet rest stage in the estrous cycle. Factors such as breed, age, size, and health condition will influence the duration of anestrous. The length of anestrous varies, lasting on average about 3–5 months. During this phase, the bitch shows no signs of heat and no sexual interest in males. Following anestrous, the heat cycle begins again.

REPRODUCTIVE CYCLE OF MALE DOG

Male dogs, like bitches, reach sexual maturity at varying ages, depending on the size and breed of the dog. Most males are sexually mature and capable of producing sperm at about 10 months of age. The hormones FSH and LH, secreted by the pituitary gland, stimulate the production of sperm (spermatogenesis) and testosterone by the testicles. Testosterone is necessary for the development and maintenance of male sex characteristics, male sexual behaviour, and spermatogenesis which occurs throughout the year.

MATING

The best rule to follow when breeding dogs is to be certain that they are physically mature. This means that both the bitch and the male dog should be 18–24 months of age, by which time the bitch should be in her second or third heat period. Since ovulation usually occurs on the second day of estrous, it is highly effective to breed the bitch as soon as she is sexually receptive to the male dog and again two days later. The bitch is usually brought to the male dog for breeding. Courtship behaviour begins with the male dog sniffing to become familiar with bitch's face and flank and licking of the vulva. When ready, the bitch presents her hindquarters to the male dog and stands still with her tail towards one side. The male dog then clasps the flanks of the bitch with his forelegs, inserts his penis into the vagina (intromission) and begins to thrust.

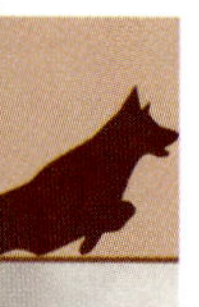

The enlargement of the bulbus glandis occurs at this time, resulting in the coital tie. With the penis firmly in place, ejaculation begins. Then with their genitalia still "locked," the male dog dismounts by placing both front feet to one side and lifting one hind leg over the bitch's back so that they are facing in opposite directions. The enlarged bulbus glandis of the male dog prevents separation from the bitch for about 5 to 60 minutes. Do not interfere with a coital tie as injury could result. Separation occurs naturally and both dogs usually wash themselves afterwards. When artificial insemination is practiced, conception rate is also equal to those attained by natural breeding. However, the kennel clubs have their regulations concerning the registration of dogs produced by artificial insemination. Therefore, before using this technique, check with the national/local kennel club for information about artificial insemination and registration of puppies.

PREGNANCY

After successful mating, the sperm cells will reach the eggs in the oviducts of the bitch within 30 seconds of ejaculation and have a viable life span up to seven days. Fertilization (union of sperm and egg) takes place in the distal portion of the oviducts and occurs a few days after mating. The resulting zygotes (fertilized eggs) begin cell division growth, and the growing organisms are then called embryos.

The developing embryos move from the oviducts into the uterus 6 to 10 days after conception and implant or attach to the uterine walls 17 to 21 days after fertilization. As they implant and their placenta develops, the embryos are then called fetuses. The fetuses are usually evenly spaced throughout the two uterine horns. The pregnancy or gestation period of the bitch lasts between 56 to 66 days, with an average length of 63 days. During this period the corpora lutea are maintained and remain functional, secreting progesterone, which is important for the maintenance of pregnancy.

To confirm pregnancy, palpation of the bitch's abdomen for the presence of evenly spaced swellings can be conducted by an experienced person between 20 and 30 days after the last mating. However, improper procedure or excessive prodding can cause a miscarriage. After confirming that the bitch is pregnant, the pregnancy or gestation period extends leading to parturition (whelping). A pregnant bitch requires additional food to support the growth of pups inside her and to produce the milk that pups will need after birth. Feed her the same amount of the usual adult maintenance diet for the first 4 weeks of pregnancy. Then gradually increase the amount of food so that by whelping time she is eating about one and one-half times her maintenance diet. Switching to a commercial dog food that is specifically formulated for pregnancy and lactation may also be considered. However, due to possible whelping problems, make sure that the bitch does not gain any excessive weight during this period. Very few physical changes occur until the fifth week of pregnancy. By the fifth week of pregnancy, the nipples and mammary glands swell and darken in colour. Between the sixth and seventh weeks, the bitch's abdomen is enlarged due to the growth of the pups. At about 8 weeks into the pregnancy, the bitch's mammary glands will enlarge considerably and milk may appear on the nipples.

WHELPING

About a week before the estimated date of parturition, the bitch should be introduced to the whelping area and the whelping box. Approximately 12 to 24 hours before labour begins, the rectal temperature drops from a normal of 101.5 °F (38.6 °C) to less than 100 °F (37.7 °C). In addition, the bitch loses her appetite, becomes restless and lethargic, and her abdomen becomes more distended. An increase in the production and secretion of the hormone, prostaglandin F-2-alpha by the placenta and uterus causes regression of the corpora lutea and a subsequent decrease in progesterone. The decrease in progesterone permits uterine contractions to effect delivery of puppies and the uterus usually returns to its normal size (involution) within 12 weeks of whelping. The labour and delivery process in dogs usually does not require human intervention, however, for emergency purposes, the following supplies should be kept in hand:

- A clean, small plastic syringe to aspirate secretions from the mouth and nose.
- A spool of dental floss to tie the umbilical cords.
- A pair of sterilized, straight, blunt-tipped scissors, in case it becomes necessary to cut the umbilical cords.
- A small bottle of iodine solution to apply to the umbilical cords.
- Several clean, laundered towels for drying the puppies.

The whelping entails three stages:

Stage I: It lasts about 6–12 hours, characterized by mild uterine contractions and displaying of external signs by the bitch such as intense nesting and constantly lying down and standing up. During this period release of relaxin hormone peaks which widens pubic bone, facilitates labour, softens the cervix and relaxes uterine musculature to facilitate whelping.

Stage II: Characterized by intense uterine contractions, which causes the expulsion of the puppy. Bitches usually deliver lying down, but some may assume a squatting position. In general, the bitch will deliver her entire litter over a period of several hours. Most puppies are born with feet and head first. The bitch should instinctively start to lick the fetal membranes away from the puppy's face, and then sever the umbilical cord with her teeth. There should be no interference with this maternal process. However, if the bitch does not act, you should step in and break the membrane with your fingers, so the puppy can breath. Similarly, the umbilical cord needs to be tied, cut, and disinfected.

Stage III: This is characterized by expulsion of the placenta. The bitch usually expels placenta within a few minutes and it is normal instinct for the bitch to eat the placentae. However, it should be made sure that the bitch has expelled placenta for each puppy. If she retains any, she may develop postpartum metritis and may need veterinary help. After that she may be shifted to dry, warm, draft-free, secluded, and quiet place. The whelping or nesting box may be constructed of a variety of materials but should be designed to accommodate the bitch fully stretched out on her side and have room to spare for the pups. The bitch should be able to step into it, but the pups should not be able to climb out. The bedding of the box should include fresh, flat newspaper laid at the bottom for fluid absorption and heavy towels, mattress pads, or pieces of carpeting laid on top of the newspaper for good traction. If necessary, a source of supplemental heat should be placed in the whelping box for the puppies, especially after the first few weeks of birth. Supplemental heat can be furnished by using heat bulbs either suspended or mounted above the floor of the whelping box. However, an area of the box should be left without supplemental heat, so the bitch and puppies can move away from the heat if they get too hot.

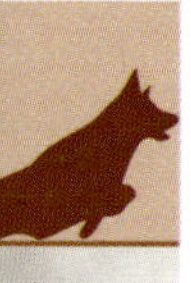

POSTPARTUM AND POSTNATAL CARES

Since the bitch's appetite returns within 24 hours after whelping, she is fed a highly palatable food, moistened with water. The bitch now needs three to four times more food than she normally does. Although the eyelids of the puppies are not open at birth, they can still locate the bitch's nipples in order to feed. This is of extreme importance since the puppies must consume colostrum (dam's first milk) within the first 12 to 24 hours after birth. Colostrum contains high levels of antibodies that are absorbed intact into the bloodstream and provides protection against infectious diseases. Hence, make sure that each puppy has access to a nipple and is able to suckle. Remember that the most important indicator of puppy health during the first few days and weeks of life is regular and normal weight gain. If a puppy does not gain weight during the first 72 hours of life, you should start supplemental feeding immediately. Commercial milk formulas, which can be obtained from pet supply stores, should be fed warm in a small bottle with a hole in the nipple. Handle the puppies daily to get them used to human contact, and change the bedding often to prevent urine burn. As you handle them, inspect for cleft palates, umbilical hernias, atresia ani (absence of anal opening), and any other abnormal conditions. At about three weeks of age, puppies should be given access to dry food mixed with warm water (gruel) in a large bowl several times a day. Gradually, the water content should be reduced so that by 4 to 6 weeks of age the puppies are meeting most of their requirements with the dry food. By this time there is less demand on the bitch's milk, and her food intake should be reduced. This initiates the process of stopping milk production and helps to normalize the bitch's food intake. After about 6 or 7 weeks of age, puppies are ready to be weaned and placed into new homes. Before sending them off, make sure that they have been treated for parasites and vaccinated as per the advice of a veterinarian.

MANAGEMENT OF BREEDING STOCK

Care and management of stud dogs and breeding bitches is an important aspect in having a healthy and disease-free litter. Hence an organized, systematic and scientific approach has to be followed for attaining desired results in breeding programme.

Management of Stud Dogs

Stud dogs are optimally exercised and well-fed with balanced diet supplemented with vitamins and minerals so that they remain in pink of health. They should be regularly dewormed and vaccinated to keep them free of any aliments/disease and optimal health is maintained. Periodic medical and semen examination must be carried out to assess the health and spermatozoa count and those found lacking must be investigated and treated. Unfit and over-aged studs must not be bred as they have poor breeding performance associated with low conception rate, leading to small litter size with low birth weight and congenital abnormalities. The studs should adhere to the laid down specifications of height and weight and should have a proven blood line so that quality pups with maximum litter size and birth weight can be produced. New blood lines with proven record may be introduced from time to time to avoid inbreeding and to obtain a good litter size of quality pups.

Stud dogs should be kept in the best possible physical condition so as to enable them to perform well during mating, which is a physically taxing activity. Regular exercise in safe and enclosed area such as paddocks or fenced yards, helps to maintain good muscle tone. All stud dogs should be housed individually with no doubling and away from the breeding bitches so as to maintain their libido at peak.

Management of Breeding Bitches

Empty Bitches

Empty breeding bitches should be housed in semi-liberty paddocks to live in harmony which not only provides space for free exercise and keeping them fit but also provides environment for exhibiting social behaviour, i.e. estrous. The bitches come in estrous between 8–12 months of age and for all purposes the first heat should be spared. After every two conceptions/whelping, sexual rest should be given for optimal breeding performance. Mating is carried out on 11th and 13th days of estrous and a tie/knot during mating is considered for better results. Bitches in anoestrus should be managed and treated. They should be given regular exercise coupled with balanced diet supplemented with essential vitamins and minerals. Specific treatment for anestrous and repeater cases should be given as per veterinarian's advice.

Pregnant Bitches

Covered/pregnant bitches are kept separate from other dogs and housed individually in separate kennels. Regular exercise in morning and evening is given during pregnancy to maintain health and to keep the muscles in tone, required for whelping. However in late pregnancy, the bitch is only given light exercise. The covered bitch is confirmed pregnant after 4 weeks of mating by analyzing the weight gain. The food given to the pregnant bitches is gradually increased from 4 weeks of gestation, i.e. extra 1/3rd ration each day by 5th weeks and extra fifty percent supplemented with calcium and phosphorous just before whelping to cater for increased nutrients required for the growth of puppies. The bitch is fed four times a day during last month of pregnancy and fresh water is made available at all times. Regular weekly recording of body weight after 4 weeks of gestation so as to monitor health. Grooming the bitch regularly during pregnancy is important as it helps to reassure her of the handler's involvement and makes it less likely that she will resent help at time of whelping.

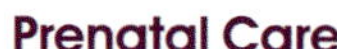

Prenatal Care

The pregnant bitches are shifted to the whelping complex 7 days prior to the due whelping date. High standard of hygiene and sanitation are maintained and the bitches are protected against extreme weather conditions. Light exercise is given till a few days before whelping. The bitches are groomed daily morning and evening taking care not to scratch sensitive abdominal area. Excess matted hairs are clipped from her vulva and mammary glands and her nipples are cleaned with a safe disinfectant just before the beginning of labour pains.

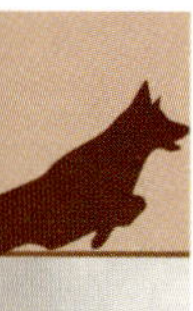

CARE AND MANAGEMENT OF PUPS

Postnatal Care

For the first 3 weeks of life the newborn puppies are totally dependent upon their mother for food and security. Ensure that they are kept warm and their mother is well-nourished, healthy, and producing sufficient milk. Sometimes, with extra-large litter, mother's milk may be supplemented with special canine milk formula. Important aspects in postnatal care are:

- Bonding with mother
- Bottle-feeding
- Cleaning up
- Monitoring weight gain
- Stimulating body functions
- Nail trimming

At 3 weeks of age, the pups are shifted from whelping room to the post-whelping room but care is taken to protect them from inclement weather. The pups are fed 5 times a day till 16 weeks of age and their feed supplemented with lactogen/cerelac and vitamins/minerals as per requirement. Pups are taken out for stool at the stool site area after every feed. At 7 weeks of age, they are transferred from breeding kennel to pups kennel. Three pups can be housed in one kennel and adequate care is taken to protect them from inclement weather by use of coolers/blowers. Pups are screened regularly for any sickness and remedial measures should be taken immediately as warranted. Deworming and vaccinations to be carried out and weekly recording of body weight should be monitored regularly.

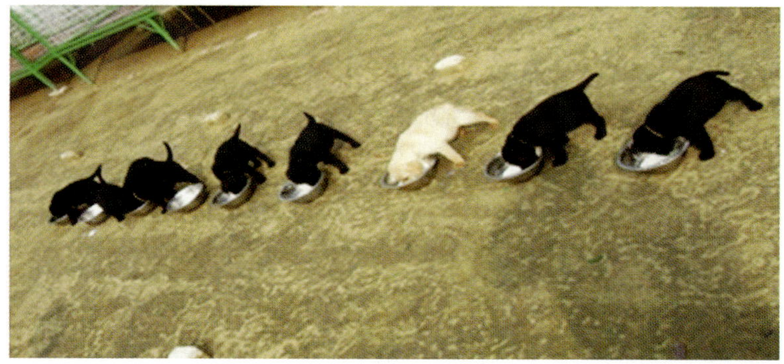

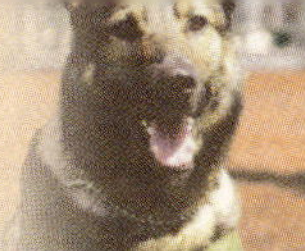

The pups should be delicately handled, groomed regularly and exposed to natural sights and sound. The pups are encouraged to socialize by eating and playing together. The critical period of growth in pups is between 2–6 months of age during which about 16–18 kg weight is gained, that is daily gain of 135–150 gm. As such, full attention is required to be focused on these growing pups so as to have high quality and optimally healthy adult dogs.

Height and weight specifications of pups/dogs

Age (month)	*GSD*		*LAB*	
	Height (cm)	*Weight (kg)*	*Height (cm)*	*Weight (kg)*
1	15–17	1.8–2.3	14–16	1.8–2.3
1½	23–27	2.5–3.4	22–26	2.5–4
2	28–32	4.5–7	28–32	4.5–6
3	33–37	7.5–9	32–37	7.5–9
4	39–43	12–15	38–42	11–13
6	46–52	20–25	44–50	18–21
9	60–62	25–27	53–54	22–24
12	62–63	27–30	53–54	25–27
Adult	63–65	30–35	54–57	28–30

After completion of 17 weeks of age and up to 24 weeks, the pups are exposed to the sights sounds and vagaries of nature. The pups are subjected for training lesson slowly and gradually. The pups are introduced to small obstacles in the agility course and encouraged/rewarded for each attempt. Feeding is now required to be carried out 4–5 times a day and their feed supplemented with essential vitamins/minerals.

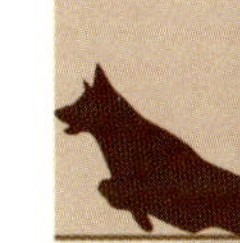

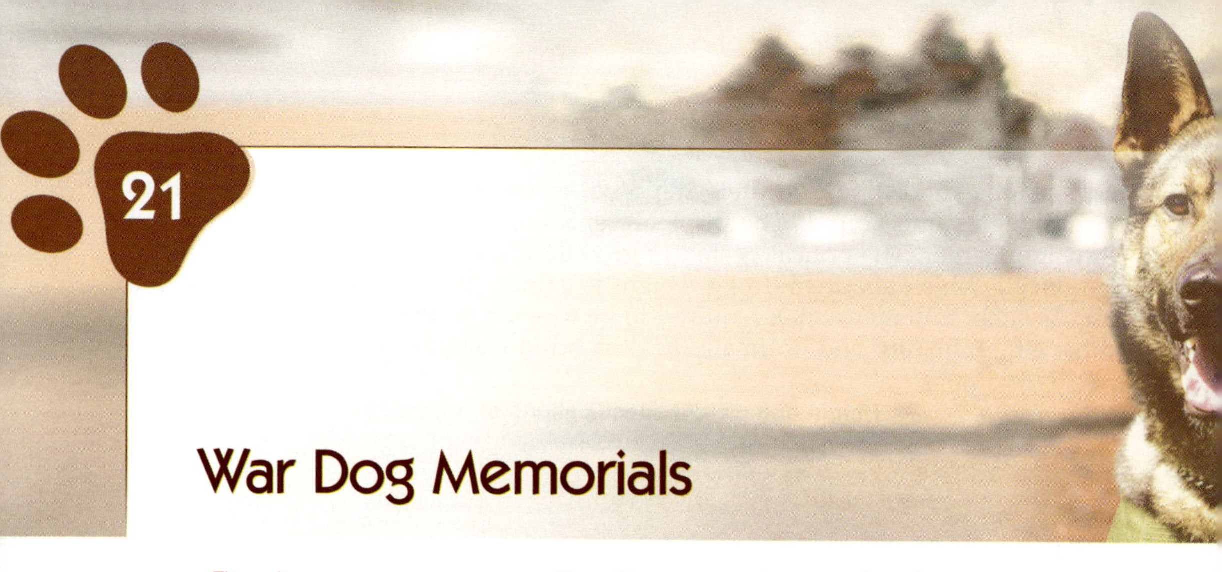

War Dog Memorials

The glamour gone, some scattered graves and memories dim remain
with their old pals across a field, they'll never treck again
but yet there's nothing they regret as they await their call
for what was done or lost or won, they did their bit—that's all.
Now as silent as the guns have fallen,
Their tired hearts resting, closed eyes of loving grace,
I ask in your quiet thoughts of honourable remembrance
you allow them, the animals to take their long awaited place.

World over, soldiers are measured for their distinguishing qualities for which they are bestowed with medals and the recognition of their country. Military Working Dogs (MWDs) also possess these qualities and faithfully served in wars for thousands of years as scouts, sentries, messengers and much more. They have served in many conflicts without compensation or recognition. Though these gallant dogs have more than earned the right to be fully recognized for their service to their countries yet appropriate national memorials were not built to recognize their profound contributions in many countries.

One of the earliest recorded memorials to dogs was after the battle between rival Greek states in the Peloponnesian War, 431–404 BC. The Corinthians used guard dogs as shoreline sentries as defence against the Athenian flotilla. According to a legend 50 war dogs leaped with open jaws at the Athenians as they crept ashore on a surprise night-time attack. The dogs fought ferociously but were all slain except one who awoke the Corinthians troops in a nearby town by barking. The Corinthians rallied and defeated the Athenians. So grateful were they that they built a monument to honour the dogs. Sorter, the surviving dog, was awarded a special collar inscribed 'Defender and Saviour of Corinth'.

After World War I, a public memorial building was erected at Kilburn, England, honouring war dogs. Its inscription reads in part "This building is dedicated as a memorial to the countless thousands of God's humble creatures who suffered and perished in the Great War of 1914–1918 knowing nothing of the cause but looking forward to final victory, filled with only love, faith and loyalty, they endured much and died for us". In 1918, a bronze statue of a German Shepherd mounted upon a 3-meter (10-foot) granite monument was built in Hartsdale, New York, to commemorate the bravery of dogs in war.

UNITED STATES OF AMERICA

Hartsdale Pet Cemetery, New York

Hartsdale Pet Cemetery, New York has been home to war dog memorial for many years in the USA. It was founded by Dr Samuei Johnson who was a professor of Veterinary Surgery at New York University. In 1896, a distressed client approached him pleading that she had no place to give an appropriate burial to her dog. Dr Johnson offered her a place in his apple orchard in Hartsdale, Westchester. This gesture was casually mentioned to a journalist friend and the complete story was published in print. Subsequently, Dr Johnson was flooded with such requests and he set aside three acres land in his apple orchard for this purpose. In due course of time, dotted with gravestones, it was looking like a cemetery and presently this is known as the final resting place for thousands of pets, many dogs of war as wells as service dogs.

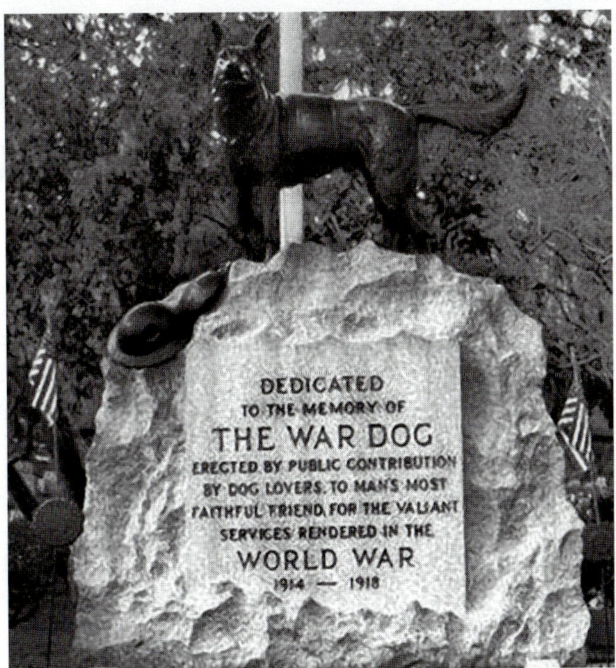
DEDICATED
TO THE MEMORY OF
THE WAR DOG
ERECTED BY PUBLIC CONTRIBUTION
BY DOG LOVERS TO MAN'S MOST
FAITHFUL FRIEND FOR THE VALIANT
SERVICES RENDERED IN THE
WORLD WAR
1914 — 1918

World War I war dog memorial, "Hartsdale Pet Cemetery", New York

US Marine Corps War Dog Cemetery on Guam

In World War II, the US Military Working Dogs returned home after the war to their former owner or new adopted one. On 21st July, 1994, a memorial was dedicated at the US Marine Corps war dog cemetery on Guam to honour the dogs who served in the Pacific theatre during World War II. In the battle for Guam (21st July to 10th August, 1944), a Doberman named Kurt saved the lives of 250 Marines when he warned them of Japanese troops ahead. Kurt is honoured by a life-sized bronze and granite statue at the memorial on Guam. Carved into the stone are names of twenty-five other Dobermans who gave their lives liberating the island and who are buried nearby. An exact replica of this memorial is located at the College of Veterinary Medicine, University of Tennessee, USA. 29 US Marine war dogs were listed as killed in action during World War II and 25 of those deaths occurred in the second battle of Guam which was fought between American and Japanese forces.

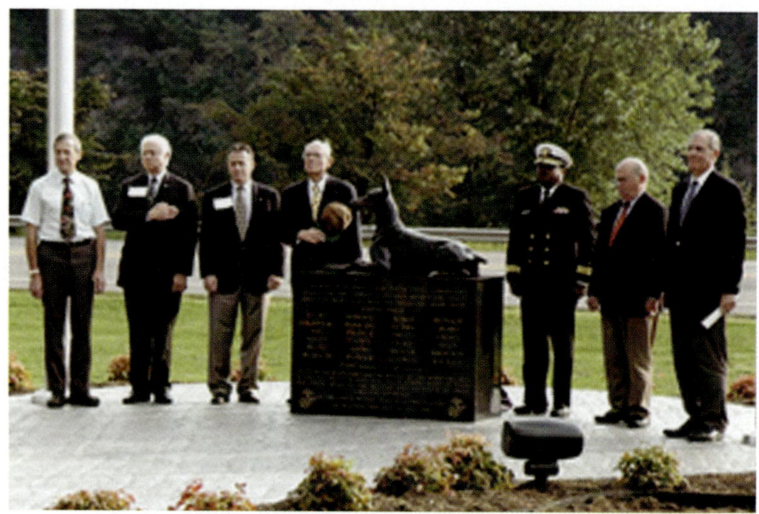

War dog memorial on Guam at College of Veterinary Medicine University of Tennessee, USA

Albama War Dogs Memorial

The first Marine dog platoon with twenty-four Dobermans and German shepherds landed on Bougainville on 1st November, 1943, moving ahead of the main body of men, looking for snipers in the jungle. Six dogs were recognized for heroism on Bougainville, with the Second and Third Marine Raider Battalions. Alabama's MWDs and their handlers had their day recently at the dedication of the Alabama War Dogs Memorial at USS Alabama Battleship Memorial Park. The memorial depicts the Alabama war dog team of LittleJoe, a German Shepherd, his handler, Charles 'Wade' Franks, and other combat patrol riflemen. The Alabama War Dog Memorial Foundation plans a service dog retirement centre as well. The four-ton granite slab supports statues depicting a war dog, his handler and other soldiers. The marble slab lists war dogs associated with handlers from Alabama. In front of the piece are boot prints made from an actual soldier's footwear, along with paw prints. Little Joe gave his life for those men on 22nd February, 1970 in Vietnam.

Military War Dogs Memorials

The Vietnam War was different in that the US war dogs were designated as expendable equipment and were either euthanized or turned over to an Allied Army prior to the US troop's departure from South Vietnam. Deeply hurt by these developments, veteran dog handlers from Vietnam War made untiring lobbying efforts and as a result the US congress approved a bill allowing the US Military Working Dogs to be adopted after their military service. A law to this effect was signed by President Bill Clinton in 2000. Jeffrey Bennett, founder and former CEO of Nature's Recipe Pet Foods, first learned about the dogs who served and the fate of so many of them and then he set out to make others aware. Based on about three years of research, he coproduced the documentary "War Dogs: America's Forgotten

Heroes," which was first aired 11 years ago on the Discovery Channel. Donations earned through this film allowed Bennett, to commission three monuments, sculptures featuring a German Shepherd and his handler. The first one was unveiled at the **March Field Air Museum in Riverside California** on 21st February, 2000. The black obelisk/column is just past the entryway B-24 bomber. Funded and sponsored by Nature's Recipe Pet Foods, the 16-foot tall granite and bronze statue depicts a soldier and a German Shepherd. It was sculpted by A Thomas Schumberg and dedicated on 21st February, 2000.

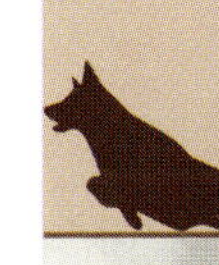

Other somber military monuments and memorials are arrayed around the grounds but the war dog memorial commands the plaza's central vantage. The sculpted soldier is half absorbed, Han Solo-like, by the slab but vigilant. His dog is alert, attuned to an impending jungle ambush or may be just a noisy weekend pass latecomer.

A bronze plaque at the base reads:

"They protected us on the field of battle, they watch over our eternal rest. We are grateful.

The war dog memorial is a tribute to all dog and handler teams that served our country so proudly."

Most touching are the tiles around the Memorial's base, tributes to individual dogs, each marked with a symbolic black paw print. Inscriptions are short and a bit cryptic, but hint at the adventures and trials these dogs must have undergone: "Hilda" My Hero Da Nang, 66B Martin" or "Team F BanMe Thout 981st MP K9 Mort 69." Other tiles salute dogs from World War II and Korea.

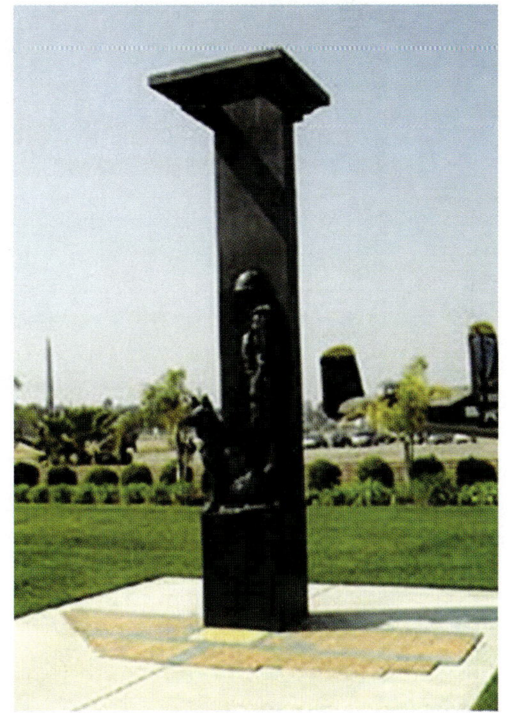

One is a stark apology: "King leaving you was sad and wrong peace. The Memorial doesn't explain, but you get the sense the remembrance of each canine, whether for valour or simple companionship, helps veteran handlers find closure on the relationship with their departed dogs."

The East Coast National War Dog Memorial (second memorial) identical to first one, was dedicated on 8th October, 2000 (Columbus Day) at the **National Infantry Museum, Fort Benning, Columbus, Georgia**.

The third one still remains to be unveiled, with the original goal to place it in Washington beside the Vietnam Veterans Memorial or at Arlington National Cemetery in Virginia which still remains an elusive dream. The proposed National War Dog Monument will be erected in the greater Washington DC area. It will proudly honour all Military Working Dogs who have served their country for the last century and into the future. The inscription will read 'In perpetual honour of the service and sacrifice of all Military Working Dogs of all armed services of all wars and peacekeeping missions since World War I.'

Military Working Dog Teams National Monument

Keeping in view the ever-growing demand for recognition of sacrifices of Military Working Dogs and their handlers in combat on national scale, the United States' first national monument to a soldier's best friend, was dedicated by the US Military at Joint Base San Antonio-Lackland, in San Antonio, Texas on 28th October, 2013. Inscribed with the words "Guardians of America's Freedom," the nine-foot tall bronze statue features four dogs and a handler. The sculpture features the four major breeds used since World War II: Doberman Pinscher, German Shepherd, Labrador Retriever, and Belgian Malinois.

Lackland is home to the US Armed Forces Centre that has trained dogs for all branches of the military since 1958. These dogs were patriots just as much as anybody else who served.

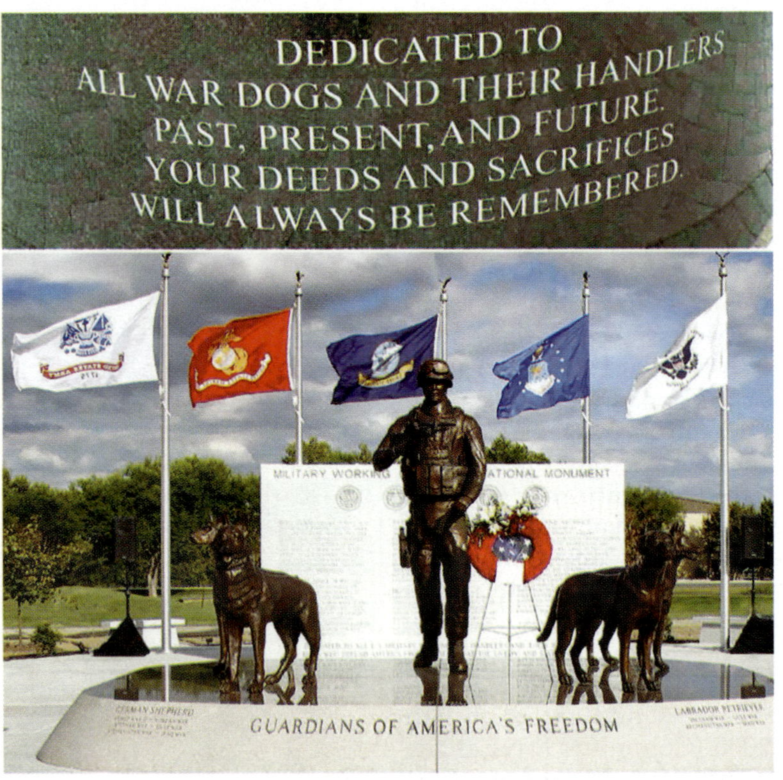
DEDICATED TO
ALL WAR DOGS AND THEIR HANDLERS
PAST, PRESENT, AND FUTURE.
YOUR DEEDS AND SACRIFICES
WILL ALWAYS BE REMEMBERED.
GUARDIANS OF AMERICA'S FREEDOM

War Dog Memorials in Small Towns

Small town tributes such as **"Guardians," a war dog memorial in Streamwood, Illinois**, are becoming more common. A war dog memorial has been unveiled in Village of Streamwood, Illinois, USA. There may be many more such regional or private memorials to war dogs across villages and towns. The bond of affection for these dogs will no doubt give rise to more over the years. Military canines make

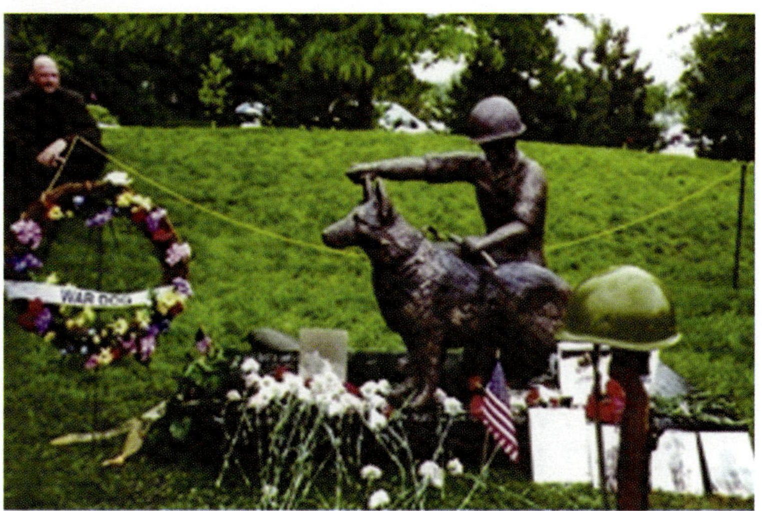

War dog memorial, Village of Streamwood, Illinois, USA

contributions every day while they serve in military. They are hardworking and do a great job of saving the lives of their handlers and the troops who walk in their footsteps. There has been many dog handlers who have turned to their dogs in the depths of war and told them things they would never say to another soldier. MWDs have been a source of friendship, family and true love to their handlers, the price they ask is a pat and a smile. While we often focus on the human cost of operations we must never forget the ultimate sacrifice made by man's best friend, the dog.

Veterans and War Dog Memorials, Houma, Louisiana

The bronze veteran and war dog statue was created in memory of the brave men, women, and animals who have fought for our freedom. The bronze statues are

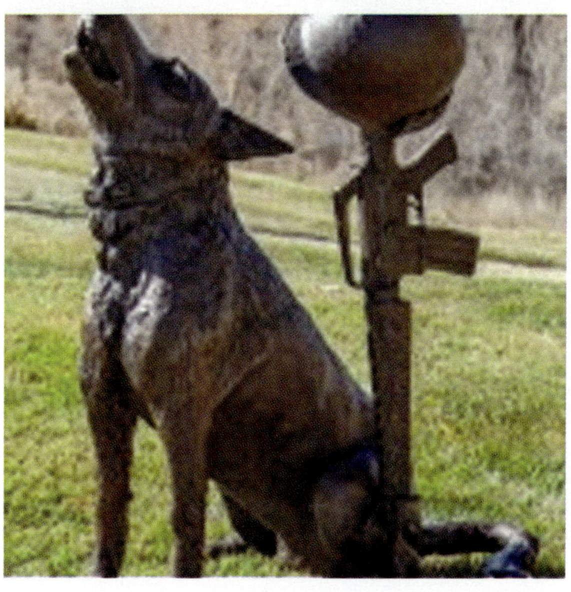

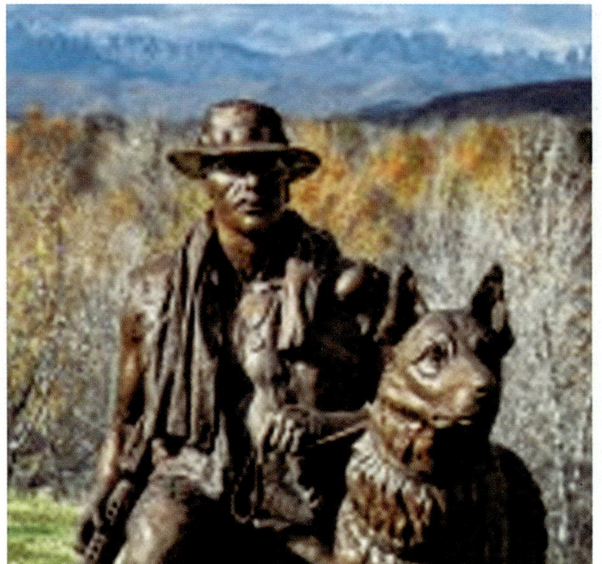

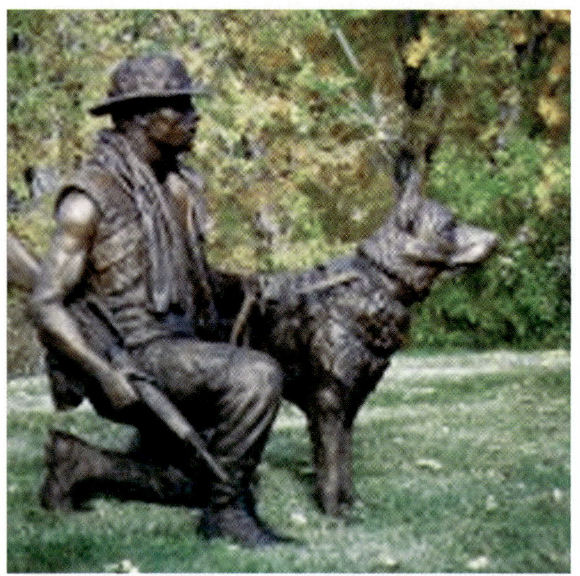

placed in Houma, Louisiana by Diane Baker. They are located at a recently opened animal adoption centre. Their unveiling was very moving with many attendees crying because of mixed emotions as they remembered all those who have served for their country.

In March, 2010, Congressman Leonard Lance (NJ-07) moved a House resolution in the United States House of Representatives which was approved and introduced by honouring MWDs of the United States for their service throughout the nation's history.

'Throughout our nation's history Military Working Dogs have made great contributions to help our military men and women accomplish their important missions,' Lance said during a speech on the House floor. 'These dogs have helped to save lives and protect our soldiers in harm's way'. Specifically, Lance's resolution recognizes the significant contributions of the MWD programme to the United States' Armed Forces, active honours and retired Military Working Dogs for their loyal service, and supports the adoption and care of these quality animals after their service. Lance said that for more than six decades, MWDs have helped to prevent injuries and saved the lives of thousands of Americans.

AUSTRALIA

The fate of Australia's war dogs, once their service came to an end in Vietnam, caused consternation in army circles and anguish to their handlers. Unlike their human counterparts, the length of duty for a tracker dog was around three years (at least one year too long, according to many handlers). This made it impossible for the dog to return to Australia when his handler's tour ended. The main reason for keeping the dogs 'in country' was the Army's reluctance to cover the quarantine costs involved.

After much discussion about the issue, and with the matter having been raised in Parliament, the Army decided in 1968 that at the end of their working lives, the dogs would be kept by the battalion as a reserve and then given as pets to European or Australian families resident in Saigon. Only as a last resort, if no home could be found, would they be destroyed. However, none of the 11 dogs who served in Vietnam was put down as suitable homes were found for the ten who survived (One dog, Cassius, died of heat exhaustion after a training run). Having to part with their dogs at the end of their tours was often the hardest thing the dog handlers had to face in Vietnam. Some likened it to losing a child. Handler, Denis Ferguson trained Marcus in Australia and served with his 'mate' during two tours of Vietnam. Ferguson applied through all the appropriate army channels to take Marcus home with him even offering to pay all the quarantine costs. The curt refusal he received and being given no reasons caused Ferguson trauma that he felt deeply. The family of Garry Polglase, the handler of Julian, had a similar experience. Polglase was accidentally killed in Vietnam in April, 1968, and his mother applied to have the dog brought home soon after her son's death. After questions were raised in Parliament, the family had conducted a public campaign that raised enough money to pay the quarantine costs of all the tracker dogs, the army confirmed its policy on the fate of the dogs and refused the request.

These refusals might have been easier to bear had the handlers been told one apparent reason for them. An army veterinary report noted that a large number of American tracker dogs in Vietnam had died from a tropical disease, thought (but not confirmed) to be transmitted by ticks. The disease, which very quickly caused massive haemorrhage in all major organs, was hard to detect and could be carried by the dogs without symptoms for some time. The report strongly recommended that no tracker dogs be allowed back into Australia, "even under strict quarantine", until the mode of transmission of the disease was discovered. By the end of 1972 the majority of Australian troops, including the dog handlers were back home from Vietnam. Most got on with their lives more or less successfully but their dogs were never far from their thoughts. Haran, a veteran dog handler felt that his dog Caesar had been forgotten as a soldier and soldiers should not be forgotten in war. There should be some sort of memory of them.

Many ex-handlers shared this feeling and it finally resulted in a permanent memorial for the dogs being erected in Australia. Presently, Australia has three war dog memorials. An Australian War Dog memorial completed with carved statue and a drinking trough for dogs, was unveiled at a ceremony on 7th April, 2001 at the Bluff, Alexandra Headland, Sunshine Coast, Queensland. This monument recognizes the enormous contribution of war dogs that saved countless lives in Vietnam. An inaugural reunion of past and present trackers in Queensland in March, 2002 further cemented the bonds between those who served with these remarkable dogs of war and highlighted their importance and rightful place in Australian Military history.

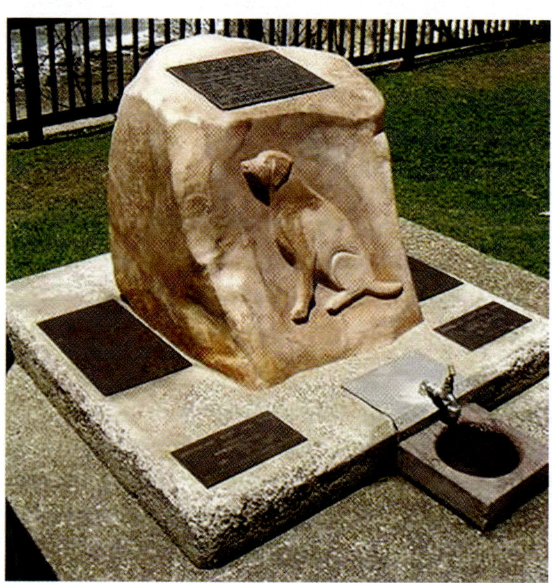

Australian war dog memorial, Alexandra Headland, Queensland

Another war dog memorial is located in Goolwa, South Australia and was dedicated in May, 2003. It is made of black marble and on the face of the memorial, etched in the stone is a photograph of a South Australian soldier with his tracking dog. The names of eleven tracker dogs that served in Vietnam from 1962 to 1972 are also listed on the memorial.

Canines in Combat-Vietnam, 1962–1972

Cassius	Tiber	Justin	Marcus
Janus	Julian	Caesar	Milo
Trajan	Juno	Marcian	

A third war dog memorial in Australia is located at Moorebank, NSW, and is dedicated to the dogs that have lost their lives on active service in Afghanistan.

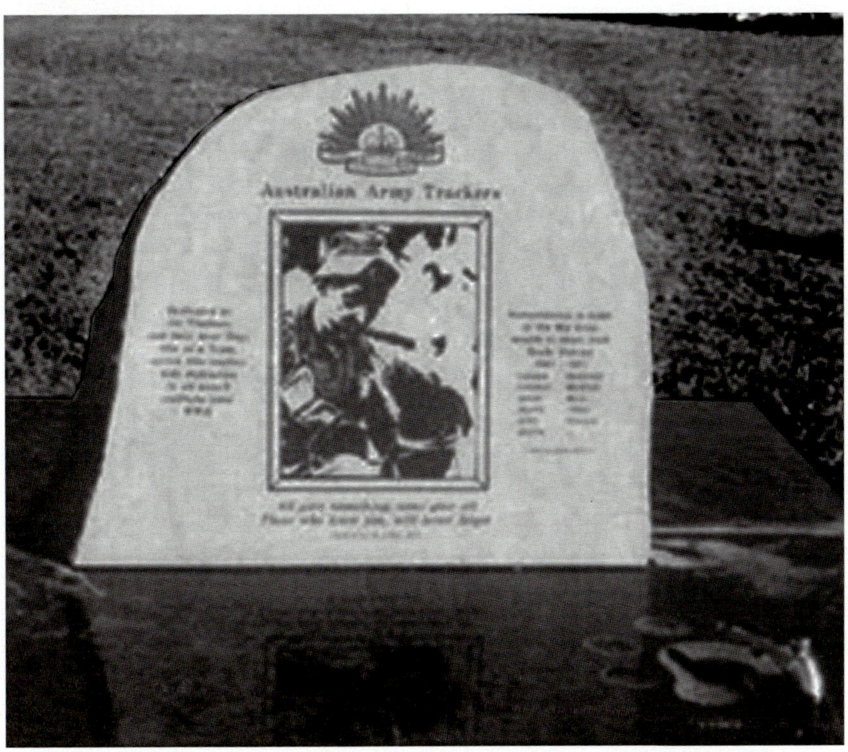

The Australian Army trackers memorial, Goolwa, South Australia

Recently a memorial for Australia's Explosive Detection Dogs Killed in Action in Afghanistan has also been unveiled in July, 2011, in a corner of the Australian recreation area named in memory of Trooper David "Poppy" Pearce. A poignant ceremony marked the unveiling of a memorial for another group of very special fallen Australians. The memorial was conceived following the deaths of Sapper Darren Smith and his dog, "Herbie", in June, 2010. Further, recognizing the loyalties of four-legged diggers, the former Chief of Defence, Air Chief Marshall AG Houston, confirmed the endorsement of 7th June to be annually commemorated as "Military Working Dog Day".

The polished metal board at the memorial features the names of the five dogs, Merlin, Razz, Andy, Nova, and Herbie along with the name of Sapper Darren Smith. Above the names is a pair of silhouetted images, one of a dog and his handler and the other of a dog sitting at rest.

It symbolizes the working partnership and mateship between the dog and his handler.

RSPCA Purple Cross Award

RSPCA Australia (Royal Society for the Prevention of Cruelty to Animals) is an Australian peak organization established in 1981 to promote animal welfare. Each state and territory of Australia has an RSPCA organization that predates and is affiliated with RSPCA Australia. The national body is funded in part by the Australian

Government but relies on corporate sponsorship, fund-raising events and voluntary donations for its income. It describes itself as a "federated organization made up of the eight independent state and territory RSPCA Societies." It defines its purpose as being the leading authority in animal care and protection, and to prevent cruelty to animals by actively promoting their care and protection. The RSPCA Purple Cross Award was implemented to recognize the actions of animals, particularly if they have risked their life to save a person from injury or death. The award was named after the Purple Cross Society, which was established after the Second World War. On 5th April, 2011, the Australian Special Forces Explosives Detection Dog "Sarbi" received the Purple Cross Award, at the Australian War Memorial.

Australian Defence Force Trackers and War Dog Association Medals

Medals have been awarded to the country's courageous canines by the Australian Defence Force Trackers and War Dogs Association (ADFTWDA). Six medals, two of them posthumous were presented to explosive detection dog (EDD) teams of two Combat Engineers Regiment at a ceremony at Brisbane's Army Barracks. Another Explosive Detection Dog called Aussie was awarded two medals for both operational service and for his five years of service in the Australian Defence Forces. The eight-year-old golden Retriever who has served in Afghanistan and the Solomon Islands, was one of six dogs to receive the medals during a ceremony at the army barracks. In 2008, the army lost three Explosives Detection Dogs on active duty in Afghanistan. Sadly, again in June, 2010, Sapper Darren Smith and EDD Herbie, were killed in action. Speaking at the occasion, Major General Ash Power said in a statement that in this case, the dogs have paid the ultimate sacrifice to the safety of Australian soldiers on operations. **A memorial at the School of Military Engineering in Sydney, where the dogs were trained, will be expanded to pay tribute to these dogs**.

The ADFTWDA issues two unofficial canine medals:

1. **The War Dog Operational Medal:** This is issued to those Military Working Dogs who have served for a minimum period of twenty-eight days in a theatre or war or an area of operations.
2. **The Canine Service Medal:** This is issued to those working dogs who have served for a continuous period of five years.

The ADFTWDA has also awarded medals to service dogs from the police, corrective services and other government agencies.

BRITAIN

"The Animals in War" memorial was unveiled on 24th November, 2004 by the Princess Royal-Patron. It exists as a memorial to the huge number of animals that have served and died under British Military command throughout history. The memorial is located at Brook Gate, Park Lane, on the edge of London's Hyde Park.

"This monument is dedicated to all the animals that served and died alongside British and Allied Forces in wars and campaigns throughout time."

"They had no choice."

On a smaller scale than memorials, some units have devised medals to honour their combat hero dogs.

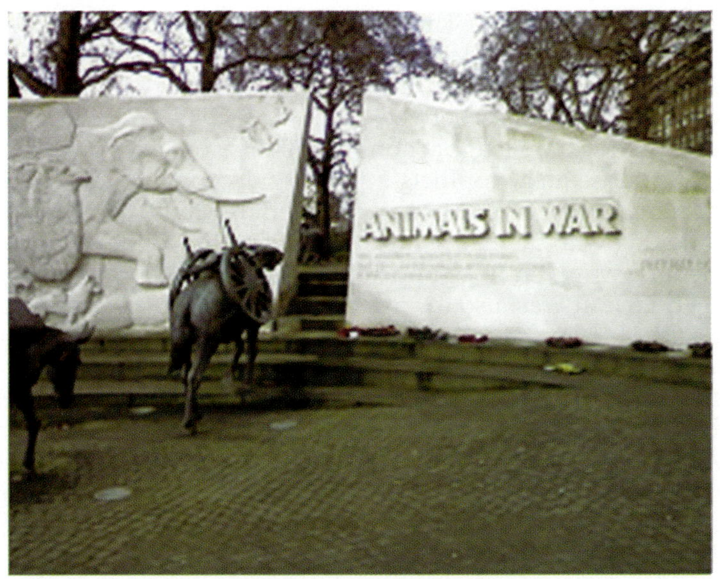

The animals in war memorial, London

PDSA Dickin Medal

Maria Dickin, the founder of the People's Dispensary for Sick Animals (PDSA), a British Veterinary Charity, instituted PDSA Medal in 1943 in the United Kingdom to honour the work of animals in the war. It is a bronze medallion bearing the words "For Gallantry" and "We Also Serve" within a laurel wreath, carried on a ribbon of striped green, dark brown and pale blue. It is awarded to animals that have displayed "conspicuous gallantry or devotion to duty while serving or associated with any branch of the Armed Forces or Civil Defence Units". The award

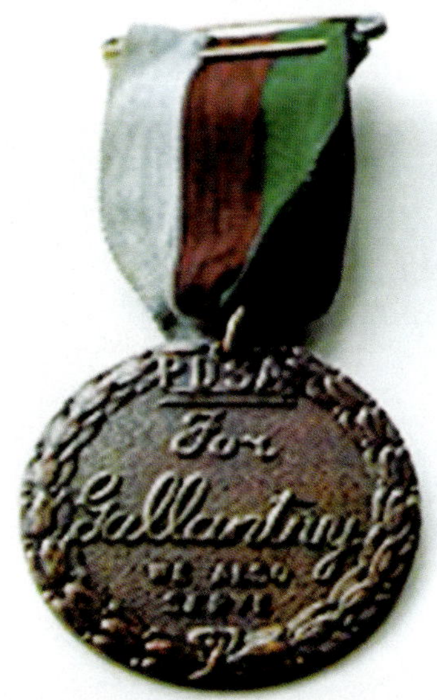

PDSA Dickin Medal

is commonly referred to as " The Animals' Victoria Cross". The award was established for any animal displaying conspicuous gallantry and devotion to duty whilst serving with British Empire Armed Forces or Civil Emergency Services. The medal was awarded 54 times between 1943 and 1949—to 32 pigeons, 18 dogs, 3 horses, and 1 cat to acknowledge actions of gallantry or devotion during the Second World War, and subsequent conflicts.

The awarding of the medal was revived in 2000 to honour Gander, a Newfoundland dog who saved infantrymen during the Battle of Lye Mun. In early 2002, this medal was given in honour of 3 dogs for their role responding to the September 11 attack. It was also awarded to 2 dogs serving with Commonwealth Forces in Bosnia-Herzegovina and Iraq. In December, 2007, 12 former recipients buried at the PDSA Animal Cemetery in Ilford, Essex, were afforded full military honours at the conclusion of a National Lottery-aided project to restore the cemetery. The first recipients of the award, in December, 1943, were 3 pigeons, serving with the Royal Air Force, all of whom contributed to the recovery of air crew from ditched aircraft during the Second World War. The most recent animal to be honoured is Sasha, a search dog serving in Afghanistan. As of April, 2014, the Dickin Medal has been awarded 65 times.

JAPAN

The "Monument to the Loyal Dogs," in Zushi, Japan, was built in memory of three German Shepherds Military Working Dogs, who served in Manchuria in 1931. These dogs were trained and deployed in battlefield under the loving care of their Zushi-born handler, Maj. Itaru Itakura who also died in action in Manchuria. His wife Shizuko moved to Zushi in 1932 from Mukden, taking with her three children and a male German Shepherd named Juri. She had worked at an elementary school in Mukden and found work in Kanagawa Prefecture teaching English and music at Zushi Practical Course Girls' High School and Zushi Elementary School. Juri died from distemper-related infection on Valentine's Day in 1932, around the same time that Nachi and Kongo were becoming household names. His remains were buried at the rear of Enmeiji Temple.

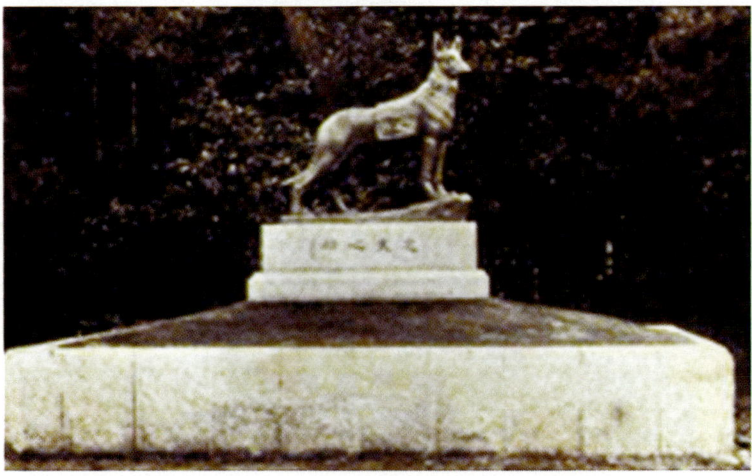

Postcard depicting the monument to the loyal dogs in Zushi

Itakura's eldest daughter Atsuko entered Zushi Practical Course Girls' High School where her mother worked in April, 1933. Principal Yujiro Arai learned of Itakura's story during the initial entrance inspection. He visited Juri's grave with children from the school and related the story of Nachi and Kongo. According to a bulletin by the Imperial War Dog Association, Arai conclude by saying:

"Even though they were non-native dogs, Kongo and Nachi lived in the Empire and were trained by a solider of the Imperial Army, working loyally to the Imperial Japanese Army; we should remember their devotion and loyalty".

Arai's words apparently stirred something in the pupils. Flowers and money started to stack up in front of Juri's grave. The head priest of the temple promised the children he would set aside a corner for the memorial, if they could raise enough money for a gravestone. The children solicited donations and handed over their own pocket money. Some kids placed a collection box outside the staff room at the school and in two days it was full. The funds totaled ¥20, approximately $75 today. The school itself had raised enough money to purchase a gravestone but the collection efforts were far from over. On 22nd April, 1933, Tokyo, Nichinichi Shimbun published a story on the children's efforts and money flooded in from the public. Very quickly, the children's coffers exceeded ¥900, or $3,350 today. With the explosion in donations, the principal founded a support committee including Enmeiji's chief priest, Zushi's mayor, the local veteran's association and Vice Adm. Kamiizumi to plan monument to faithful hounds.

Toshio Aoyanagi, a young engraver, won the commission to produce a bronze statue in Juri's image. But with Juri already deceased, Aoyanagi was forced to use a dog from Tokyo named Hirumoa, probably from the name Gilmore. In contrast to the obedient canine his image would represent, Hirumoa which was reportedly a very difficult model but after a year of labour, Aoki finished the double-sized mould of a German Shepherd standing tall with his messenger pack. On 9th July, 1933, the three heroic dogs of Japanese Army were commemorated by opening of the

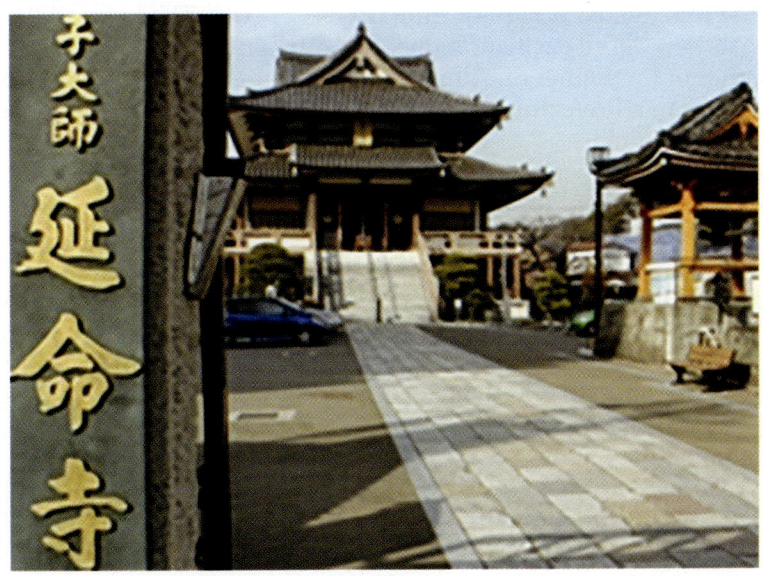

Entrance to Enmei Temple in Zushi in 2014

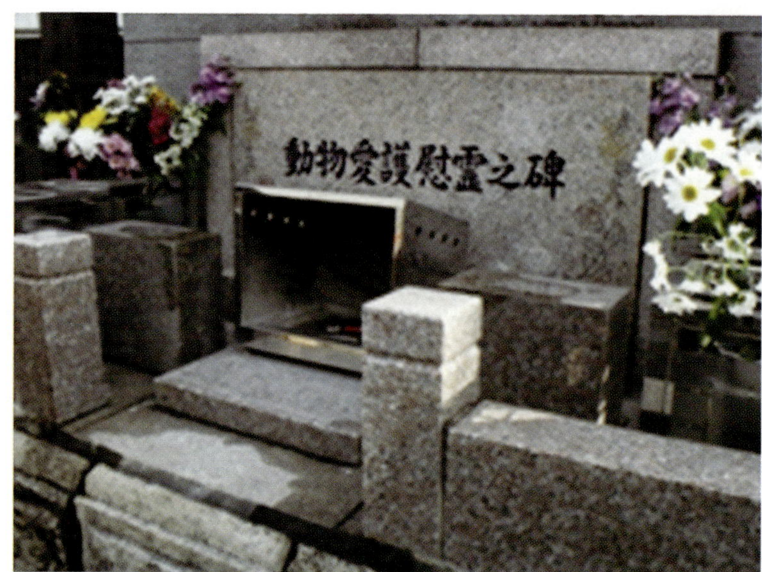

The Monument to the Protection of Animals at Enmei Temple as it stands in 2014

"Monument to the Loyal Dogs" at Enmei Temple in Zushi. Itakura's widow, Army Minister Sadao Araki and former minister of war and soon-to-be Commander of the Kwantung Army, Gen Jiro Minami all attended the ceremony along with other political and military dignitaries plus more than 2,000 schoolchildren who had raised the funds to erect the statue. The students sang a song in the dogs' honour called "Nachi and Kongo's War Feat."

Juri's remains were also placed in the memorial alongside the remains of "Kongo" and Nachi, retrieved from Peitaying.

However, the monument in Enmei Temple did not survive the war. Aoyanagi's bronze statue was melted down for military use in 1939. The memorial was rebuilt in 1958 with its new, more pacifistic name, "Monument to the Protection of Animals."

In the corner of the Enmei Buddhist Temple grounds in the coastal city of Zushi in Japan's Kanagawa Prefecture, stands a stone cenotaph that reads "Monument to the Protection of Animals."

The inscription dates back to 1958, although the incense still burns for the ashes of three dogs interred here more than 80 years ago.

ISRAEL

In Israel, a vivid symbol of the relationship between Unit Oketz's warriors and their dogs is the unit's canine graveyard, formed to honour the memory of the dogs that fell in the line of duty. The cemetery at the Oketz Military Base in central Israel is the final resting place of 60 four-legged recruit heroes. It bears testimony to the increasingly significant role that dogs have come to play in the ranks of the military. Amid the tombstones stands a large sculpture of a dog and handler with an inscription reading: "Walk softly, for here lie soldiers of Israel." Unit policy is that any dog that loses his life in the line of duty receives a military funeral. Every year on the eve of Independence Day, a remembrance ceremony is held for the dogs that have died in action.

War Dog

High on a hill overlooking the sea,
Stands a statue to honour and glorify me.
Me and my mates that have all gone before,
To help and protect the men of the war.
I am a war dog, I receive no pay,
With my keen, sharp senses, I show the way.
Many of us come from far and around,
Some from death row, some from the pound.
I am a member of the canine pack,
Trained for combat and life on the track.
I serve overseas in those far off lands,
Me and my master working hand in hand.
I lift my head and look across the land,
Beside my master, I await his command.
Together we watch as we wait in the night,
If the enemy comes, we are ready to fight.
In the plantations of Nui Dat I do camp,
The smell print of the VC, to track, as I tramp.
"Seek 'em out boy!" my master does call,
Through the vines of the jungle, together we crawl.
I remember the day we were trapped underground,
With military wildfire exploding all around.
My master and I packin' death through the fight,
Comforting each other till the guns went quiet.
My master's tour of duty has come to an end,
Vietnam he will leave, I will lose a good friend.
No longer will we trudge through the jungles of war,
The canine, the digger, the memory will endure.
Now the years have passed and I patiently wait,
For God to receive me through His celestial gate.
Where I'll roam in comfort for evermore,
He'll keep me safe from the ravages of war.

— Santina Lizzio

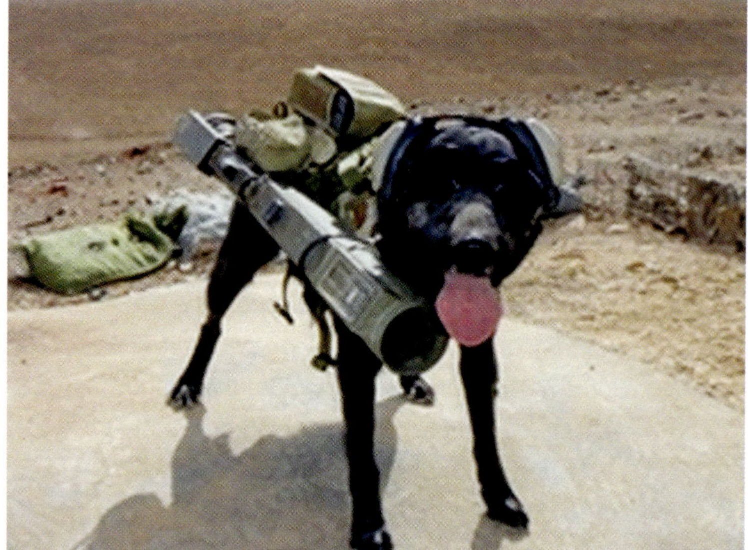

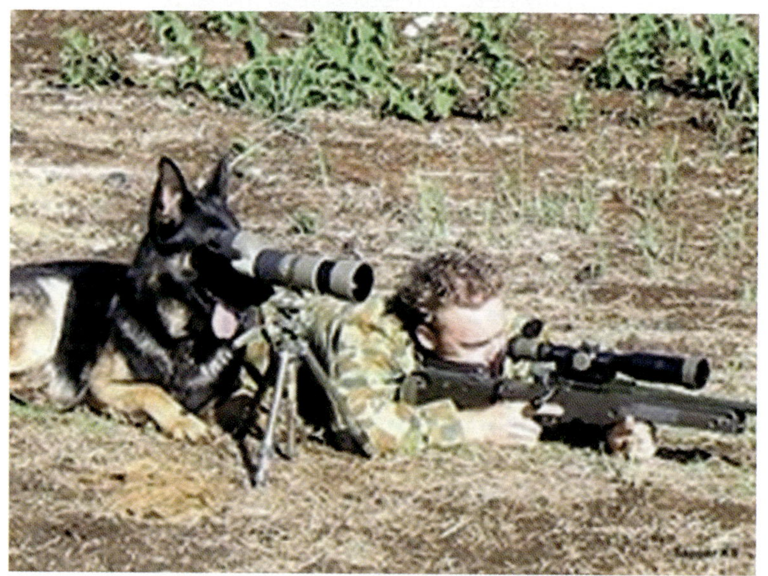

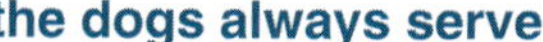

the dogs always serve

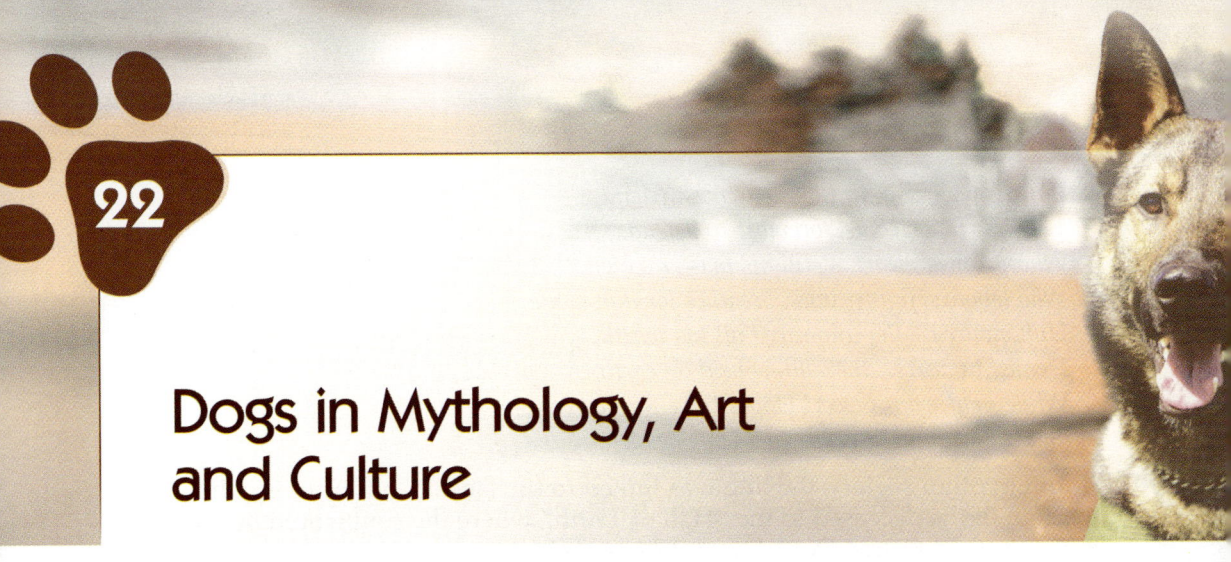

22

Dogs in Mythology, Art and Culture

"The one absolutely unselfish friend that man can have in this selfish world, the one that never deserts him, the one that never proves ungrateful or treacherous, is the dog ... He will kiss the hand that has no feed to offer. When all other friends desert, he remains."

... George G Vest in a speech in the US Senate, 1884

MYTHOLOGY AND DOGS

An ancient Greek philosopher and critic of social mores, Diogenes of Sinope, was known to be living with many dogs. It used to be thought that the dog originated somewhere in the fertile crescent, but Finnish genetic researcher Savolainen, in his analysis of the mitochondrial DNA (mtDNA) of a great variety of dogs from around the globe, demonstrated that their domestication must have taken place in East Asia. This transformation from wolf to dog is thought to have occurred more than 27,000 years ago. Without dogs, it seems unlikely humans would have been able to spread throughout the world, nor would civilization had developed as quoted in "Dogs That Changed the World, Nature, PBS, 2008".

Even before the written word, dogs had been a part of the history of human beings. The ancient temple of Gobekli-Tepe in Turkey dated to at least 12,000 years BCE, has provided archaeologists with evidence of domesticated dogs. Natufian Grave (Circa 12,000 BCE) discovered in Ein Mallaha, Israel, that an old man was buried with a puppy. The Epic of Gilgamesh from ancient Sumeria (2150–2000 BCE) mentions that Goddess Innana had seven prized hunting dogs in the famous descent of Innana, the Goddess goes down into the underworld where her husband Dumuzi, keeps domesticated dogs as part of his royal retinue. In an article in the New York Times magazine atheist Natalie Angier quoted Frans de Wall, a primatologist at Emory University:

"I have argued that many of what philosophers call moral sentiments can be seen in other species. In Chimpanzees and other animals, you see examples of sympathy, empathy, reciprocity and a willingness to follow social rules. Dogs are good example of a species that have and obey social rules; that is why we like them so much, even though they are large Carnivores."

Lord Byron, the English poet in his famous poem epitaph to a Dog in 1808 expressed his thought as under:

But the poor dog, in life the firmest friend,
The first to welcome, foremost to defend,
Whose honest heart is still his master's own,
Who labours, fights, lives, breathes for him alone,
Unhonoured falls, unnoticed all his worth,
Denied in heaven the soul he held on earth—
While man, vain insect! Hopes to be forgiven,
and claims himself a sole exclusive heaven.

In Egyptian society, the dog was linked to the Jackal God, Anubis, who guided the soul of the deceased to the "Hall of Truth" where the soul would be judged by the great God Osiris. Domesticated dogs were buried with great ceremony in the temple of Anubis at Saqqara, a town in northern Egypt; site of the oldest Pyramids. The idea behind this seemed to be to help the deceased dogs pass on easily to the afterlife known in Egypt as the "Field of Reeds," where they could continue to enjoy their lives as they had on earth. Dogs were highly valued in Egypt as part of the family, and when a dog would die, the family, if they could afford, would have the dog mummified with as much care as they would pay for a human member of the family. Great grief was displayed over the death of a family dog and the family would shave their eyebrows as a sign of this grief. Tomb paintings of the Pharaoh (the title of the ancient Egyptian kings) Rameses the Great (one of 12 kings of ancient Egypt between 1315 and 1090 BC), depict him with his hunting dogs. The dogs were often buried with their masters to provide this kind of companionship in the afterlife. We even know many ancient Egyptian dog names from leather collars as well as stelae. They included names such as Brave One, Reliable, Good Herdsman, North-Wind, Antelope, etc. Other names come from the dogs colour, such as Blacky whereas some dogs were given numbers for names such as "The Fifth". Many of the names seem to represent affection, while others convey merely the dog's abilities or capabilities. The dog was an important part of Egyptian society and culture. Enlilbani, a king from the Old Babylonian first dynasty of Isin, commemorated the temple to the Goddess Ninisina. A dog cult did exist in this area being important to the "Cult of Ninisina". More than 30 dog burials, numerous dog sculptures and dog drawings were discovered when the area around this Ninisina temple was excavated. Dogs were also closely associated with the "Gula cult" who used them in taking oaths and even referred them as a divinity. In Isin, Mesopotamia, a temple was named e-ur-gi7-ra which translates as "dog house".

In ancient Persian culture, dogs were one of the preferred means of disposing of corpses. This is the likely reason why they were, and still are, in some places considered to be especially unclean. It is not solely because they may have eaten carrion that they are avoided, but also because it is often thought that evil spirits readily associate with dead bodies. However, dogs were seen as important members of the Persian family during the pre-Islam era, and received a lot of attention in Zoroastrianism. Work with ancient texts has emphasized the sacred importance of dog cults in fifth century BC during the Persian and Hellenistic periods in the Grecian, Phoenecian, and Mesopotamian world. This was considerably highlighted by the discovery of the ritual burial of thousands of dogs in the eastern Mediterranean (Israel and Lebanon). The dogs, it seems, had always held a supernatural significance for man and it is an ancient dog cult we witness in man's close association with the animal.

In Zoroastrianism, the dog is regarded as an especially beneficent, clean and righteous creature which must be fed and taken care of and is praised for the useful work it performs in the household. The legal books of Avesta (the Zoroastrian Holy Scripture archives) divided the dog into two kinds, i.e. the "house" dog to protect the owner's home and the "herd" dog, having the function to protect cattle. The relationship between man and dog is an important one according to the Avesta documents and man has to be grateful to the dog for protecting him and his possessions.

It was also believed that dogs have a special connection with the afterlife, i.e. the "Chinwad Bridge to Heaven" is said to be guarded by dogs in Zoroastrian scripture, and dogs are traditionally fed in commemoration of the dead. Respect for the dog, is a common injunction among Iranian Zoroastrian villagers. Detailed prescriptions for the appropriate treatment of dogs are found in the Vendidad which is a subdivision of the Zoroastrian Holy Scripture Avesta. The faithful are required to assist dogs and harsh punishments are imposed for harm inflicted in various ways on domestic as well as stray dogs. Often, help or harm to a dog was equated with help or harm to a human. The killing of a dog, was considered to lead to damnation in the afterlife. A homeowner was required to take care of a pregnant dog that lies near his home at least until the puppies are born and preferably old enough to take care of themselves. If the homeowner does not help the dog and the puppies come to harm as a result, "he shall pay for it the penalty for willful murder", because "Atar (Fire), the son of Ahura Mazda, is believed to be watching over a pregnant dog as he does over a woman". It is also a major sin if a man harms a dog by giving him bones that are too hard and get stuck in his throat, or food that is too hot, so that it burns his throat. Giving bad food to a dog was considered as bad as serving bad food to a human. The believers are required to take care of an injured dog and should try to heal him in the same manner as they would do for one of the faithful.

According to the Vendidad and in traditional Zoroastrian practice, dogs are allotted some funerary ceremonies akin to those of humans. In the Vendidad, it is stated that the spirits of a thousand deceased dogs are reincarnated in a single otter ("water dog"), hence the killing of an otter is a terrible crime that brings drought and famine upon the land and must be atoned either by the death of the killer or by the killer performing a very long list of deeds considered pious, including the healing of dogs, raising of puppies, paying of fines to priests, etc. Zoroastrian believe in "Sagdid" (dog sight) a funeral ceremony, in which a dog is brought into the room where the body is lying so that be can look on it. There are various spiritual benefits thought to be obtained by the ceremony. It is believed that the original purpose was to make certain that the person was really dead, since the dog's more acute senses would be able to detect signs of life that a human might miss. A "four-eyed" dog, that is one with two spots on its forehead, was preferred for Sagdid because of the belief that the dogs have special spiritual virtues and a dog's gaze is considered to be purifying and drive off contaminating *Asuras* (demons) away from the corpses.

However, the traditional rites involving dogs have been under attack by reformist Zoroastrians since the mid-19th century, and they had abandoned them almost completely by the late 20th century. Even traditionalist Zoroastrians tend to restrict such rites to a significant extent nowadays.

In Christianity, the deuterocanonical Book of Tobit mentioned that a dog faithfully accompanying Tobias (Tobit's son) and the angel Raphael on their journeys. Jesus told the story of the poor man lazarus, whose sores were licked by street dogs for healing. The Catholic Church recognizes Saint Roch (also called Saint Rocco), who lived in the early 14th century in France as the Patron Saint of dogs. It is said that he caught the plague while doing charitable work and went into the forest expecting to die. There, he was befriended by a dog who licked his sores and brought him food, and he was able to recover. The feast day of Saint Roch (16th August) is celebrated in Bolivia as the "Birthday of all dogs". A dog was named Saint Guinefort who received local veneration as a Saint at a French shrine from 13th to 20th centuries.

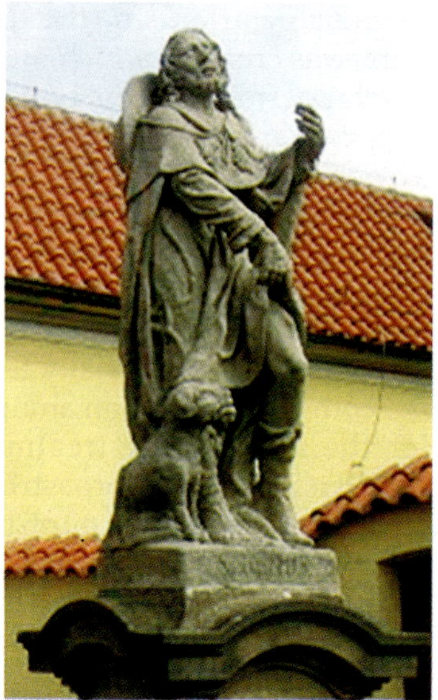

Statue of Saint Roch with his dog

In Islam, it is uncommon for practicing Muslims to have dogs as pets since majority of both Sunni and Shia Muslim jurists consider dogs to be ritually unclean. However, there are a number of traditions concerning Muhammad's attitude towards dogs. He said that the company of dogs, except as helpers in hunting, herding, and home protection, voided a portion of a Muslim's good deeds. On the other hand, he advocated kindness to dogs and other animals.

Many Muslim theologians have argued that the dog is not an unclean animal based on the inclusion of a dog among the "Seven Sleepers" as recorded in the 18th Verse of the 18th Chapter of the Quran which reads:

"Thou would have deemed them awake, whilst they were asleep, and we turned them on their right and on their left sides: their dog stretching forth his two fore-legs on the threshold: if thou had come up on to them, thou would have certainly turned back from them in flight, and would certainly have been filled with terror of them (Surah Al Kahf, Qur'an: 18)".

GREEK MYTHOLOGY AND DOGS

In Greek mythology, the dogs are not only considered "man's best friend," but also favourite pets of the Gods. They are not as overpowering as Hercules, but their presence is far more consistent. Dogs find themselves in many of the Greek tales. Here they often serve a similar role as they do in our own society, but their symbolic value increases ten-fold. Three dogs stand above the rest and each represents a particular canine virtue we all cherish, loyalty, perseverance and determination.

The dog appears in Greek literature early on in the figure of the three-headed dog Cerberus who guarded the gates of Hades. One example of this is the Caeretan black-figure hydria vase of Hercules and Cerberus from circa 530–520 BCE. The art work is presently displayed in the Louvre Museum in Paris, France. In Greece, as in ancient Sumeria, the dog had been associated with the Goddess in that both the Goddesses Artemis and Hecate kept dogs. Artemis had hunting dogs while Hecate had black Molossian dogs. The philosophic school of Cynicism in ancient Greece takes its name from the Greek for 'dog' and those who followed this school were called 'Kynikos' meaning, dog-like, in part because of their determination to follow a single path loyally without swerving. The dogs were considered messengers of the Gods, and it was thought that they could smell out diseases. Special healing dogs, were kept in temples to comfort the sick and dying, and to lick their wounds which sometimes caused a miraculous recovery, and thus dogs were associated with the healing process. Their divine patron was Hermanubis (Hermes + Anubis) with the head of a dog on the body of a man.

The famous dogs mentioned in Greek mythology are described below:

Argos

The most famous dog story from ancient Greece, however, is that of Argos, the loyal friend of king Odysseus of Ithaka (a Greek Island to the West of Greece) during the period circa 800 BCE. When Odysseus fighting in Trozan war left the fallen Troy (an ancient city in Asia Minor) for his beloved home of Ithaca, most people in Ithaca assumed him dead. His wife, the ever faithful, "Penelope", his earnest son "Telemachus", and eternally faithful dog "Argos", never gave up hope that Odysseus will return home. For twenty years, Odysseus braved the high seas, and finally his determination was rewarded. Odysseus, at first, enters the town unnoticed, in a beggar's disguise so that he could not be recognized by the hostile suitors who were trying to win Odysseus's wife "Penelope's hand in marriage". As they were talking, a dog that had been lying asleep raised his head and pricked up his ears. This was Argos, whom Odysseus had bred before setting out for Troy. In the old days he used to be taken out by the young men when they went hunting wild goats, or deer, or hares, but now that his master was gone and he was lying neglected full of fleas on the heaps of mule and cow dung that lay in front of the stable doors, till the men should come and draw him away. He was in poor condition after Penelope's suitors had kicked him on the ass.

As Odysseus approaches his home, the old dog, Argos takes notice of him. Poor Argos had been exiled from the house and was now living in squalor. On seeing Odysseus, he drops his ears, and wags his tail in greetings to his master. Odysseus notices the dog straight away but could not return the greetings to his beloved dog Argos, as it would have disclosed his identity. By seeing the hound's faithfulness, Odysseus moved to tears. Composing himself and without being noticed by others he asked:

"Eumaeus (first mortal that Odysseus meets in Ithica) what a noble hound that yonder on the manure heap: his build is splendid, is he as fine a fellow as he looks or is he only one of those dogs that come begging about a table and are kept merely for show?" Eumaeus answered that this hound "belonged to him who has died in a far country. If he were what he was when Odysseus left for Troy, he would soon show you what he could do. There was not a wild beast in the forest that could get away from him when he was once on his tracks. But now he has fallen on evil times, for his master is dead and gone, and the women take no care of him. Servants never do their work when their master's hand is no longer over them. For Zeus (supreme God of ancient Greek mythology) takes half the goodness out of a man when he makes a slave of him."

So saying he entered the well-built mansion, and made straight for the riotous pretenders in the hall. Argos, having remained faithful to the end, lets out a cry and passed into the darkness of death, now that he had seen his master once more after twenty years. Argos has become the very symbol of faithfulness.

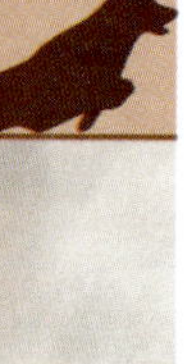

Laelaps

Dogs hardly ever sit and wait patiently as they are doers and constantly on the go. If the dog sees cat or little squirrel while on walk, the owner holding the leash had to hold on tight and be on guard. This characteristic has been noticed for centuries. Dogs are determined and if they set their mind to chase something, there is almost no way to break their will and they will only decide when they are going to give up a chase. Some dogs seem to be willing to run for eternity.

One such dog was Laelaps as mentioned in Greek mythology. When Zeus (supreme God) was a baby, a dog, known as the "golden hound" was charged with protecting the future King of Gods. This may have been the same dog, Zeus later gave to Europa. Zeus had fallen deeply in love with the beautiful Europa, and when given the chance stole her away to the Island of Crete. There he tried to seduce her by giving her three gifts: Talos, a giant bronze creature (perhaps more accurately a robot), a javelin that never missed, and Laelaps, a dog that never failed to capture its prey. Europa eventually gave the dog to Minos, King of Crete (largest Greek Island). Later on, Minos gave the great dog Laelaps to Procris as a reward for saving him from a deadly disease. The dog was soon sent to capture the Teumessian fox, a giant fox that could never be caught. This created a paradox, for the dog always caught its prey, and the fox could not be caught. The chase went on until Zeus grew weary and simply turned both into stone, frozen forever in the chase.

Cerberus

The most fearsome dog in Greek mythology is the great three-headed Cerberus. Like many dogs, Cerberus was a watch dog but what he chose to guard was not something as pleasant as our homes. He watched Hades, the ancient Greek God of the underworld and although he allowed many people to enter, he didn't let anyone leave. He had three heads and a snake as a tail. In most works, the three heads each respectively see and represent the past, the present, and the future. Some other sources suggest that the heads represent birth, youth, and old age. Each of Cerberus' heads is said to have an appetite only for live meat, and thus allow only the spirits of the dead to freely enter the underworld, but allow none to leave. Cerberus was always employed as Hades' loyal watch dog, and guarded the gates that granted access and exit. However, a few were able to escape on entering Hades. Somehow, Orpheus (a legendary musician in Greece) lulled Cerberus to sleep by playing soothing music and Hermes could also do the same by using water from the Lethe (a river in Hades). The most famous of all was Hercules (a hero noted for his strength in Greece) who did not use such subtle methods since he had been given 12 labours, as penance for an act of terrible violence by king Eurystheus. The last of these was to capture Cerberus and bring him to the land of the living without using weapons. This most dangerous and difficult task was in recompense for the killing of his own children.

After having been given the task, Hercules went to Eleusis (a town in Greece) to be initiated in the Eleusinian mysteries (secret rites) so that he could learn how to enter and exit the underworld alive and in passing absolve himself for killing centaurs (a creature half man and half horse). He found the entrance to the underworld at Tanaerum (a Peninsula in Southern Greece having a big cave). He traversed the entrance in each direction and passed Charon (ferry man). Whilst in the underworld, Hercules met Theseus and Pirithous. The two companions had been imprisoned by Hades for attempting to kidnap Persephone (daughter of Zeus). Hades had organized a pretended hospitality and invited them to sit in chairs of forgetfulness and they were permanently trapped. Hercules pulled Theseus and Pirithous from their chairs. However, Pirithous desire to have the wife of a God for himself, was so intense and insulting that he was doomed to stay behind.

Finally, Hercules found Hades and asked permission to take Cerberus to the surface, to which Hades agreed if Hercules could overpower the beast without using weapons. Finally, in a fierce fight, Hercules was able to overpower Cerberus and he sling the beast over his back, dragging it out of the underworld through a cavern entrance in the Peloponnese (southern Peninsula of Greece), brought him to Eurystheus and gained immortality.

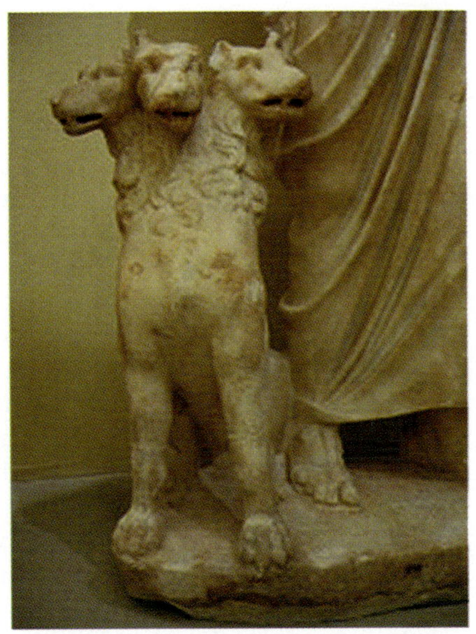

Cerberus, the three-headed guardian

Sirius

Sirius was not originally a dog. The name comes from a Greek word meaning "glowing" or "scorcher." It is associated with dogs because it is the brightest star of the constellation Canis Major, the "Great Dog." Ancient Greeks also thought this star affected dogs negatively. Dog days of summer comes 6 weeks after the solstice and the Dog Star, Sirius, appears in the night sky of the Northern Hemisphere. It was once thought that this bright star contributed to the heat characteristic of the beginning of August.

THE BUDDHISM AND DOGS

Animals have always been regarded in Buddhist thought as sentient beings and according to the Mahayana school, animals possess Buddha nature, and therefore, potential for enlightenment. The doctrine of rebirth held the view that any human could be reborn as an animal and any animal could be reborn as a human. An animal might be a reborn dead relative, as such, through their series of lives might come to believe that animal may also be a distant relative. Buddha expounded that sentient beings currently living in the animal realm had been our mothers, brothers, sisters, fathers, children and friends in past rebirths. One could not, therefore, make a hard distinction between moral rules applicable to animals and those applicable to humans and ultimately humans and animals were part of a single family. The Chinese scholar Tiantai taught the principle of the Mutual Possession of the Ten Worlds which meant that all living beings have buddha-nature 'in their present form'. In the 'Devadatta chapter of the Lotus sutra, the Dragon King's daughter attains Buddhahood in her present form thus opening the way for both women and animals to attain Buddhahood. The Jataka stories which tell about past lives of the Buddha in folktale fashion, frequently involve animals as peripheral or main characters and it is not uncommon for the Bodhisattva (the past-life Buddha) to appear as an animal as well.

The first Buddhist monarch of India, Asoka, included in his Edicts an expression of concern for the number of animals that had been killed for his meals, and expressed an intention to put an end to such killing. He also included animals with humans as the beneficiaries of his programmes for obtaining medicinal plants, planting trees and digging wells. In his fifth Pillar Edict, Ashoka decrees the protection of a large number of animals that were not in common use as livestock. He advocated protection of young animals and mother animals still feeding their young from slaughter and bans a number of other practices hurtful to animals.

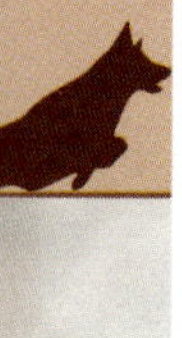

In East Asian Buddhism and particularly in Tibet and China, the release of animals, particularly birds or fish into their natural environment became an important way of demonstrating Buddhist pity. In the later Ming dynasty, societies "for releasing animals" were created, which built ponds in which fish that were redeemed from fishermen for this purpose were released. It is increasingly recognized that animal release has the potential for avoiding negative environmental impacts.

Many Buddhists believe people with negative karma are reborn as dog who are not intelligent enough to raise their karma on their own and they essentially have to remain dogs until their negative karma has worn off. Eventually, they will get another chance to become human again and can work on reaching Nirvana. The important idea to get is that karma does not work the same way for animals as it does for people because they are not able to affect their own karma. In Australia, a Tibetan Buddhist master came to help family pets on the path to enlightenment and many other Buddhists feel very strongly about animals deserving Buddhist rights and treatment. Care for all living things is a central tenet of Buddhism. So Lama Zopa Rinpoche, a Buddhist master taught by the Dalai Lama, blessed about 100 cats, dogs, even mice and mud crabs. Lama Zopa believes that animals don't have as many opportunities as humans to attain happiness. The master feels that animal blessings are a way for Buddhists to create compassion. Basically, loving animals are good for the soul and there are stories of dogs arriving regularly at the Buddhist temple and being treated as spirits, wishing to embrace the religion. After all, they have expressed a desire to take part in the ceremony and may have the opportunity to do the same on two legs in another life.

Lama Zopa advises pet owners to expose them to holy objects, recite prayers to them and bless their food. In Thailand's capital, Bangkok, they have gone one step further and begun offering Buddhist funeral rites to pets. Dogs live entirely in the moment with a limited memory of the past and do not seem to spend much time pondering in future. To a dog only the now is important, the love that surrounds him, the pleasure in a meal or a game of fetch. Some people argue that there is much to learn about proper living from a dog.

The following tales gives us more insight about the relationship between the Buddishts and their dogs.

The Guilty Dog

One evening, after the king had spent the day travelling in his magnificent carriage, the three pairs of horses were led back to the stables to be fed and watered. However, due to some oversight, the vehicle was left untended in the courtyard. During the night it rained and the fine leather harnesses were softened and began to exude a spicy, powdery odour that proved irresistible to the palace dogs. They tugged, gnawed, scrabbled and chewed and when just a faint glow appeared on the eastern horizon, they tip-toed away to curl up in their usual places. In the morning, the syces and stablemen could not believe their eyes. With cold feet and trembling hands, they went to tell the happening to the king. After listening the details, the king was furious. It is not known as to how the people responsible were to be punished, but he called for the death of every single dog in the vicinity. All the dogs in the city, pets and pye dogs alike, knew what would be the consequence of the actions of the royal hounds and so they fled to the outskirts to join the packs that lurked in the woods. At any moment, they expected the king's enforcers to come and exterminate every one of them for something they had not done. The lead dog, believed to be Buddha in a previous lifetime, put his own fear aside and calmly with great dignity, went to talk to the king. He was so imposing that the guards made no move against him. As he approached, the king asked, "How is it that you are still alive? The great dog prostrated his head on the carpet between his paws, rose again and replied "I have come on a mission of mercy, your Highness". Why are you determined to put to death every dog in the kingdom? It is not possible that they all had a bite of the royal livery. There is certainly not enough leather on six bridles and harnesses for every single dog here. "The king replied", Dogs chew royal property, dogs die". "Highness, you have always been a most just ruler. The guilty ones deserve a punishment, that is true. Which dogs did the chewing?" The noble hound continued, "Maharaj, is it right for all to suffer for the wrongs of only a few?" Your response to this question will surely cause deep reflection by those in your own household, not to mention your ministers and even your many loyal subjects of high and low degrees." After a brief hesitation, the king said, "If you can show me the guilty parties, I will spare the other animals". The skillful dog responded, "It is known that dogs eat grass to scour their stomachs, therefore, let all the dogs eat kula grass. This will make them cough up what is in their bodies, and then we will find the guilty parties". "It seems that most of the dogs have fled," said the king. "Only the royal hounds remain and how can royal dogs be compared to common curs?" but let us see if the kula grass is effective. We will try it on them first "the royal dogs were fed kula grass and they coughed it up along with little bits of gilded leather".

The king was amazed, and he reflected on his spontaneous angry response. He put an immediate stop to the dog hunt. He even halted the destruction of wild dogs (except those known to kill cattle). As their penance, every year the royal dogs had to serve all the others pets, pye dogs and even those that lived in the forest, at a great feast in the city centre. So it happened that a great king learned the virtue of restraint, justice, courage and compassion from Tathagata, who in that lifetime was living in the animal realm as a lead dog.

Asanga and the Dog

Asanga yearned to have direct experience of the future Buddha, Maitreya. He slowly learned patience through guidance, practice and extraordinary experience. Once, after he had been meditating for 12 years, he left the cave and encountered a poor dog lying ill by the wayside. It was near death, its lower body covered with maggot-infested sores. His meditations had helped him to develop great compassion, and so Asanga was moved to ease the animal's suffering. Naturally, he thought of removing the maggots, but he realized that if he did that with his fingers, he might injure them. Therefore, without injuring any maggot but yet to relieve the dog,

Asanga's solution was to crouch down and gently skim off the maggots with his tongue. The moment he did that, the dog disappeared and Bodhisattva Maitreya appeared in his place. Asanga said, "I have longed to see you all these many years and why have you chosen this moment to appear to me?" Maitreya replied, "I have always been with you, but before now, you were not able to see me. It was necessary for you to purify your mind and develop your compassion sufficiently before it was possible for this to happen." To demonstrate the truth of what he had just said, the Bodhisattva whose name is Maitreya or loyal friend asked Asanga to pick him up, put him around his shoulders and take a stroll through the neighbouring village. Once there, no one noticed anything unusual at all except for one old woman, who asked, "What are you doing walking around like that with a sick dog on you?" Of course, no one saw Maitreya and most noticed nothing out of the ordinary at all.

This tale from the biography of Asanga, who was a Brahmin from Peshawar (ca. 300–370 CE), makes a lesser and a greater point: "There is neither clean nor unclean, repugnancy comes from learning". More importantly, whatever we experience, all of reality, depends only on the state of our mind.

Asanga is considered the founder of the Buddhist approach called Yogachara, especially the branch known as *chittamatra* or consciousness only.

The Dog Yogi

Kukuripa was one of the Mahasiddhas (one of the 84 greatest yogis) and one of Tilopa's teachers. He stayed not far from Pullahari in Western Magadha, where he lived on an island "in a poison lake" surrounded by dogs. One of the female dogs reveals herself as a Dakini, saying that she is instrumental in his "Realization" and he has descended from paradise to rejoin her in the cave. When she caught sight of her beloved master, she leaped and pranced with joy. But no sooner did Kukuripa set down and began to scratch her favourite spot just behind the ears, she vanished from sight and wreathed in a cloud of glory stood as a radiantly beautiful Dakini.

The Himalayan Dog

The largest and best known place in the Himalayan region is Tibet. Outside the realms of geography and political science, the word "Tibetan" is often used in broadest sense. There is a proverb saying that happiness is being accompanied when someone travels with a dog. Also, dogs are believed to be a superior type of animal possessing of a nature close to that of humans. Some gompas or monastic institutions keep and care for them in the belief that dogs are monks who could not maintain their commitments and continued contact with the Buddha's teachings.

One Lama even said that if someone disturbs you while you are at your practice, ask them not to do it again. However, if a dog want something, attend to its needs.

CHINESE MYTHOLOGY AND DOGS

In Chinese mythology, there are many myths about dogs. It refers to those myths found in the historical geographic area of China and these include myths in Chinese and other languages, as transmitted by Han Chinese as well as other ethnic groups, of which fifty-six are officially recognized by the administration of China (Yang 2005: 4). Dogs are an important motif in Chinese mythology and include a particular dog which accompanies a hero. The dog is one of the twelve totem creatures for which years are named. The first grain which allowed current agriculture is believed to have been provisioned by a dog. Even certain ethnic groups claims of having a magical dog as an original ancestor. In the study of historical Chinese culture, many of the stories that have been told regarding characters and events which have been written or told of the distant past have a double tradition: one which traditionally presents a more historicized and one which presents a more mythological version. This is also true of some accounts related to mythological dogs in China. Ritual burials of dogs in China is also well-known.

Wolfram Eberhard points out that compared to other cultures it is "striking " that Chinese literature rarely has given names for dogs. This means that in the context of Chinese mythology, often a dog will play an important role, but it will not be given a proper name and rather being referred as "dog". As Chinese grammar does not require the use of definite or indefinite articles or marking for singular or plural number, there may be ambiguity whether the reference to dog means "Dog" (proper name), "dogs", "a dog", "the dog", "some dogs", or "the dogs".

Zodiacal Dog

For thousands of years, a twelve-year cycle named after various real or mythological animals has been used in Southeast Asia. This twelve-year cycle which may be referred as the "Chinese Zodiac" associates each year in turn with a certain creature, in a fixed order of twelve animals, after which it returns to the first in the order which is the Rat. The eleventh in the cycle is the Dog. One account is that the order of the beings-of-the-year is due to their order in a racing contest involving swimming across a river, in the so-called Great Race. The reason for the dog finishing the race second from last despite generally being a talented swimmer is explained as being due to its playful nature. The dog played and frolicked along the way, thus delaying in completing the course and reaching the finishing line. The next Year of the Dog in the traditional Chinese sexagenary calendar is from 19th February, 2018 to 4th February, 2019 (Year of the Yang Earth Dog). The personalities of people born in dog years are popularly supposed to share certain attributes associated with dogs, such as loyalty or exuberance.

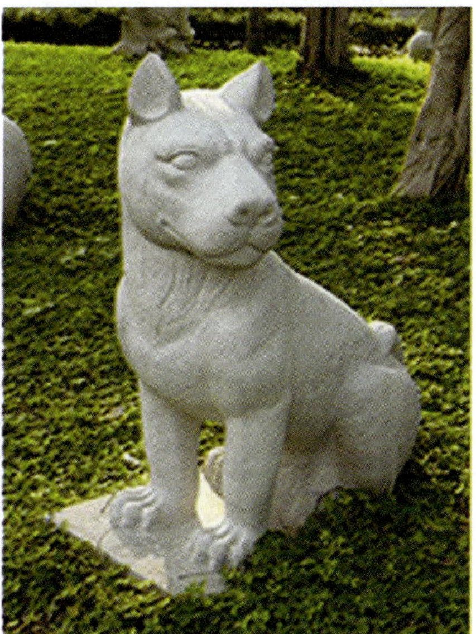

The dog statue is one of the 12 Chinese Zodiacal creatures portrayed in the Kowloon Walled City Park in Kowloon City, Hong Kong.

However, this would be modified according to other considerations of Chinese astrology, such as the influences of the month, day and hour of birth, according to the traditional system of Earthly Branches, in which the zodiacal animals are also associated with the months and times of the day (and night), in twelve (two-hour) increments. The Hour of the Dog is 7–9 pm, and the dog is associated with the ninth lunar month.

Panhu

There are various myths and legends in which various ethnic groups claimed to have had a divine dog as a forebear. One of these is the story of Panhu. The legendary Chinese sovereign Di Ku has been said to have a dog named Panhu. He helped him win a war by killing the enemy general and bringing him his head and ended up with marriage to the emperor's daughter as a reward. The dog carried his bride to the mountainous region of the south, where they produced numerous progeny. Because of their self-identification as descendants from these original ancestors, Panhu has been worshiped by the Yao People and the Shui People, often as King Pan, and the eating of dog meat tabooed (Yang 2005: 52–53). This ancestral myth has also been found among the Miao People and Li People (Yang 2005: 100 and 180).

Earlang's Dog

Earlang has been said to have a dog. In Journey to the west. Earlang's dog helps him in his fight against Sun Wukong, biting him on the leg. Later, Sun Wukong, Earlang, and their companions fight a nine-headed insect monster, which the small hound of Earlang defeats by biting off its retractable head which pops out of its torso and the monster then flees, dripping blood. It is believed that this is the origin of the nine-headed blood-dripping bird, its descendent.

Tiangou

Tiangou also called "Heavenly Dog" has been said to resemble a black dog or meteor, which is thought to eat the sun or moon during an eclipse, unless frightened away.

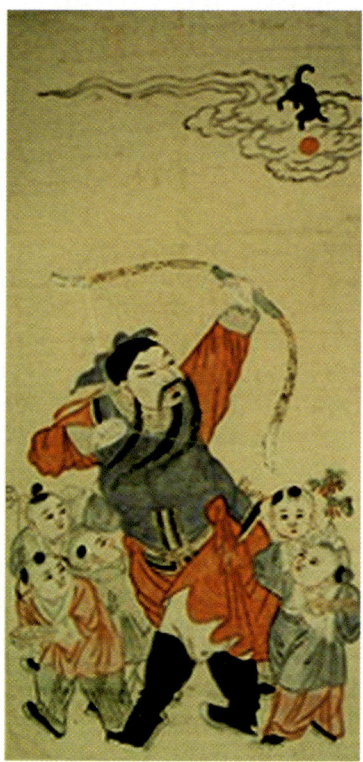

The immortal Zhuang shooting at the Tiangou

Seed Grain Dog

According to the myths of various ethnic groups, a dog provided humans with the first grain seeds enabling the seasonal cycle of planting, harvesting, and replanting staple agricultural products, by saving some of the seed grains to replant, thus explaining the genetic origin of domesticated cereal crops. This myth is common to the Buyi, Gelao, Hani, Miao, Shui, Tibetan, Tujia, and Zhuang peoples (Yang 2005: 53). A version of this myth collected from ethnic Tibetan people in Sichuan tells that in ancient times the grain was tall and bountiful. Rather than being duly grateful for the plenty, the people even used it for personal hygiene after defecation. This practice angered the God of Heaven so much that he came down to earth to repossess it all. However, a dog grasped his pant leg, piteously crying and moving God of Heaven to leave a few seeds from each type of grain with the dog. These seeds provided the seed stock of today's crops. Thus it is said that because human owe their possession of grain seed stocks to a dog, people should share some of their foods with dogs (Yang 2005: 53–54). Another myth of the Miao people, recounts the time of the distantly remote era when dogs had nine tails, until a dog went to steal grains from heaven and lost eight of its tails to the weapons of the heavenly guards while making its escape but grain seeds stuck onto its surviving tail. According to this, when Miao people hold their harvest celebration festival, the dogs are the first to be fed (Yang 2005: 54). The Zhuang and Gelao peoples have a similar myth explaining why it is that the ripe heads of grain stalks are curly, bushy, and bent, just so as is the tail of a dog (Yang 2005: 54).

Paper Dogs

In northern China, dog images made by cutting paper were thrown in the water as part of the ritual of the Double Fifth (Duanwu Festival) holiday, celebrated on the fifth day of the fifth lunar month, as an apotropaic magic act meant to drive away evil spirits. Paper dogs were also provided for protecting the dead (Eberhard, 2003: 80).

Foo Dogs

Numerous statuary of Chinese guardian lions exist, which are often called "Fu Dogs" "Foo Dogs", "Fu Lions", "Fo Lions", and "Lion Dogs". Modern lions are not native of China, except perhaps the extreme west area. However, their existence was well-known and associated symbolism and ideas about lions were widely familiar. In China, artistic representations of lions tended to be dog-like and the 'lion' which we see depicted in Chinese paintings and in sculpture, bears little resemblance to the real animal but plays a big part in "Chinese folklore"(Eberhard, 2003: 164). The reasons for referencing "guardian lions" as "dogs" in Western cultures may be obscure but the phenomenon is well-known.

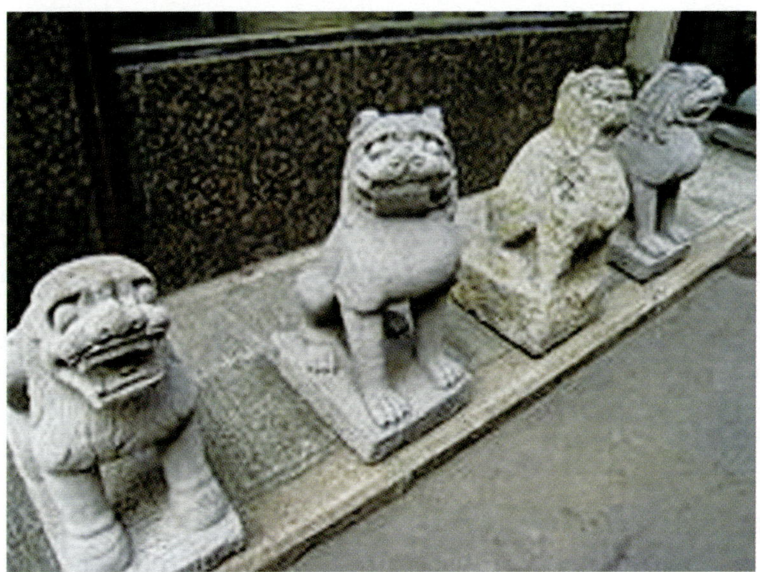

Chinese stone statue of "lions", showing pronounced dog-like features

Despite any myth from China about dogs, real and legendary dogs have been familiar throughout China since prehistorical times, unlike certain exotic animals such as lions or other creatures whose real attributes may often only have been known indirectly. Dogs also feature in various historical and legendary accounts or stories found in the extensive literary records of China, although in some cases the lines between myth and ancient history are uncertain.

TIBETAN MYTHOLOGY AND DOGS

Generally, the dogs of Tibet are not classed by Tibetans as being of a certain breed but rather by size and function. Although the distinctive features of the various kinds are recognized a dog is preferred according to how closely it resembles to the one believed to have accompanied the Buddha. Those animals resembling lions are said to be rakshasas in disguise who could regain their enormous size and ferocious character for the protection of the Master and the Dharma.

Tibetans living in the traditional manner did not traffic in dogs since they were held in such high esteem and only considered them fitting as gifts. An especially fine dog might also be given to a monastery or to an individual lama as a donation. Damchi ("tied dog") is the term for a guard dog and how various types of dog behave depends on how they are treated. The dogs that are left loose to guard compounds and monasteries are often fierce. If you are thinking of choosing a Tibetan name for a dog, find out how the name is actually pronounced. "Tashi" (auspicious one) is possibly the most popular name for a Tibetan dog. "Yangchen" (melodious sound) is suitable for a dog that enjoys its own voice. As in any cultural context, it would not be considered respectful to choose the names of venerated figures.

White Dogs

It was a custom of Iroquoian people to use a white dog as a sacrificial scapegoat, though they have often been considered unlucky. In the Treasury of Good Sayings, a Bon Cehronicle of Tibet, the coat of a white dog was dressed with a poisonous substance by a son of King Trikum's widowed queen called Rulakye. When it went home to the Bon ruler Lonam, who had held the throne for 13 years, he could not resist patting the dog and so he subsequently died.

Dogs of Fo

Bronze or ceramic guardian or temple dog figures are not really dogs at all, though they may be referred to as "Foo dogs" or "dogs of Fo (Buddha)". They are an evolution of the lions that support Buddha Shakyamuni's throne. One Chinese eclipse myth tells how it is a celestial dog that continuously tries to swallow the sun, and the male of the pair of Fo dogs is usually shown playing with a splendid ball. There is a relatively rare type of dog of the Spitz family that resembles a Chow. It is called the Foo, and was bred to resemble the guardian lion or T'ien Kou, the celestial dog. Also known as the "Sacred Dog of Sinkiang" or "Chinese Choo Hunting Dog," it may derive its common name from the ancient city of Foochow.

JAPANESE MYTHOLOGY AND DOGS

The Japanese word for "dog" is "inu". You can write "inu" in either hiragana or kanji but the kanji character for "dog" is quite simple. Typical Japanese dogs include Akita, Tosa and Shiba breeds and the onomatopoeic phrase for a dog's bark is wan-wan.

In Japan, the dog is believed to have been domesticated as early as the Jomon period (10,000 BC). White dogs are thought to be specially auspicious and often appear in folk tales (Hanasaka Jiisan, etc.). In the Edo period Tokugawa Tsuneyoshi, the fifth shogun and ardent Buddhist, ordered the protection of all animals, especially dogs. His regulations concerning dogs were so extreme that he was ridiculed as the Inu Shogun. A more recent story is the 1920s tale of the chuuken (faithful dog), Hachiko who met his master at Shibuya station at the end of every workday. Even after his master died at work, Hachiko continued to wait at the station for 10 years and he became a popular symbol of devotion. After his death, Hachiko's body was put in a museum, and a bronze statue of him was erected in front of Shibuya station.

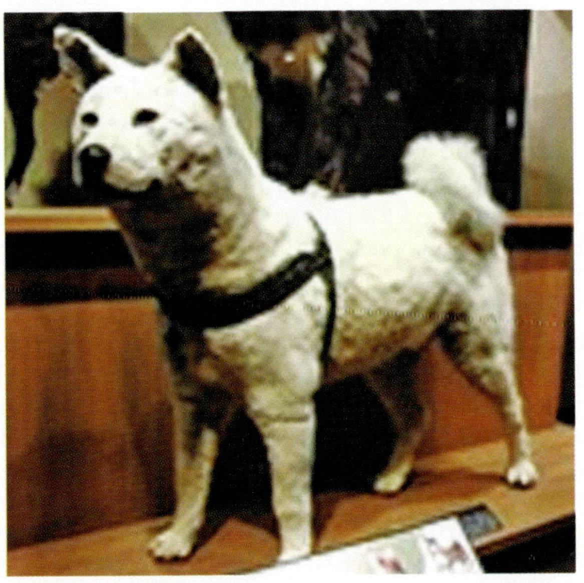

Hachikō exhibited at the National Museum of Nature and Science in Ueno

Critical phrases referring to inu (dogs) are as common in Japan as they are in the West. Inujini (to die like dog) is to die meaninglessly and to call someone a dog is to accuse him or her of being a spy or dupe. "Inu mo arukeba bou ni ataru (when the dog walks, it runs across a stick)" is a common saying and it means when you walk outside, you could possibly meet with an unexpected fortune.

According to Japanese folklore, there is a darker side of pet spirituality in Shinto religion, known as the Inugami, which literally translates to dog God. Inugami are dark dangerous spirits which are conjured up through dark rituals involving the sacrifice of a common pet dog. In a way similar to shikigami, these rituals allow the dog's tortured spirit to be under the control of whomever summoned it. The Inugami can then be used by its owner to do their bidding and curse other people or even possess them and bring misfortune. The idea of this type of spirit could be linked to the fact that traditionally, pets in Japanese culture were kept for utilitarian purposes as opposed to companionship. Japanese traditional folk religion and Buddhism have significantly influenced the death rites of pets, and their memorialization thereafter.

To some extent, western culture and christianity have also made an impact, however, the aspects present in such procedures vary across Japan and rely heavily upon the beliefs, traditions, and circumstances of each individual family. Traditionally, pets were not often considered to be members of the family. Although there are some examples of pets being memorialized and given posthumous names during the mid-nineteenth century but only a few records of such efforts that exist have been attributed to the elite samurai class. During that time most dogs and cats were considered community residents and did not inhabit any one individual home. Upon a community animal's death, folk tradition required that special care be taken of the deceased animal's remains, in order to protect the entire village from vengeful spirits. The concept of vengeful spirits comes from the belief that "small animals such as cats and dogs were believed to be able to travel freely between the here-and-now and the afterworld and possess the power to wreak spiritual vengeance (tatari) on people". In order to ensure that the living would not be harmed and in some instances to enlist good luck or protection from the animal spirit, special procedures were required, such as burial in a specific location of significance or inclusion of certain items within the animal's grave. If the correct process was followed, the village could rest assured that they would not be troubled by the deceased spirit.

Buddhist practices, specifically ancestral memorialization directly influenced the death rites and rituals performed for pets in Japan. However, "there are no scriptures specifically for animals, let alone pets" in Buddhist doctrine. Thus memorialization of pets is left open to diverse interpretation and one central disagreement among spiritualists revolves around the Buddhist cycle of rebirth. Some individuals claim that it is indeed possible, through proper care during life and correct memorialization after death of a beloved pet, he may eventually be reborn as a fellow human, thus making enlightenment achievable, whereas others feel that pets are only capable of being reborn as pets. Often, Buddhist clerics tend to allow families to decide for themselves what process they would like to follow. As different temples interpret the rites in different ways, they often combine various elements or omit some entirely.

Over the last few decades, pet cemeteries have increased in popularity, particularly within crowded urban areas. In rural areas, many pets are buried directly in the ground "in the hills outside the village creating a harmony between the decay of the pet's body and the fading away of memories and grief". In more urban metropolitan areas, pet owners generally choose cremation for their lost companions and can also choose to inter them in individual or communal graves or display the remains in columbariums. On occasions pet owners request to be buried with their deceased pets and some choose to conduct the rites just as they would be conducted for a human. In contrast with the traditional folk beliefs, the majority of pet owners no longer believe that the spirits of their deceased pets will cause them harm as a result of their choice of memorialization. Moreover, the rites and rituals serve as a means of easing the grief and loss of the living. As a result, "the significance of animal funerals in Japan has shifted from prayer for the animal soul to a way of expressing grief by the pet owner". Deceased pets are now more commonly remembered as members of the family, and are often memorialized at the family altar and become a part of the family's ancestry.

In contemporary society, elements of western thought and christianity have also become interwoven into burial practices of deceased pets. One example of this influence is found in the image of a "Rainbow Bridge," a concept very much like the western ideal of heaven. The Rainbow Bridge is described as a utopian space where the deceased pet's spirit remains until the death of their owner, at which time both spirits travel together into the realm of heaven. This concept further emphasizes the growing familial connection between pets and their owners in contemporary Japan.

CELTIC MYTHOLOGY AND DOGS

The dog appears frequently in celtic mythologys, everywhere from personal names to the companions of Gods to beasts both of good and ill omen. Indeed, though we have a large number of references to dogs from a multitude, it's almost impossible to pin down the precise mythological nature of this animal. Perhaps this is because the dog represents both the loyal companion and at the same time presents us with a shadow of its ancestor, the wolf. Dogs were the favourite animals of Fionn MacCumhaill, who was the great mythological warrior and celebrated hero in Irish literature and his two hunting dogs, Bran and Sceolaing were almost as famous as Fionn himself. The most famous dog-named in Cu Chulainn in Celtic mythology is Cu Chulainn (literally the Hound of Chulainn). This mythological hero of the epic Tain Bo Cuailgne Setanta, is better known by his nickname 'Cu Chulainn'. He earned this nickname after he killed Chulainn's favoured yet fierce guard dog in self-defence. He then offered to take the place of the hound until a replacement could be reared. As per the tale, Setanta was semi-divine and his birth name was derived from the name of the early Scottish tribe, the Setantii. When Setanta was seven years old, he was being looked after by Royal Court. Once the Royal Court departed to visit the wealthy Chulainn at his lonely mansion and as the procession begin to leave, the boy decided to stay behind to play with Hurley and thought of reaching at Chulainn-mansion later in the night. The guests at Chulainn's mansion carouse and make merry as they know that they are protected from attack by Chulainn's giant and ferocious hound. But later that night they hear a fearful howling and a sickening crunch. Arriving late, the boy, Setanta encountered the dog and slayed. Though the guests cheer at Setanta's deeds, Chulainn was saddened by the loss of his faithful hound. Setanta reassures him that he will raise another pup to be his defender, but till such dog is trained, he will act as Chulainn's guardian. Thus Setanta adopted his hero's name Cu Chulainn.

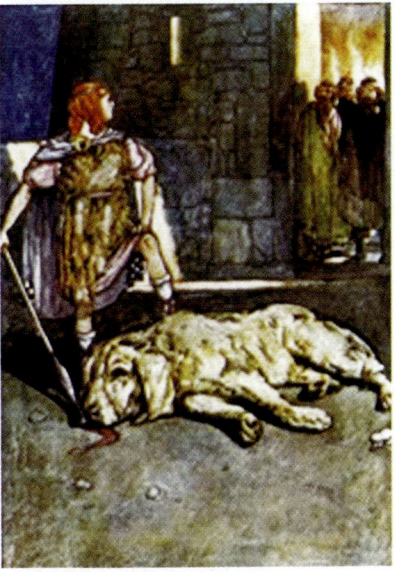

"Cu Chulainn (Setanta) Slays the Hound of Chulainn"

Dogs also appear in the iconography of a number of Celtic deities. The attributes here are very complex or at least they are very broad. They are often seen to accompany hunter deities with examples being the image of a God found at Le Touget in France, which shows a man with a hare held in his arms and a Hound by his side. Another image from London shows a Hunter God with a bow and quiver (case of holding arrows) and a dog by his side. The association of Hounds with hunting is obvious and the dog might have had a role in protecting his master from the wild beasts.

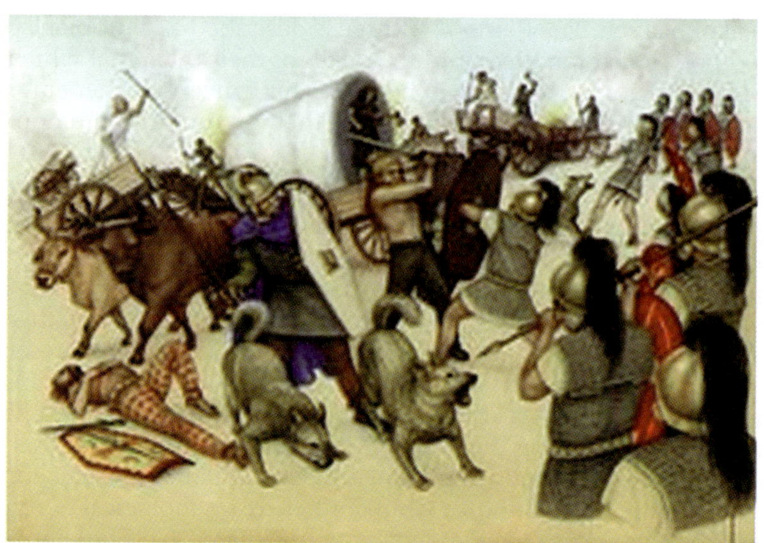

Depicting dogs with Celtic warriors

Known as "man's best friend", dogs have a strong social intelligence that leads to their close relationship with humans and unique ability to fit into the human household. This human relationship with dogs is steeped in Irish history and mythology. The dogs were also known to accompany Gods and the Goddess. In the relief from her shrine at Zierikeeze, Goddess Nehalennia, being the guardian of sailors on their crossings of the North Sea and probably represents a protective animal. The same protective presence may also account for the depiction of a dog who accompanies the Gaulish God Cissonius who may, himself be a protector of travelers. The Gaulish hammer God, Sucellus is also often associated with a dog as he seems to have been a deity of prosperity and well-being and his canine companion may well represent the guardian of home and health. Though the iconography of Sucellus is very complex and a relief from Varhely in Dacia (modern Romania) shows the hammer God accompanied by what seems to be a three-headed dog.

Dogs are also frequent companions for the Celtic Maters (Mother Goddesses). At Trier in Germany many statues and depictions of single mother Goddess with lapdogs have been recovered. The Goddess Epona is also sometimes associated with a dog, though, this is undoubtedly related to Epona's role as a psychopomp, a transporter of souls. Other female deities such as Aveta and Sirona are also depicted with lapdogs or accompanying canines. Both Goddesses are deities of healing and childbirth and this leads us to another aspect of the dog cult, the healing aspect. This may be originally from the healing properties of canine saliva and the way a dog licks at a wound to clean it. This healing aspect may also be a part of the cult of the God Cunomaglus (Great Hound Lord) who is known from an inscription at Nettleton Shrub in Wiltshire (a country in southwest England). He is the only Celtic deity with the word 'dog' explicitly in his name and his association with Apollo by Interpretato Romana indicates that this God may have had both healing and hunting aspects. A small intaglio found at Risingham (Northumberland, England) and depicting the God Cocidius shows the Warrior God as a hunter with

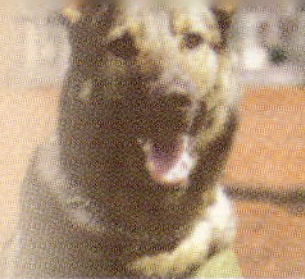

a rabbit and accompanied by a dog. Again we may have the intermingling of a hunter and warrior aspects, both attributes of the hunting dog. Thus we come full circle in terms of the attributes of the Celtic dogs.

In Celtic belief, the dog seems to possess a hunting, healing and otherworld connotation. The iconography of the sacred dog is extremely ancient in Celtic mythology. However, dogs are referred very frequently in both the Cymric and Irish tales but a very few are explicitly named. Rare examples of such dogs are Bran and Sceolang, the hounds of Fion MacCumhaill, Cafall, the hunting dog of Arthur, Drudwyn the hunting dog of Culhwch and Failinis the dog of Lug Lamfhota. Apart from canines that are essentially benign in nature, there are much darker canine incarnations, believed to be portents of death and destruction in folklore. In this class of beast we have the Cymric Cwn Annwn. There is also the Cymric Gwyllgi (mad dog), the Moddey Dhoog and Mauthe Dhoog of Manx folklore and the Crom Dubh, Coinn Iotair and Saidhthe Suariaghe of Ireland.

There has been a very long mythological association between dogs and death in the British Isles and beyond. The ki du (black dog) of Brittany considered to accompany re-incarnations. Iron Age graves have been excavated to reveal the skeletons of hounds, alongside tools, valuables and the bodies of their supposed human owners. The folklore and legends of the Celts and similar stories from other people, particularly the Germanic, Scandinavian and some Latin cultures, the sighting of an underworldly black dog can be a harbinger of death. This may well have been originally based on dogs' unerring ability to find carrion. Many Cymric battle poems speak of both hounds and ravens feasting on the flesh of the battle dead. Interesting corroboration for the associations of dogs with the netherworld come from excavations of Celtic burials where many dogs have been interred with their masters. An interesting example of multiple dog burial was found in a 65 metres deep well at Muntham Court, Sussex (a country of Southern England).

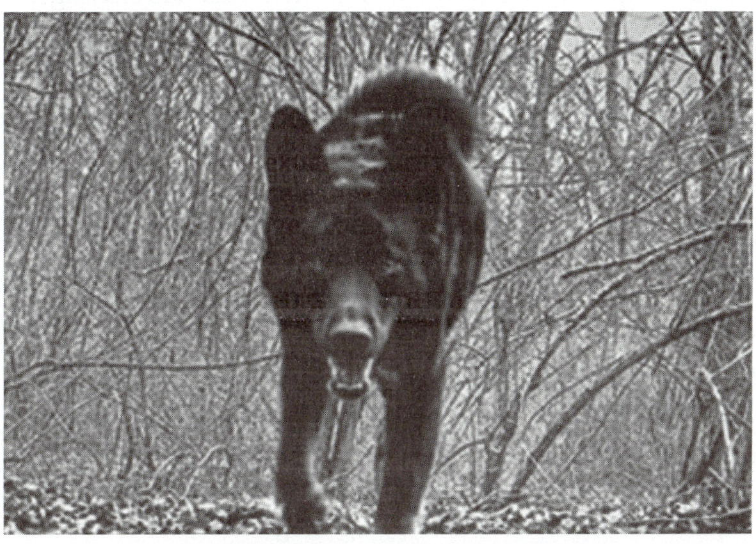

Celtic mythological underworldly black dog

In Wales, the situation is even more complex and sometimes seeing the black dog is far preferable than encountering a variant that is pure white. In the lonely lanes and mountain fords, the Gwyllgi and the Cwn Annwn roam, while, elsewhere, whole packs of ghostly dogs chill the air with their barks and yelps. But what does it mean for those who meet them?

Some of the famous otherworldly dogs of Wales are described below:

Gwyllgi

In Welsh, 'gwyll' means 'twilight', while 'gwyllt' means 'wild'. Either word has been proposed as the source of the Gwyllgi's name. The last part 'gi' is a mutation of 'ci', which simply translates as 'dog'. The twilight dog or the wild dog, it matters little when it is spotted because those seeing it have more pressing matters on their mind. This black dog is described as being like a large mastiff and considered an omen of an impending death. There is no way it could be mistaken for that natural dog, as the eyes give the Gwyllgi uniqueness. There is a distinct glow to them, variously described in the legends as being like stars or burning coals. This blazing stare bores into the poor individual who is doomed to die soon or else lose a loved one and the traditional haunt of these hounds is country lanes. In Marchwiel, near Wrexham, Lon Bwbach Ddu (Black Spectre Lane) is believed to refer to sightings of such a creature but were not confirmed. Tour guides tell of a Gwyllgi inside the mansion of Plas Teg, near Mold and mostly seen in the Regency Room which is also said to be the most haunted spot of the house. Paranormal investigator, Richard Holland, heard more recent stories of these dogs, seen in Anglesey and Ruthin. The first mention of Gwyllgi in a written text occurred in the southern county of Glamorgan, while their prevalence is believed to be throughout Wales.

Cwn Annwn

Before Christianity brought concepts of Heaven and Hell to evangelized Wales, its population believed that death took them to Annwn. That was envisaged as an island somewhere in the west, surrounded by sea. The poems of the famed Celtic Bard, Taliesin, describe Annwn (or its alternative name of Caer Sidi) as a paradise place of eternal youth. There are fountains providing the best food and drink. It was a wonderful afterlife, ruled over by mythical figures like Morgan le Fey or Gwyn ap Nudd (underworld God) who blurred the line between fairies and deities. It is from this otherworld that the Cwn Annwn get their name with cwn being the plural of 'ci', i.e. dogs. These creatures tended to move in a pack, though it was possible to glimpse one on its own. They are pure white and their ears may be edged with red. Their eyes, like the Gwyllgi, shine preter naturally and it is said that the farther they are away, the louder their bark whereas they are almost silent when nearby. They are believed to convey souls to Annwn and the reason they were often feared more than the black dogs, was due to this destination though originally, the Cwn Annwn were welcomed as escorts or a honour guard. Another name for them was Cwn Mamau (Hounds of the Mothers) as they were believed to be sent by the ancestors but as Wales was converted to Christianity, these dogs became associated with firstly with the fairies and then to the devil. Annwn was linked, with a little help from priests and saints, with hell. A sighting of them meant that Heaven was denied to the hapless person about to die.

The Ghostly Pack of Wepre

Apparently unrelated to either the Gwyllgi or Cwn Annwn are a pack of former family pets which have been seen on several occasions in the grounds of Wepre Park, wherein the Freme family established a pet cemetery for generations of their hounds. Over the years, local people have sometimes reported the strange behaviour of their own living dogs, during walks in that park. Typically, their pet will suddenly cower with its ears back and its fur on end, then it will pull its owner anxiously back to the main gate indicating to leave right now. For some dog-walkers, the incident is a little more hair-rising as they also hear the barking of a large pack of hounds and then they will see them. The dogs are pure white and arrive in all breeds and sizes ranging from large hunting dogs to tiny lap dogs. They are the spectral family pets out for one last run.

The Hunter

One of the more recent additions to the legends, stories and tales of wild dogs includes variations on the "Hounds of Hell" theme. This may be referred to as "The Hunter" or "The Hunt." According to legend, a pack of massive, all black or pure white hounds runs ahead of a mounted horseman, the Hunter. These dogs often have loud baying voices that sound like thunder, coupled with glowing red or bright orange eyes. The hounds as well as the hunter, may be seen together or apart and their aim is to find and consume lone travelers found on the road.

Aboriginal Americans and Dogs

According to a Native American legend, the dog freely chose to become a companion to man. This legend has the virtue of being romantic, and in a way true, at least according to some scientific theories. No one can determine exactly when the Native Americans welcomed the wolf into their homes and slowly developed it as domesticated dog, but every dog loving person in the world owes them a debt of gratitude. The little information that is available comes from archeology and anthropology. By studying ancient canid bones along with Native American pottery, ceramic, jewelry and cave art, some theories on the role of the dog have emerged. Most researchers agree that more than 27,000 years ago, a change slowly began to occur in the wolf populations. Some continued to thrive but others began to spend more time with people. It is possible that some wolves tended to be a little more playful than others. These wolves were not tolerated in the structured wolf pack but this type of wolf went well with people. Perhaps shunned by their peers, these more friendly dogs entered the camps of the Native American. These dogs still looked to a leader for guidance and felt more comfortable knowing their place within a hierarchy. For this reason, the dog readily became an intricate part of the life of Native Americans.

It seems logical that the Native American welcomed the dog into his home and community. Over a period of time, the dog was bred for qualities, they needed. These dogs were considered as a part of the family and were even given names based on their appearance, personality or characteristics. Some excelled at hunting while others were excellent protectors. Before Europeans introduced the horse to North America, the dogs where used as a method of transportation, pulling carts and carrying heavy loads. When the Native Americans left their homes to hunt, they departed knowing that the dogs would protect their wives, mothers, children and even livestock. If someone was lost, the keen sense of smell of dogs was used to search and find the missing person. The bravery, courage and loyalty of dogs sealed a place for them in the annals of American tribal life. The importance of the dogs in tribal life can be found in the various myths and legends passed on from generation to generation. The legend of the dog's decision to join man is one example, explained in beautiful prose by Joseph Bruchac in his two books, "Dog People" and "Native Dog Stories". For the most part, tribes revered the dog and included them in religious ceremonies, believing the dog helped people navigate the journey to the afterlife. A few tribes, however, considered the dog to be the symbol of promiscuity and filth. Today, the Native American dog is a distant cousin of the original. Many people feel that the true Native American dog was likely driven to extinction due to interbreeding with wolves and various imported European breeds. As the early settlers migrated across the country, they were forced on to reservations and the dog's popularity and population suffered. Whether the true Native American dog (also called the Plains Indian dog or Navajo dog) still exists is in dispute. Many Native Americans contend that the breed has wholly ceased to exist, in spite of attempts to re-establish the breed.

Dogs usually play the role of loyal helpers and friends of men in Native American folklore, just as they do in most other world mythology. Many folktales have to do with the proper treatment of dogs. People who are kind and generous to their dogs are often rewarded, while people who abuse, disrespect, or even annoy dogs are harshly punished. They were also raised for food in some tribes which is not necessarily incompatible with the theme of respect since some other animals such as buffalo and bears were also regularly eaten by Native Americans, though highly respected and had taboos governing their treatment. Occasionally dogs were represented in the Native American folktales with negative traits such as being gullible, easily distracted, or even a tattletale but in general people at large considered them a symbol of friendship and loyalty. They were also occasionally used as clan animals in some Native American cultures. Tribes with Dog Clans include the Menominee tribe and the Ottawa tribe. The dog was also the symbol of several warrior societies of the Great Plains such as the Crazy Dog Society of the Crow tribe (Bishkawaalaaxe in the Crow language) or the highly respected Dog Soldiers of the Cheyenne (Hotametaneo'o or Hotamitanio in Cheyenne also known as the Dog-Men or Dog Warriors). To Cheyennes, the dog represents fierce guardianship and self-sacrificing. Although, Prairie dogs are not prominent animals in Native American mythology and most often they appear in legends as food items, yet to the Cheyenne tribe, Prairie dogs were a symbol of corn and were honoured in several ways. Southwest tribal cultures like the Navajo and Apache believed that Prairie dogs had spirit power over water and rain. In Plains, legends often associated Prairie dogs with carelessness and foolishness but they also represented humility. Prairie dog medicine was used for healing in some Plains tribes such as the Sioux and some Sioux tribes also have a Prairie Dog dance among their tribal dance traditions.

There are no descendants of ancient aboriginal American dogs left, except for the few northern breeds and perhaps the Mexican hairless/chola and the chihuahua.

Native American cultures are rich in myths and legends that explain natural phenomenon and the relationship between humans and the spirit world. Native

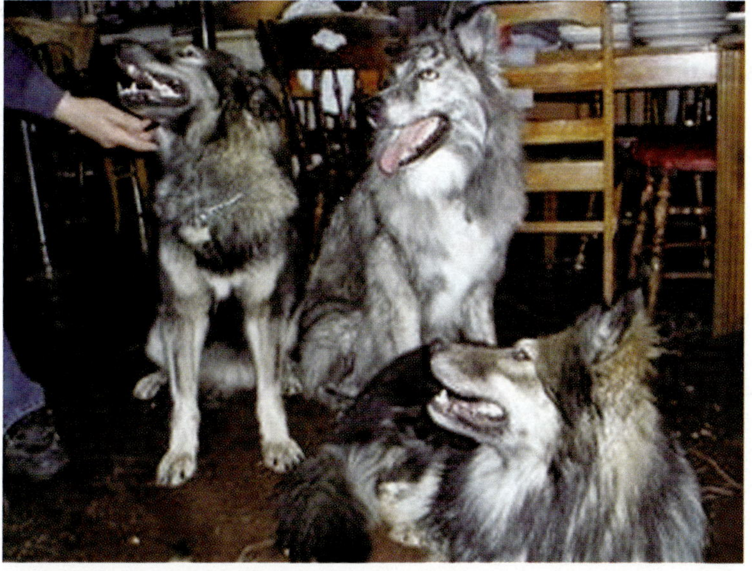

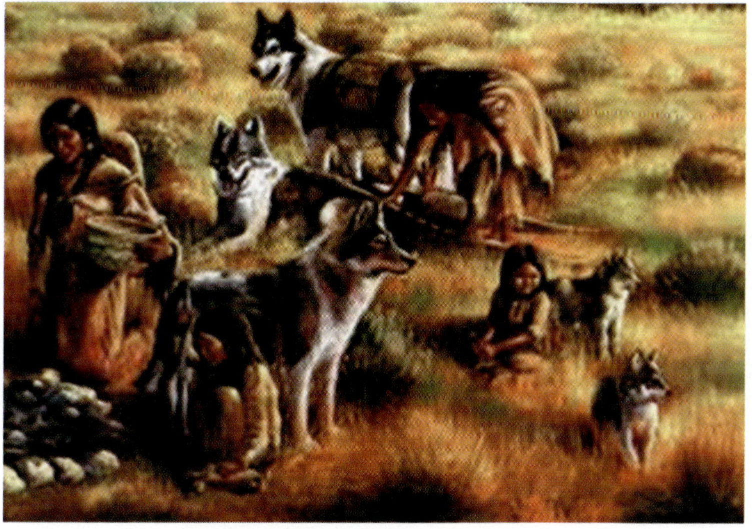

Dogs of Native American tribes

American cultures are numerous and diverse. Though some neighbouring cultures hold similar beliefs, others can be quite different from one another. The most common being, the creation myths, that tell a story to explain how the earth was formed, and where humans and other beings came from. Others may include explanations about the sun, moon, constellations, specific animals, seasons, and weather. This is one of the ways that many tribes have kept and continue to keep their cultures alive. These stories are not told simply for entertainment, but as a way of preserving and transmitting the nation's, tribe's particular beliefs, history, customs, spirituality and traditional way of life.

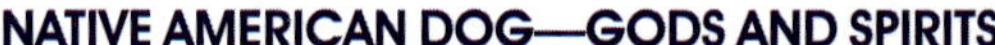

NATIVE AMERICAN DOG—GODS AND SPIRITS

Mahakh (Aleut)

The traces of Native American tribal religion are evident in the people of the Alutian islands (southwest of Alaska). The Russian invaded the islands in 18th century and then transferred to the USA in 1867. They believe in a high God Aleuxita-Aqudax. One of the legends was a dog mother named Mahakh. A form of shamanism is part of their religion. Drum plays a great part of the ritual along the symbol.

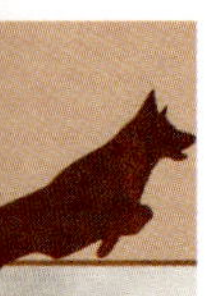

Poko Kachina (Hopi)

Dogs figure amongst the clan names of Red-Greasewood (Bow phrathry) which was known for warfare and used to hunt with bow and arrow. Hopi Bow clan believed to be inherently associated with the stars, especially the winter constellation of Orion and Pleiades. One funerary practice, highlights the canine and hundreds of dogs were ritually buried between 400 BC and 1100 AD in northern New Maxico and on the New Maxico-Arizona border. This suggest that dogs played a key role in the spiritual beliefs of ancient American tribals. These grave dogs, which is in the aried climate became naturally mummified, are believed to serve as escorts in the spirit's afterlife journey through the underworld.

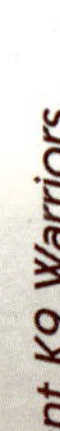

NATIVE AMERICAN TALL TALE

The tall tale is a fundamental element of American folk literature and its origin is linked to the bragging contests that often occurred when men of the American frontier gathered. A tall tale is a story with unbelievable elements, related as if it were true and factual. Some such stories are exaggerations of actual events, others are completely fictional tales set in a familiar setting. They are usually humorous or good-natured. Many myths exaggerate the exploits of their heroes but in tall tales the exaggeration looms large to the extent of becoming the whole of the story. While dogs act as key characters in many stories and myths, one culture appears to repeatedly emphasize the bond between man and man's best friend. These tribes across the country have passed along numerous tales featuring our four-legged friends tales of courage, loyalty, creation, and lifelong friendships.

NATIVE AMERICAN FOLKLORE

There are many different kinds of stories. Some are called "Hero Stories" which are the stories of people who lived at one time and who were immortalized and remembered through these tales. There are "Trickster Stories", relating to the different trickster figures of the tribes (Saynday for the Kiowa, Coyote for the Navajo and so on) and spirits who may be either helpful or dangerous. There are also tales that are simply warnings against doing something that may harm in some way. Many of these tales have morals or some form of belief that is being taught. This is how the things were remembered.

Black Dog

Somewhere at the junction of the prairie and the maka sicha (the badlands), there is a hidden cave and nobody has been able to find it. Even now, with so many highways, cars and tourists, no one has discovered this cave. There lives a woman so old that her face looks like a shriveled up walnut. She is dressed in rawhide, the way people used to be, before the white man came. She has been sitting there for a thousand years or more, working on a blanket strip for her buffalo robe. She is making the strip out of dyed porcupine quills in the ancestor's style, before the white traders brought glass beads to this turtle continent. Resting beside her, licking his own paws and watching the old woman all the time is Shunka Sapa, a huge black dog. His eyes never wander from her. The teeth of old woman are worn down to little stumps as she often used them to flatten so many porcupine quills. A few steps from where the old woman sits, working on her blanket strip, a huge fire is kept going. She lit this fire a thousand or more years ago and has kept it alive ever since. Over the fire hangs a big earthen pot, the kind some Aboriginal people used to make before the white man came with his kettles of iron. Inside the pot, wojapi (berry soup, sweet and red) is boiling and bubbling. That soup has been boiling in the pot for a long time, ever since the fire was lit. Every now and then the old woman gets up to stir the wojapi in the huge earthen pot and she is so old and feeble that it takes a while to get up and hobble over to the fire. The moment her back is turned, Shunka Sapa, the huge black dog starts pulling the porcupine quills out of her blanket strip. This way she never makes any progress and her quillwork remains forever unfinished. The Sioux people used to say that if the old woman ever finishes her blanket strip threading with the last porcupine quill to complete the design, the world will come to an end.

LATIN AMERICAN DOG MYTH

South and Central American wild dogs have played a large role in various myths and legends. In many ancient cultures dogs, both wild and semi-domestic, were seen as guides to the afterlife. Dogs, typically black or very dark in colour were often believed to carry or guide the newly dead souls across a large body of water or a river to the afterlife. People that had been abusive or cruel to dogs would be given a poor guide or a dog that was so dark that it would lose the human soul in the water, ensuring that it would remain forever outside of the afterlife.

Wild dogs or semi-feral dogs, as believed in Maya culture, have brought fire to humans. The Aztecs believed that one of their most powerful and important Xoloti was a huge dog, often seen in legend as a fire and lightening God. It is a direct reference to Xoloti that the Mexican hairless dog is currently known in its native land as Xoloitzcuintli. Although they were also believed to escort the dead to the afterlife. They were also used as sacrifices and even as meat in specific religious ceremonies. There are many local legends and myths about sorcerers and witches that can transform themselves into large black-coloured dogs. These dogs may hunt livestock in the area at night, returning to their human form in the morning hours. These witch dogs are known as a nahual, and may also steal valuables and riches in dog form since they are believed to have the intelligence and understanding of a human.

AUSTRALIAN ABORIGINALS AND DOGS

A major role of dingoes in aboriginal society seems to have been their use as pets, when a woman who had recently lost her child or was barren or beyond the age of child-bearing, would carry a dingo pup wrapped round her waist and at night a dingo might also serve as a blanket. Dingoes were also used in hunting and traditionally dogs had a privileged position in the aboriginal cultures of Australia. They are an important part of rock carvings and cave paintings such as "Dingo speared for food" is depicted at Burrup Peninsula rock art in the Pilbara region of Western Australia adjoining the Dampier Archipelago near the town of Dampier. The Burrup peninsula is a unique ecological and archaeological area. It contains the world's largest and most important collection of 'petroglyphs'—ancient aboriginal rock carvings which date back as far as the last ice age about 10,000 years ago. Present day's concern around the ecological, historical, cultural and archaeological significance of the area has led to a campaign for its protection, causing conflict with industrial development on the site.

There are ceremonies (like a keen at the Cape York Peninsula in the form of howling) and stories connected to the dingo, which were passed down through the generations. The male dingo is connected to holy places, totems, rituals and dreamtime characters. There are stories that dogs can see the supernatural, and warn against evil powers. There is evidence that dogs have been buried together with their owners to protect them against evil even after death. Most of the published myths hail from the western desert and show a remarkable complexity. In some stories, dingoes are the central characters, in others only minor ones. In some stories, it is an ancestor who created humans and dingoes or gave them their current shape. There are also stories about creation, socially acceptable behaviour and explanations why some things are the way they are. There are myths about shape shifters (human to dingo or vice versa), "dingo-people", and the creation of certain landscapes or elements of those landscapes like waterholes or mountains. The dingo is also considered responsible for death.

Dingoes have been on the Australian continent for the past 4000 or so years. It is thought that they were brought to the mainland by Asian seafarers with whom the aboriginal people had extensive trade links. During this time dingoes have been woven into the fabric of aboriginal life, law and culture. Little distinction is usually made between dingoes and more recently introduced dogs when applying beliefs and law. Aboriginal people in contemporary society own dogs for a variety of reasons. They served the following role:

Companion: As for most societies, this is particularly the case for the elderly and children. It is also noted here that elderly people, possibly because of a stronger need to obey law and culture, tend to give their dogs greater attention than younger people in communities. It is common for older women to give large amounts of their own 'meals on wheels' (food) to their dogs. Older people also tend to accumulate dogs in far higher numbers than younger people.

Physical protector: The level of protection offered by dogs serves an important role for the family.

Hunter: Many dogs are known as the "good kangaroo dog" or the "good goanna dog". These dogs are prized for their hunting prowess and strategic breeding of their lines occurs.

Source of warmth: "Two, three and four dog nights" are still in practice in many aboriginal communities where due to relative poverty, there is often not enough warm bedding to go around when the temperature drops.

Spiritual protector: Dogs continue to be seen as protectors from spiritual interference as "Sorcery" remains a very real threat in contemporary tribal life in northern Australia. Dogs howling, barking or indeed being silent through the night are often interpreted in relation to the spirit world.

Dingoes, and now dogs, are regarded as sacred animals to some extent. They are incorporated into aboriginal society via formal inclusion into family units and certain dogs are given "skin" names. This automatically positions the dingo into society, granting them status such as parent, grandparent, aunt, child, etc. In some cases dogs are considered important enough to attend rituals, acting as fully-fledged lawmen. In certain areas dogs are also believed to be direct reincarnations of ancestors.

Dogs are also incorporated into creation and "dreaming" knowledge. The dreamtime or dreaming is that part of aboriginal culture which explains the origin and culture of the lands and its people. There are many dog dreaming sites located around the Australian continent. Each has its own and often interconnected story of creation and movement of the dingo through the country. Stories are told covering areas over thousands of kilometres and across different language groups. Ceremonies that are based around the dingo and dog continue to be practiced across northern Australia with relevant songs, dances and these stories remain very much intact.

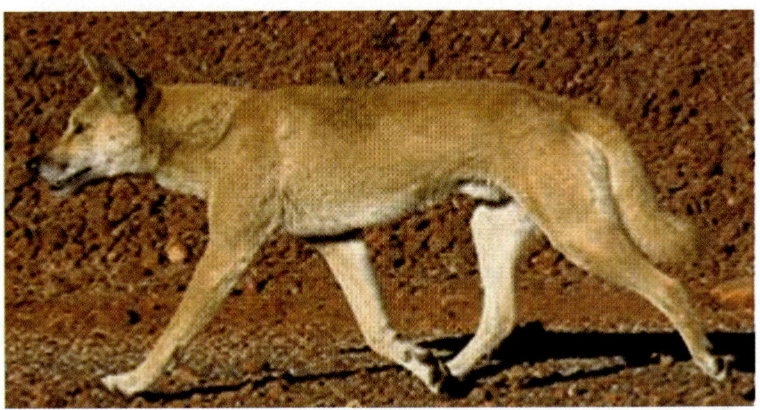

Australian Dingo

In other myths there are advice and warnings to those who do not want to follow the social rules. Stories can show the borders of one's territory or the dingo in it might stand for certain members of the community, for example, rebellious dingoes stand for "wild" members of the tribe. The dingo also has a wild and uncontrollable face in other stories and there are many stories about dingoes that kill and eat humans, for example, the Mamu, who catches and devours the spirit of every child who roams too far from the campfire. Other stories tell of a giant devil dingo from which the real dingoes originate. The dog is thereby depicted as a homicidal, malicious creature that apart from the lack of a subtle mind, is similar to a trickster since it plays the role of a mischievous adversary for other mythological beings. Many of them fall victim to blood-thirsty dogs or escape them. Here individual beings have a significant meaning too or sometimes become part of the landscape. Even the actions of these dogs result for instance in the creations of stones and trees from flying around bones and meat or ochre from the spilled blood.

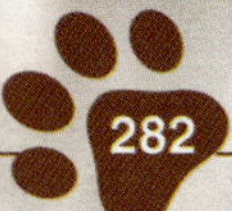

Giant Dog Gaiya

The mythology of giant dogs is found all across Australia and there is one story from the far north of Australia. Mornington Island off Cape York Peninsula which has been related by Dick Roughsey of the "Lardil people". He said that there were two dog dreamings sites, one on Mornington Island itself and the other on the smaller Denhan Island. His version differs from the myth found on the mainland.

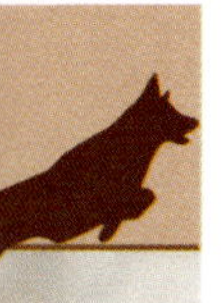

In Dick Roughsey's version, an old grasshopper woman, Eelgin, came from the west with the giant dog, Gaiya. They both hunted humankind for food. Once when Gaiya was out hunting two young men, butcherbird brothers came to the old woman's camp. They spoke to Eelgin, before becoming alarmed and running off. Gaiya returned and the old woman sent him after the two butcher-bird brothers and he followed their tracks, loping after them with giant strides across Cape York Peninsula and drawing nearer and nearer. Finally, the butcherbirds decided to ambush the giant dog at a place called Bulinmore, a big rocky pass through the hills. The dog came along and behind him came the old grasshopper woman, hobbling along with a stick. The butcherbirds began spearing Giaya and kept on until he was dead. They then called for all the people of the country to come and have a meal of cooked dog, then cut off the tip of his tail (in which his spirit resided) and gave it back to the old woman. The angry spirit bit Eelgin on the nose before the butcherbirds came down and killed her. They then sent her spirit to a place near Barrow Point, where she became a large rock. The marks that Gaiya's spirit made when biting her can be seen on the noses of all grasshoppers. The body of the giant dog was divided up by the sawman, Woodbarl, the white cloud, asked for the kidneys, head and all the bones. Later he took the bones and also the skin to the top of a mountain where he made two small dogs which would be friends of humanity.

In the mainland version, as related by Tulo Gordon of the "Giuugu Yamidhirr people", the butcherbird brothers are replaced by the two magpie brothers and the old woman is replaced by a carpet snake, and thus connects up with the Melatji dog myths across the continent in the Kimberley region of Western Australia. The magpie brothers do not kill the giant dog or the carpet snake but simply forbid them to kill human beings. The lonesome howl of the dingo is a cry of repentance for the killing and eating of human beings.

AUSTRALIAN ABORIGINAL LEGENDS

There are many different aspects and interesting oddities in the relationship between the aboriginal peoples of Australia and the wild dingoes. In many cases semi-feral or almost domesticated dingoes were kept by different tribes in order to ward off demons and spirits from the camp sites and tribal areas. The dingo was seen as a guardian of the people, sent to keep supernatural spirits at bay but is also seen as a gluttonous trickster that is not to be trusted.

There are several legends of how dingoes were trusted by other beings or Gods to help in their endeavours. Almost unilaterally in these legends, the dingoes which are almost always represented by a pair, take the prize for themselves, resulting in a punishment. One legend tells of how the dingoes lost their bark. In this legend two dingoes paired up with a hawk that had found two large yams. The dingoes indicated that they would guard the yams while the hawk went to find fire from a human village to cook the food. The hawk returned only to find the dingoes had eaten the yams and cursed them by taking away their bark.

In a more modern urban controversy which started on 17th August, 1980, on Chamberlain family with their three young children were camping at the famous Ayers Rock in Australia. During the night, the mother Lindy awoke and started screaming that a dingo had entered their camp and taken a nine-week-old baby girl named Azaria. There had been prior attacks by dingoes in the area but nothing as significant as this. A trial was held and the mother was convicted of the murder of the child, even though there were tracks and some evidence that a dingo had been present. The body of the child was not found. Several years later in 1987, another inquest was held and the original verdict was overruled. The mother was released from jail with a settlement of $1.3 million. Although dingos do attack humans occasionally, there has not been another child attack of this nature and the mystery around the infamous phrase "A dingo ate my baby" still exists.

HINDUISM AND DOGS

In Hinduism, dogs has a major religious significance among the Hindus in Nepal and also some parts of India, particularly in Mithlanchal, North Bengal and Sikkim. As per the belief, dogs guard the doors of heaven and hell and they are worshiped on "Kukur Tihar", "Day of the Dog," which falls on the 2nd day of Diwali in India. It is called "Tihar" in Nepal, a five-day festival that falls roughly in November every year. On this day, dogs are applied tika (the holy vermilion dot) and garlanded generally with marigold flowers.

The purest native form of Indian dog is an elegant animal called the "Santhal Hound". Hindus venerate them in their association with a particular deity, such as the owl (Uluka) associated with goddess Lakshmi. However the ordinary street dog is known as a pye dog, or pariah which is considered an animal outcaste.

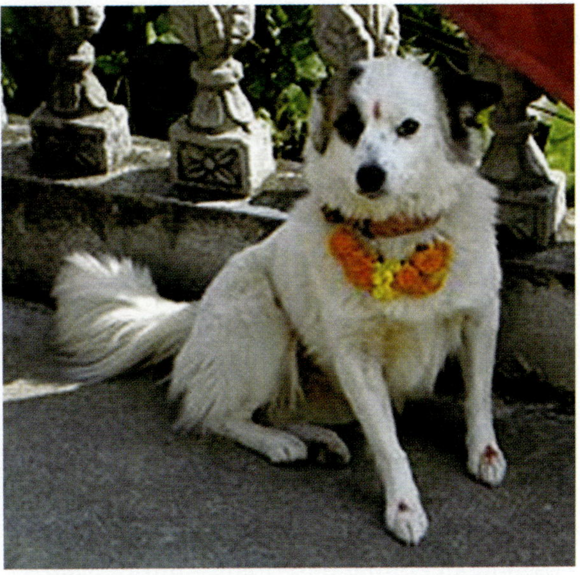

A dog after being decorated in Kukur Tihar festival

Outside the emergent Indian middle class, where dogs are kept as pets or as status symbols, the dog is generally considered unclean and a pest. But there is also an ancient tradition of respect for canines. For example, "Since 1927 a dog had been following the retinue of the Matha, a Hindu saint, in this case the 68th Shankaracharya, Chandrasekharendra Sarasvati of Kanchi. He was a strange dog, an intelligent animal without the least trace of unclean lines. He would eat only the food given to it from the Matha. The Acharya would therefore enquire every evening if the dog had been fed. When the camp moved from one place to another, the dog would follow, walking underneath the palanquin, and when the entourage stopped so that the devotees of the way side villages could pay their homage, it would run to a distance and watch devoutly from there, only to rejoin the retinue when it was on the move again.

One day, a small boy hit the dog and the dog was about to retaliate but sensing the brawl, the officials of the Matha blindfolded the dog and took him to a distance of twenty-five miles and left there in a village. But strange as it may seem, the dog returned to where the Acharya was, even before the person who had taken it away could return. From that day onwards the dog would not eat without the Acharya's darshana and stayed till the end of its life with the Matha.

In Mahabharata, it is mentioned that Yudhishthira had approached heaven with his dog, therefore among many Hindus, the common belief exists that caring for dogs can also pave the way to heaven.

The most famous mythological dog in Indian context was Sarama:

Sarama

The female dog of Lord Indra, a Vedic God, is believed to be a divine dog as mentioned in Rig Veda. This dog is said to have pursued and recovered the cows stolen by Asuras and hidden in the nether world of Patala. it is also believed that two offsprings of Sarama became the watch dogs of Lord Yama, the Hindu God of death. Both these ferocious dogs (Sarameyas) guard the road to Yamaloka. Sarama is a female dog and is considered as the mother of all dogs.

There is also a belief that Lord Yama himself took the form of a dog while guiding Yudhishthira, one of the Pandavas, to Swargaloka. Yudhishthira insisted that he be allowed to enter Swarga (the heaven) with his Shvan (dog). When both of them entered the heaven, the dog transformed itself into Yama. Lord Bhairava, the guardian deity to the abode of Lord Shiva, is believed to have a dog as his vahana and as such Bhairava is usually depicted with a dog and feeding and caring of dogs is believed to be a way of showing our devotion to the deity. Bhairava Temple in Delhi had the tradition of worshipping dogs which is now a long and little known history.

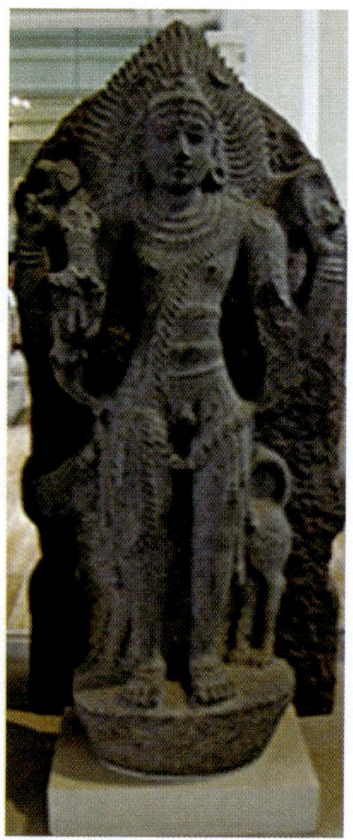
Lord Bhairava with dog as his vahan

Deities like Rudra, Nirriti and Virabhadra are associated with dogs, and an epithet describing Rudra as *Shvapati*, meaning "master of the dog". Shiva, in his aspect as Bhairava, had a dog as a vahana (vehicle) as mentioned in the Mahabharata. Khandoba, a deity, is associated with a dog on which he rides. Lord Dattatreya, the incarnation of holy Trimty—Brahma,Vishnu and Shiva is followed by four faithful dogs,which is considered to symbolize the four Vedas as his mastery over them.

In religious ceremonies, dogs are considered to be a link between us and our ancestors. Special offerings are given to dogs, along with the cow and the crow, so as to remember and invoke the blessings of our ancestors. Some people even buy dogs to free them of the "dosha" in "Shani" and "Rahu". It is believed that feeding a black dog on specified days is good for Saturn but the difficult part is finding a black dog on the specified day. As a result many people keep them as pets. Some astrologers and palmists also believe that dogs have a great importance in astrology. People are advised to feed black dogs if their Saturn is weak while feeding white dogs cures their Venus.

In spite of these narratives, in Hindu mythology, dog is also considered by some people as the most inauspicious of animals, to be kept away from wedding altars and holy sites. A howling dog becomes a harbinger of bad luck. Infact, even the sight of a dog is considered to bring bad luck because dogs are associated with death that is why, the sarameya are the companions of Yama, God of death. They are not with civilization but with the wilderness that is why they are associated with mendicants, like Dattatreya. The dog is the mount of Bhairava, the fearsome form of Shiva which mocks our territorial instinct. Yudhishthira was not allowed to enter heaven with the dog. Such literal interpretations may be convenient but may not be correct for many. Logically speaking, a dog should be the symbol of devotion in Hinduism, yet Hindus worship Hanuman, the Monkey-God, as the perfect devotee. Mythic stories and symbols are a code and a medium through which the ancestors are communicating profound messages. When Dattatreya, the mendicant walks with four dogs around him, it indicates his perfect detachment. The dogs follow him but he does not lead them.

The Indian attitude towards dogs is traced through the Vedas, Epics, Puranas, Dharma shastras and Niti shastras. Dogs had a utilitarian role in pre-Vedic and Vedic times. There were herd dogs, watch dogs and hunting dogs, and dogs were used as beasts of burden. But by the time of the Mahabharata, negative associations had begun to creep in and the change in the attitude towards the dog in India may probably be linked with the progressive decline of the traditional Vedic Gods, Indra, Yama and Rudra (who were associated with dogs), and the elevation of Vishnu, associated with an increase in Brahamanical influence which might have lead to looking down of dogs in that era.

DOG OF RAMAYANA

After returning to Ayodhya, Lord Rama began to rule and assisting him in this task were Sage Vashishtha, along with other sages, advisers and ministers. Every day, Lakshmana's (Lord Rama's younger brother) job was to go outside the court to check and see if there was anyone with a complaint. Normally, there weren't any complainants as Rama's rule was such that there were no diseases, the earth yielded plenty of food and evil disappeared fearing the king's wrath.

On one such day, Lakshmana found that there was no one outside the court. "Go back and look again," said Rama. Lakshmana returned to the main gate and found

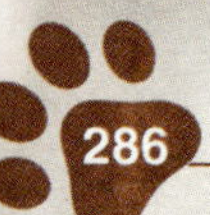

a dog barking away. "What do you want?" Lakshmana asked the dog. "If you have something to tell the king, come with me". "I can't come with you," said the dog. "Dogs are not allowed inside temples, palaces and the houses of Brahmins. Those are the residing places of Gods like Agni, Indra, Surya and Vayu. We aren't allowed there". But Rama gave special permission to the dog to approach the court. The dog had marks of a beating on its head. "What is your problem, dog?" Rama asked. "A Brahmin named Sarvarthasiddha was looking for alms and has beaten me without any provocation," replied the dog. On Rama's orders, the Brahmin was summoned. "Why have you beaten this dog?" asked Rama. Brahmin replied that I was hungry and was roaming around, looking for alms, and this dog was blocking my way. I asked him to move but he didn't. So I beat him replied Sarvarthasiddha. "I'm guilty. Please punish me. If I am punished, I will no longer have to fear about going to hell". Rama consulted his advisers and ministers like Bhrigu, Angirasa, Kutsa, Kashyapa and Vashishtha. Their advice was unanimous that according to the Shastras (Scriptures), a Brahmin shouldn't be punished. "But you have promised," said the dog. "You promised to set right my complaint. Please make this Brahmin the Kulapati of Kalanjara". Strictly speaking, a Kulapati was a small ruler and his job was to feed ten thousand sages and study under them. Kalinjara or Kalanjara is in the Bundelkhand region of India. Anyway, this seemed fair enough, because Sarvarthasiddha wasn't exactly being punished. He was sent off to Kalanjara, riding on an elephant. "You have given him a boon instead of punishing him," remarked the ministers. "Not quite," responded Rama. "Ask this dog". On Rama's instructions, the dog related his story as per the Sangraha Ramayana Uttara kanda (Verses 3.10 to 3.20) and its translation is reproduced here.

"I used to be the Kulapati of Kalanjara," said the dog. "I served Gods and Brahmins and spent my time ensuring everyone's welfare. I ate after everyone else had eaten. I shared my property with everyone else but having been a Kulapati, I am now destined to this dog's life. That Brahmin is cruel and quick to anger. He will now become a Kulapati and the next forty-nine of his descendants will spend their lives in hell. If you want to make certain that an individual and his friends, sons and animals go to hell, make him a Kulapati". So by giving that position he is liable to commit sins and go to hell. Having related his story, the dog went off to the holy city of Varanasi, resolving to starve himself to death there and thus perform penance.

DOG OF MAHABHARATA

The great cultural epic to significantly feature the dog is Mahabharata of ancient India (Circa 400 BCE). The epic relates towards the end of the tale of King Yudhishthira who ruled over Hastinapura for thirty-six years after the war (battle of Kurukshetra). He established an ideal rule and ensured all round peace and tranquility. Now he had become completely disenchanted with worldly things and decided to go to the Himalayas and beyond to engage himself in deep austerities and give up his life in bliss. His four brothers and their wife Draupadi also decided to accompany him. The Pandavas threw their weapons into the river and began the ascent to Swarga, Indra's heaven on Mount Meru but a dog began to tag along with them. As they neared the summit, first Draupadi was left behind because of her attachment to Arjuna and then one after the other (because of each person's pride, hunger, love or other kind of attachment) four Pandavas fell dead. The only survivors remained, the Yudhishthira and the dog.

Now Shakra (Indra's private name) appeared in his gleaming chariot. "Embark in my chariot and come with me to Swarga." But when Yudhishthira went to take his seat in the vehicle, the dog also hopped in. When they reach the heavenly gates of Swarga, Shakra invited the pious, truthful Yudhishthira to came in. I do not want to be there alone, said Yudhishthira. Shakra assured him that he would see his brothers and Draupadi, already there. Yudhishthira then says, "Lord of Past and Present, this dog who was so devoted to me should also enter." Indra replied, "You have acquired immortality and all the joys of heaven today; leave the dog behind." The man said, "Lord of a Thousand Eyes, what may be the use of such bliss, if it rejects one who is so devoted to me?"

"Even for such bliss, I could never leave one who is terrified, devoted to me, needs my help, weak or begs for his life. I could never abandon such a one." Shakra again informed him, "whatever blessings or benefits a dog can observe, the heavenly daughters will take way. So renounce the dog and attain the joys of heaven. You went on without your own brothers so why won't you give up the dog?"

But Yudhishthira said, "As long as they were alive, I did not renounce them. To abandon the dog would be like injuring a friend, or like frightening someone under my protection." Yudhishthira was shocked that so loyal and noble a creature as this dog would not be allowed into heaven, as such, he preferred to remain with his dog on earth or was ready to even go to hell, than enter into a place which would exclude his dog.

Then Indra relented and praised the man for the mercy he demonstrated towards the animal. He admitted them together to Swarga as an example to others. Just then, Dharma "with his golden hair" emerged from the dog's form and blessed the man. Some say that this Dharma is the one who is the man's father and that he had come to test Yudhishthira's loyalty and was pleased with his son's conduct. Others say that it is the Dharma-rajah who is Yama, Lord of Death but many others say that Dharma stands for the law of the universe itself.

This was a unique case of a mere mortal reaching the heavens bodily. In some versions of this tale the dog is then revealed to be the God Vishnu, the preserver who has been watching over Yudhishthira all his life, thus linking the figure of the dog directly to the concept of God and the loyalty of the dog is depicted as the devoted figure to his master, whether that master returns the devotion or not.

SANTHAL HOUND: THE DOG OF ABORIGINAL SANTHAL TRIBE

The Santhal Hound is named after the Aboriginal Indian Santhal Tribe, among whom it is found in the Hazaribagh district of northern Jharkhand in India. It has been used by these tribes exclusively for hunting in a survival economy as well as in a ritual context in the annual hunts of the tribe called Desom Sendra which have an association with the forest Goddess Chandi, similar to the Arcadian huntress Diana with her hunting dogs. The Santhals call the dog Seuta and Kukur and sometimes affectionately Tuio which means jackal. The mixture of black or white in the breed may be taken as a mongrel admixture and is absent in the true type found in the jungle villages. The dog is an affectionate inmate of the Santhal household in Hazaribagh. It is a pure indigenous dog with no wolf or Nordic/Spitz in its DNA. The tests of samples of hair of the Santhal Hound for DNA were done at the Royal Institute of Technology in Stockholm by Dr Peter Savolainen in 2000 and it has been confirmed that Santhal Hound is a representative of the indigenous Indian dog. It is similar to the New

Guinea Singing Dog and Dingo of Australia, belonging to the so-called Indo-Polynesian Group. These dogs would have found their way over to Australia with Austronesians crossing by sea about five thousand years ago.

The Manjhi Santhals though being animists, do not exactly worship the God Shiva, yet they continue ancient tradition of depicting the Forest God and his two dogs, Bhairav and Bhairavi in stone relief carvings in Shiva temples. There may also be some further indications of continuity as the dog appears in the Sohrai ritual harvest paintings of the Kurmi and Ghatwal tribals of the same area, tracing its origin to a Mesolithic society. The Oraon tribals of Hazaribagh have a tradition of their God Dharmes being accompanied by his two dogs, Bhowra and Bhowri. Santhal Hound is found in all tribal-inhabited regions in Assam and West Bengal (Singur). The Santhals and other tribal groups in Jharkhand such as Santhal Parganas in Hazaribagh, Singhbhum district in Ranchi and Khonds and Saoras in Phulbani and Eastern Ghats in Odisha also keep such dogs. In Chhatisgarh, these dogs are found among the Maria and Muria Gonds in Bastar and in the Maikal Hills among the Baigas.

The myth of the horned dog is prevalent in the tribes of Hazaribagh also as they believe that in ancient times dogs wore horns (sihare diring paraiyare). This is a living tradition among the nomadic Birhor hunter–gatherers of Hazaribagh who believe that the jackal's (master of the pack) howling to the moon made him to shed his horns on a moonlit night and was then called "Pharao". The dog is depicted in the local art sometimes wearing a ritual collar similar to the Egyptian Anubis, the collared dog of Australian aboriginals from the rock art of the Kimberley ranges and the horned Sinaitic dog of the rock art of the Sinai Peninsula. In Africa, this type of dog is found among a variety of nomadic hunting tribes in East Africa, Wanderobo tribe in the Belgian Congo, Pigmy and Bantu tribes in the Sudan and Zaire and Zande tribes in Central African Republic. In South Africa, it appears in the Bushman rock art of the Drakensberg ranges of Kalahari desert in Namibia and Botswana. In Israel, it appears as the Canaan Dog/Israeli Sheep Dog.

Lord Krishna in Bhagavad Gita (5–18): "Sages see with an equal eye, a learned and humble Brahmin, a cow, an elephant, or even a dog or an outcaste".

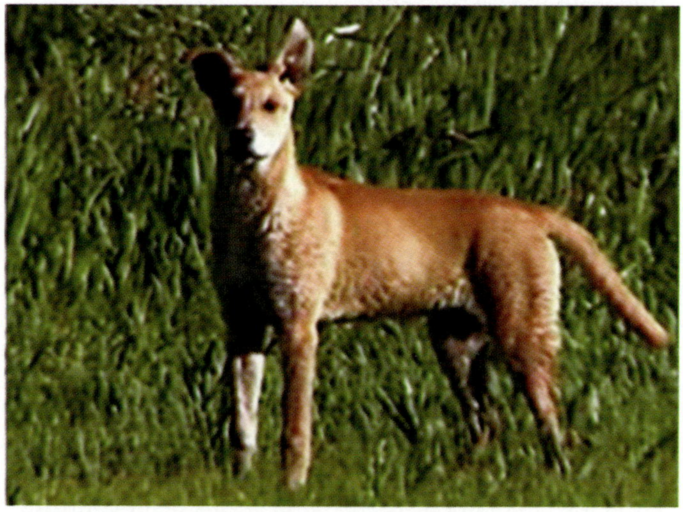

Santhal Hound

DOGS IN ART AND CULTURE

Cultural depictions of dogs extend as far back as 4500 BC when dogs were portrayed on the walls of caves and tombs, children's toys and ceramics. The hunting dogs of those days were generally portrayed. Subsequently, the representation became more elaborate as individual breeds evolved and the relationships between human and canine developed further. Hunting scenes were popular in the middle ages and the renaissance. Images of dogs were often carved on tombstones to represent the

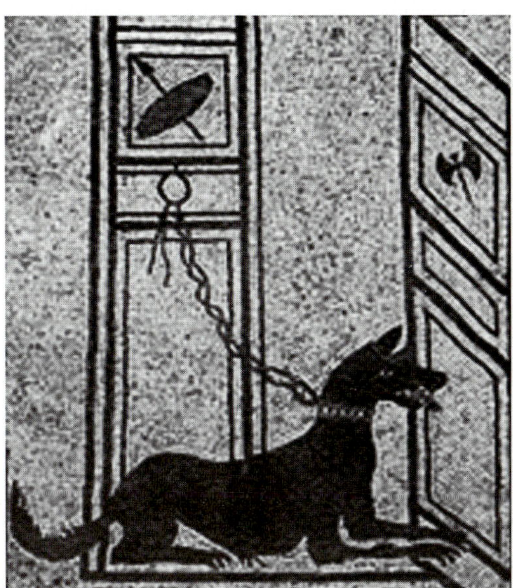

Cavev-Canem watch dog

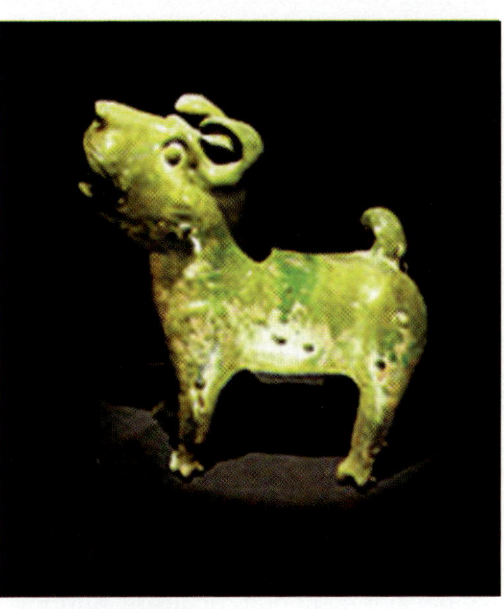

China Green glazed pottery dog

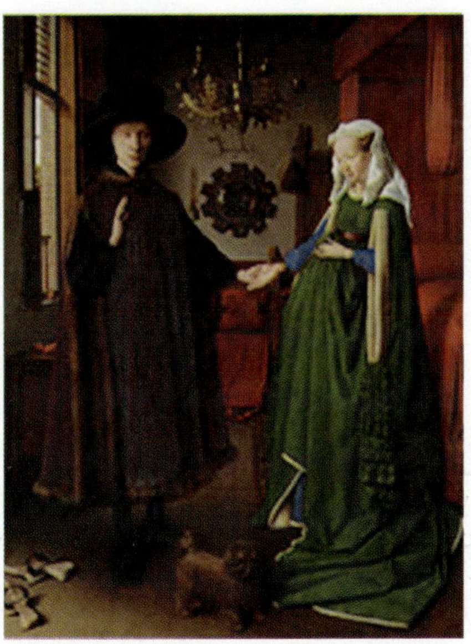

Jan Van Eyck's The Arnolfini Wedding (1434)

deceased's feudal loyalty or marital fidelity. Dogs were depicted to symbolize guidance, protection, loyalty, faithfulness, watchfulness and love. A dog, when included in an allegorical painting, portrays the attribute of fidelity personified. In a portrait of a married couple, a dog placed in a woman's lap or at her feet can represent marital fidelity. If the portrait is of a widow, a dog can represent her continuing faithfulness to the memory of her late husband. An example of a dog representing marital fidelity is present in Jan van Eyck's "Arnolfini Portrait," an oil painting on oak panel dated 1434 by the early Netherlandish painter Jan Van Eyck. It is a small full-length double portrait which is believed to represent the Italian merchant Giovanni di Nicolao Arnolfini and his wife, presumably in their home in the Flemish city of Bruges. It portrays a wedding scene where the people invited to witness the ceremony can be seen in the convex mirror at the back and the mirror symbolizing the eye of God. In those times, it was enough that two witnesses were present to make a wedding legal. A little dog is seen in the picture symbolizing in the iconography faithfulness, devotion or loyalty, or can be seen as the couple's desire to have a child.

Though generic dogs had been depicted in paint and carved in stone for millennia but as dogs became more domesticated, they were shown as companion animals, often painted sitting on a lady's lap. Dog portraits became increasingly popular in the 16th and 17th centuries. Many wealthy women in the court had lap dogs as companions. In that case the dog could reflect wealth or social status. Thus paintings of specific dogs mostly favoured the lapdogs and hunting hounds of royalty. Hunting in the medieval period was a sport exclusive of the aristocracy and was considered an essential part of court etiquette and it was a way of showing bravery and chivalric virtue. As such, in medieval and renaissance art hunting scenes were common topics. Subsequently, animal domestication became relatively widespread and even after the development of agriculture, hunting was usually a significant contributor to the

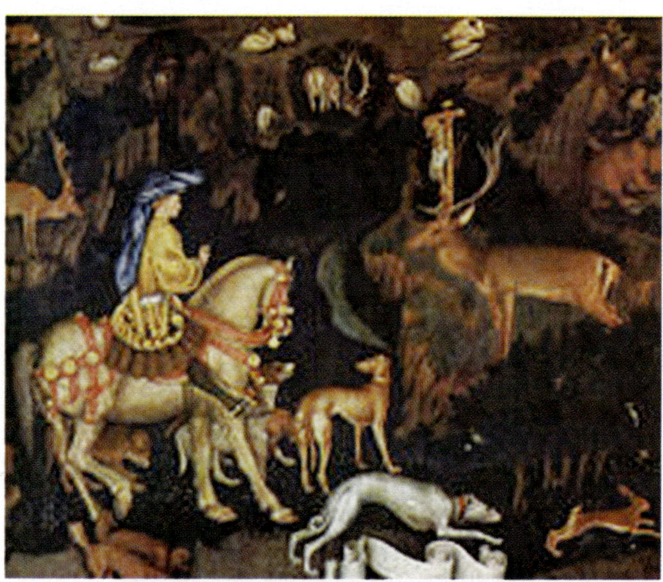

Hunting scene with dogs, Pisanello (1395–1455)

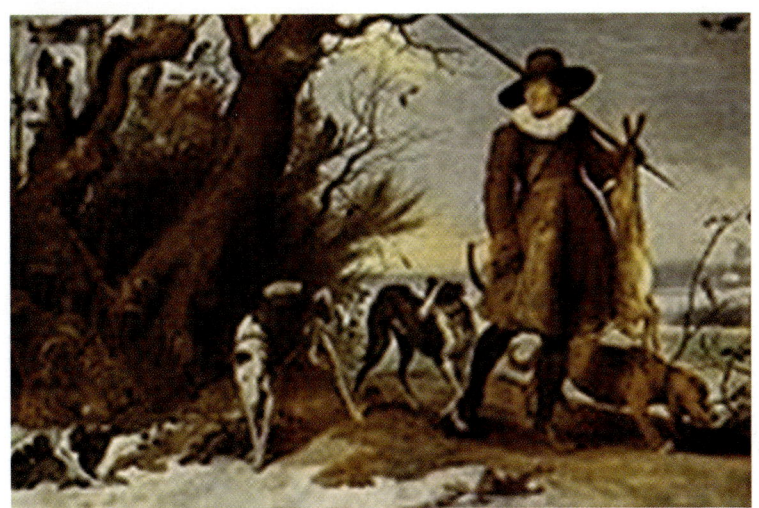

Jan Van Wildens, hunting scene with a pack of dogs

human food supply. Hunting also filled a practical necessity, assuring food for the tables of the nobility and nobles spending their money on packs of specially bred hounds were not unusual. However, hunting was forbidden to servants, peasants and also the Roman Catholic Church clerics in those days. Thus hunting dogs were very often the company of the highest social class of that society. Gaston Phoebus (30th April, 1331–1391), the 11th Count of Foix and Viscount of Bearn, was one of the greatest huntsmen of his day and hunted his entire life. He died of a stroke while washing his hands after returning from a bear hunt. He wrote a book on hunt titled "Livre de Chasse" between 1387 and 1388. In this book, he described different stages of hunting various types of animals, the animal behaviour and advice to less well-off gentry about how to enjoy hunting without bankrupting themselves. He was even sympathetic to the peasant poachers because he considered that they too have the hunting instinct. This book is the classic treatise on medieval hunting and has exquisite miniatures illustrating the hunt, in one manuscript.

The 17th and 18th centuries saw a boom in portraiture of pups. Emperor Joseph I, as a child with a Cocker Spaniel, Louis XV's daughter with a large book and a tiny Papillon, the Princess Royal and Prince William around 1770 with a Shih Tzu and George III's wife Queen Charlotte with a Maltese in one portrait and a Spaniel in another. When William III, after whom Williamsburg is named, moved from Holland to London to rule Great Britain, he brought along Pugs as favoured pets and symbol of the Netherlands. William Hogarth's, an English painter, printmaker, pictorial satirist, social critic, and editorial cartoonist who was credited with pioneering western sequential art, loved his dog so much that the tough little Pug "Trump" become a part of his self-portrait.

In monarchies, the aristocracy is a class of people who either possess hereditary titles granted by a monarch or are related to such people and thanks to the specific connection of the aristocrats with the hunting dogs, they were often shown as symbols in heraldry for visually identifying a person where the fighters were in armour. Later coats of arms remained popular in other ways such as impressed in sealing wax on documents, carved on family tombs and flown as a banner on

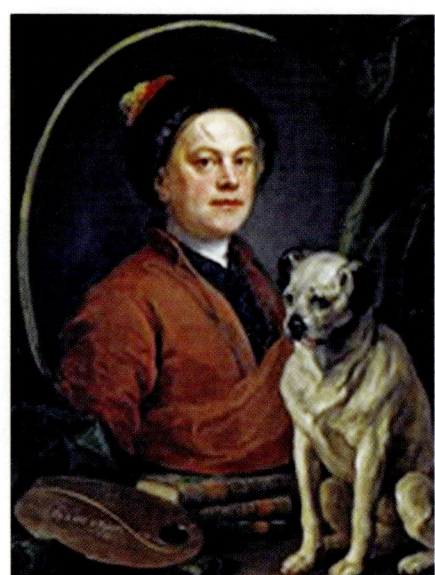

William Hogarth Painter and his Pug, 1745

country homes. From the beginning of heraldry, coats of arms have been executed in a wide variety of media, including on paper, painted wood, embroidery, enamel, stonework and stained glass.

For the purpose of quick identification, heraldry distinguishes only seven basic colours and makes no fine distinctions in the precise size or placement of charges on the field. Coats of arms and their accessories are described in a concise jargon called blazon. This technical description of a coat of arms is the standard that is

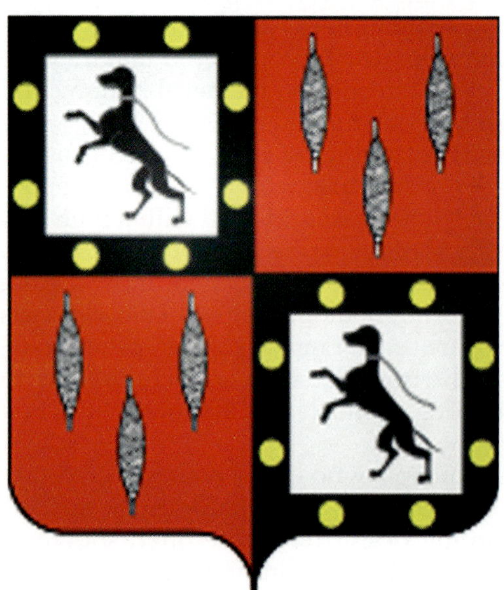

Coats of arms of the French commune d' Arreau

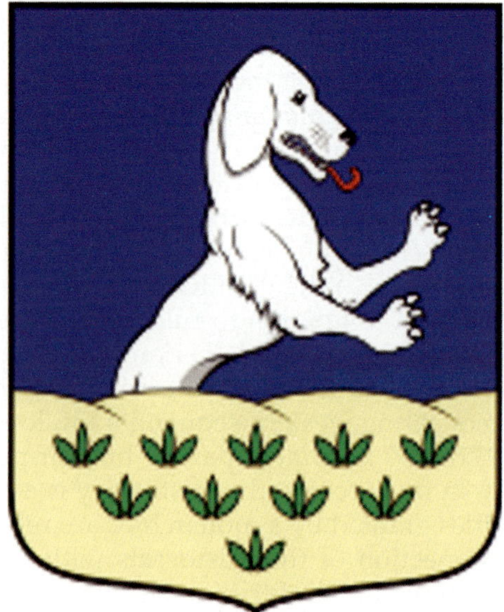

Coats of arms of the Hungarian town Ebes

adhered to despite whatever artistic interpretations may be made in a particular depiction of the arms. A charge is any object or figure placed on a heraldic shield or on any other object of an armorial composition and any object found in nature or technology may appear as a heraldic charge in armory. Charges can be animals, objects or geometric shapes. Dogs of various types, and occasionally of specific breeds relates with the specific meaning such as courage, vigilance, loyalty and fidelity. Three encaustic tiles dating from the 15th century featured a white hound, the Talbot family crest and the inscription "Sir John Talbot" (the 1st Earl of Shrewsbury) in part of a set of four and these tiles originally might have been used on a church floor. The term Talbot is used in heraldry to refer to a good-mannered hunting dog. The Talbot dog always depicts the Talbot coat of arms and is the original hound used as an English heraldic symbol. It is portrayed in the family crest of several noble German and English families.

The relationship between people and dogs kept evolving and an animal perhaps initially valued for its service was becoming man's best friend signifying a turn through the long transition. The Romans had a proverb, "cave canem"—beware of the dog. In 1613, Cervantes wrote the dialogue between Scipio and Berganza, a novel about two Spanish dogs. Later in the century, the French fabulist Jean de La Fontaine wrote "The Little Dog," a lengthy poem about a man who is changed into a woman's pet. In the mid-1700s, Francis Coventry penned "The History of Pompey the Little: the Life and Adventures of a Lap-Dog". Chapter four of the humorous novel is titled "Our hero becomes a dog of the town and shines in high-life". In his 17th century diary, Samuel Peppys tells the story of travelling on a barge with Charles II and that of a dog, the King loved, fouled the boat. Charles II was so devoted to his canines that he let them distract him during meetings, leading a courtier to growl "God save your Majesty but God damn your dogs." In 1738, Benjamin Franklin could write, "There are three faithful friends, an old wife, an old dog and ready money." Lord Byron penned an inscription for a monument to a dog in 1808 that read in part as follows:

"The poor dog, in life the firmest friend, the first to welcome, foremost to defend."

Age by age, canines claimed more and more of man's love. 18th century newspaper ads featured on the story of the evolution of the relationship between men and dog. Elsewhere in the era there were elegies for deceased dogs, paintings of Pointers and Pugs, careful breeding and a philosophical declaration about the rights of dogs under the law. Through the millennia, dogs have borne burdens, herded livestock, drawn sledges, carried messages, tracked fugitives, retrieved game, and guarded their owners. The relationship evolved from a purely practical "you help me; I feed you," to mutual affection.

As the time passed, development could be seen in the use of dogs as main characters in literature. In 1825, Sir Walter Scott wrote, "Recollect that the Almighty who gave the dog to be companion of our pleasures and our toils, hath invested him with a nature noble and incapable of deceit." Dogs were also limned on their own most notably by George Stubbs, an English painter whose 18th century portraits of horses and dogs were considered best of show by many critics. Stubbs reflects in art what was evolving in science, says Malcolm Warner, a senior curator with the Kimbell Art.

Museum in Fort Worth, Texas. Similarly, Descartes had argued that when you hear an animal cry out in pain, it's like a machine's noise when its gears go wrong.

In the 18th century, there was a huge improvement in scientific knowledge and people began to think of animals as creatures with feelings and personalities comparable to people. Stubbs filled a need to capture those personalities on canvas. The results were images of Mouton, a Barge dog, the Spaniel Fanny, Turk and Crab, a duke's Pomeranian and Terrier, etc. Amongst the other painters specialized in this genre, was Thomas Gainsborough, who put dogs into his portraits.

In France, Jean-Baptiste Oudry, a rococo painter, engraver, and tapestry designer, particularly well-known for his naturalistic pictures of animals and his hunt pieces depicting game, exhibited a painting "Bitch Hound Nursing Her Puppies" in 1753.

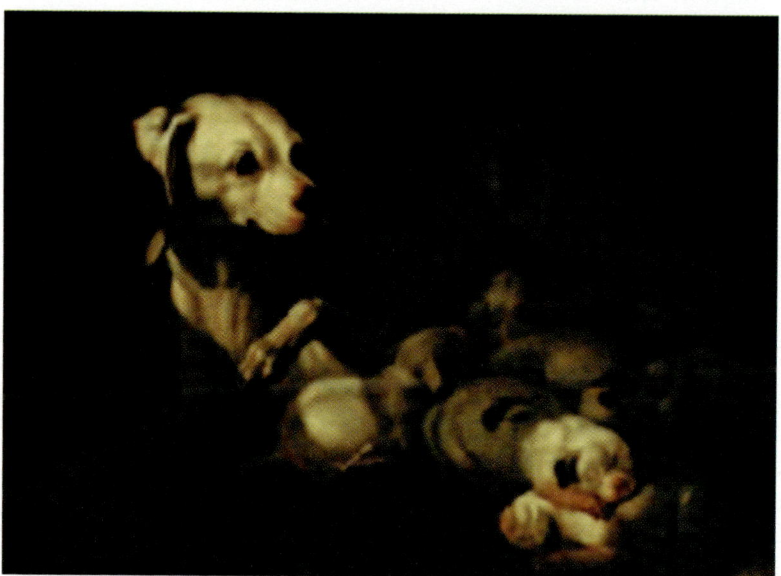

It has been credited by one modern critic as pinpointing "the moment when that all embracing empathy between man and dog was first recorded so fully and so tenderly in a canine environment." Dogs became so beloved that their deaths elicited elegies. One of the first came from Matthew Prior in 1693 to mark the loss of "True," a pet of Queen Mary II:

Envious Fate has claim'd its due,
Here lies the mortal part of True.

John Gay published "An Elegy on a Lap Dog" in 1720:

He's dead. Oh lay him gently in the ground!
And may his tomb be by this verse renown'd.
Here Shock, the pride of all his kind, is laid;
Who fawned like man, but ne'er like man betray'd.

In 1775, Williamsburg's Virginia Gazette printed "On the Death of a Lady's Dog":

Thou, happy creature, art secure
From all the troubles we endure.

One reason this attentiveness to dogs arose during the 1700s is the enlightenment, which made it more acceptable to engage in humanitarian activities, whether for people or animals, says Stanley Coren, author of "The Pawprints of History: Dogs and the Course of Human History". It seems, there was a deep philosophical shift in 18th century that led people to think of animals as having a value in their own right. Previously, they had been more or less thought of as an object in terms of their usefulness to mankind. During the enlightenment, as scientists learned more about animals, "people became more sensitive to animals' pain and that merged into a feeling that they were individuals with personalities and emotions." There was another factor in this shift, the rise of an affluent middle class. "They could express their status in purebred dogs. Once dogs were in the parlour and out of the yard, affection grew for these beasts and they were treated more as family members.

Robert Fountain, co-author of Stubbs' "Dogs: The Hounds and Domestic Dogs of the Eighteenth Century", credits the growing attentiveness to dogs to the ambitions of the upwardly mobile to become country gentlemen and improve their social standing by participating in field sports whether they enjoyed it or not. The expanding love of humans for canines was endorsed by philosophers, playwrights, poets, and preachers. Alexander Pope said that "histories are fuller of examples of fidelity of dogs than of friends." This is not to say that all dogs lived such a dog's life as bull and bearbaiting were still popular in this century. Packs of dogs were turned into a ring to harass larger animals by biting them in vulnerable spots and holding tenaciously to their snouts, called "pinning the bull," a specialty of bulldogs. The events were common in many countries and they attracted thousands of fans. What disturbed people further was not just bull baiting and cruel owners but animal experimentation and vivisection. One of the most acclaimed surgeons of the time, Dr John Hunter conducted research in 1755 on artificial respiration in hope of finding a way to revive people who had drowned. His experiment involved using bellows to repeatedly resuscitate a dog and cutting its sternum open to see how its lungs and heart were responding. A footnote by philosopher Jeremy Bentham in 1789 has become what Warner terms "a landmark in the history of animal rights", indeed and turned up in modern day literature from groups like "People for the Ethical Treatment of Animals". Bentham wrote:

"A full-grown horse or dog is beyond comparison, a more rational as well as more conversable animal than an infant of a day or a week or even a month old. But suppose they were otherwise, what would it avail? The question is not, Can they reason? Nor can they talk? But can they suffer? Why should the law refuse its protection to any sensitive being? The time will come when humanity will extend its mantle over everything which breathes.

In Japan, in the middle of the 17th century, a Shogun who was born in a Year of the Dog, instituted laws of compassion to protect canines. He decreed that anyone mistreating a dog would face capital punishment. As in the human world, dogs were divided by class with recognized breeds and coddled pets lording it over Mongrels and Strays, while the traits of colonial dogs were invoked in assertions of superiority over indigenous people and their curs. Japanese emulated the same prejudices and favoured western breeds over local varieties until the 1930s when the rising tide of nationalism boosted the status of Japanese dogs. The elevation of national breeds owes much to the venerated Hachiko whose statue outside

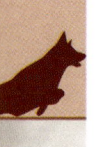

Shibuya Station is certainly one of the most popular meeting spots in the world. The present statue is not the original as the same was melted down during the war to make spare train parts, but it remains faithful to the controversial prototype.

Hirokichi, the self-appointed promoter and guardian of "purebred" Japanese dogs, raised funds for the original statue and insisted on depicting "Hachiko" with both ears upright, arguing this is how a pedigree should look. The artist refused and Hachiko's floppy left ear was immortalized. Ear controversy also surrounded the casting of "Saigo", Takamori's statue unveiled in Ueno Park in 1898. Saigo was being rehabilitated into a national hero and exemplar of samurai spirit despite his fateful rebellion against the national government since this favourite was a western dog with large floppy ears.

Returning to the story of Hachiko, every day he met his master Saito in front of Shibuya Station and kept coming for nine years even after the professor died in 1925. Saito met Hachiko and mobilized media attention for a dog that embodied unswerving loyalty, duty and desirable traits in the wake of the 1931 Manchurian Incident. In this feverish climate Hachiko's romanticized story was published and the Education Ministry included it in texts to inculcate patriotism. Unlike most national heroes, Hachiko actually lived to see his statue unveiled a year before he died in 1935, but he was probably unaware of the snarling going on behind the scenes concerning his floppy ear or role in promoting imperial devotion. Indigenous dogs were transformed into accessories of empire as Saito redefined them as repositories of national character and played an instrumental role in the official recognition of seven Japanese breeds during the 1930s. Interestingly, the Tosa breed of dog was not one of this first batch of Japanese pedigrees because it was a cross-breed with the Western Mastiff, a decision that speaks volumes about prevailing anxieties.

In England, during the late 19th and early 19th centuries, one of the leaders in the movement to safeguard animals was an Irish Protestant who campaigned in Parliament for Catholic emancipation and the care of animals. Richard Martin, born in 1754, was nicknamed "Trigger Dick" for shooting of a dog. But Martin later became known as "Humanity Dick" for his efforts on behalf of farm animals which led not only to laws but to the founding of the Royal Society for the Prevention of Cruelty to Animals in 1824. This organization was originally founded without the "royal" prefix by a group of 22 reformers led by Richard Martin MP, William Wilbarforce MP and the Revered Arthur Broome in "Old Slaughter's Coffee House", St Martin's Lane, near the Strand in London and marked by a plaque on the modern day building at 77–78 St Martin's Lane. The society was the first animal welfare charity to be founded in the world and brought sixty-three offenders before the courts. It was granted its royal status by Queen Victoria in 1840 to become the "Royal Society for the Prevention of Cruelty to Animals (RSPCA)" as it is today. In the late 1830s the society began the tradition of the RSPCA inspector which is the image best known of the organization today. The RSPCA lobbied Parliament throughout the 19th century, resulting in enacting a number of new laws. The Cruelty to Animals Act 1835 amended Martin's Act and outlawed baiting. In 1876 the Cruelty to Animal Act was passed to control animal experimentation. In 1911, Parliament passed Sir George Greenwood's Animal Protection Act and since that time the RSPCA has continued to play an active role, both in the creation of animal welfare legislation and in its enforcement. An important recent new law has been the Animal Welfare Act 2006. RSPCA centres, hospitals and branches operate throughout England and

Wales. Such acts on Prevention of Cruelty to Animals are now in vogue in all countries of the world.

Another sign of interest in dogs in the 1700s was the development of breeding techniques in the natural way, mixing and matching dogs through mating to get the characteristics they sought. Although the first official classification of English breeds was done in 1570 by John Caius in De Canibus Britannicis or Of English Dogges. Among other types, he identified Blood Hounds, Terriers, otter Hounds and Maltese. During the 18th century, an era of taxonomies and catalogues, Buffon and Linnaeus expanded on Caius with Linnaeus listing such animals as the Shepherd's Dog, the Pomeranian, the Iceland Dog, the Lesser Water Dog, the Mastiff, and the Barbet. It was on such stock that breeders went to work to improve toy Poodles for my lady, clench-jawed Bulldogs for Bull Baiters, faster Grey Hounds for racing aficionados, and dotted Dalmatians for carriage drivers.

Established landowners became more and more preoccupied with breeding better livestock, faster horses and hounds and dogs better suited to the changing style of shooting as the accuracy of firearms increased. The rise in fox hunting in both England and its American colonies spawned a need for a medium-sized hound with the stamina to follow prey for miles, a keen nose for scent and a bark that could summon his master from a distance. One of the leading 18th century breeders of Fox Hounds was Hugo Meynell who outlined the breed's traits and kept strict records to produce offspring that could keep up with foxes. Fox Hounds came to Virginia in 1738 with Lord Fairfax and the breed fascinated a Fairfax familiar George Washington, later President of America, whose pets had names like Sweet lips, Venus and True Love. Washington's diaries are crammed with notations about riding to the hounds. One January, he spent eight days pursuing foxes and often he "caught nothing". His love of canines was so strong that during the Revolutionary War, he bothered to return a stray Terrier to its owner, British General Howe, along with a note that read: "General Washington does himself the pleasure to return a dog, which accidentally fell into his hands."

In 1772, Washington's friend Bryan Fairfax said that the American General was so discerning, he could pick out the inferior pups from what others considered "superexcellent dogs." In 1789, Thomas Jefferson, later president of America, while returning from his stint as ambassador to France, imported "Shepherd's Dogs" for Monticello and later presented Washington with puppies. For his part, Washington fixated on perfecting the English Fox Hound. To that end, he built kennels at Mount Vernon where he could create "a superior dog, one that had speed, scent and brains." Washington's experiments led to the American Fox Hound breed which is lighter, taller, and faster than its British cousin.

In 19th centaury, the dog depicted in 1831 by Sir Edwin Henry Landseer, an English painter well-known for his paintings of animals, particularly horses, dogs and stags, painted a Newfoundland called "Bob" who was found in a shipwreck off the coast of England. The dog found his way to the London waterfront where he became known for saving people from drowning, a total of 23 times over the course of 14 years. For this, he was made a distinguished member of the Royal Humane Society, granting him a medal and access to food throughout life. The Newfoundlanders with white patches are now recognized as a breed of their own, as a "Landser." The painting was described by The Art Journal as being "one of the best and most interesting publications of the year" and "Mr Thomas

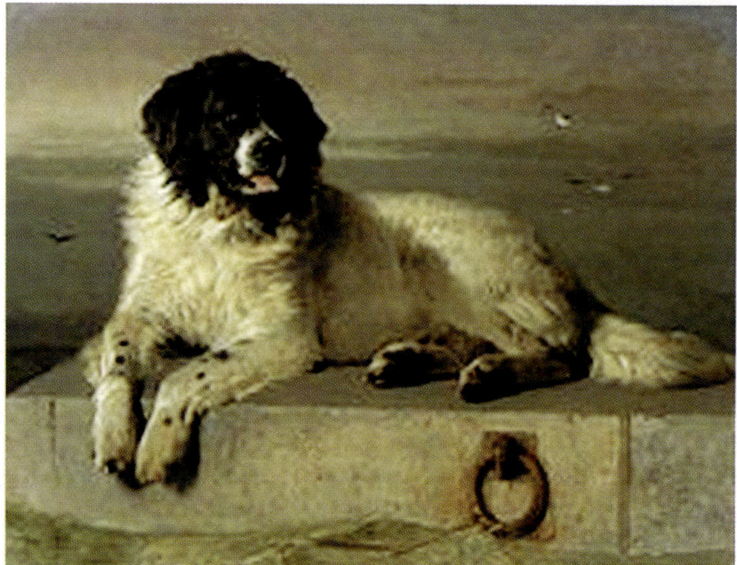

Bob, a distinguished member of the humane society

Landseer's first great effort in this department of the art." A 19th century copy of the painting by George Cole, an English landscape painter, was sold by auctioneers Bonham for £7,200 in March, 2007.

The picture was entitled "A Distinguished Member of the Humane Society".

The Royal Humane Society was founded in England in summer of 1774. It is a British charity which promotes life-saving intervention. Two English physicians, William Hawes and Thomas Cogan involved in publicizing the power of artificial respiration to resuscitate people who superficially appeared to have drowned, brought fifteen friends each to a meeting at the Chapter Coffee-house, St Pauls, Churchyard, and founded the Royal Humane Society for the Recovery of Persons apparently drowned and for rendering first aid in cases of near drowning. Gradually, branches of the Royal Humane Society were set up in other parts of the country, mainly in ports and coastal towns where the risk of drowning was high and by the end of the 19th century the society had upwards of 280 depots throughout the UK supplied with life-saving apparatus. The earliest of these depots was the Receiving House in Hyde Park, on the north bank of the Serpentine, which was built in 1794 on a site granted by George III. Hyde Park was chosen because ten thousands of people swam in the Serpentine in the summer and ice-skated in the winter. Boats and boatmen were kept to render aid to bathers, and in the winter ice-men were sent round to the different skating grounds in and around London. The society distributed money-rewards, medals, clasps and testimonials to those who save or attempt to save drowning people. It further recognized "all cases of exceptional bravery in rescuing or attempting to rescue persons from asphyxia in mines, wells, blasting furnaces, or in sewers where foul gas may endanger life."The Royal Humane Society established commonwealth branches in Australia in 1874, in Canada in 1894, and New Zealand in 1898.

Since its foundation the Royal Humane Society has made more than 85,000 awards. However, financial rewards are no longer given nor does the society give advice on how to save life. Presently, the awards granted include bronze, silver and gold medals and testimonials on Vellum or Parchment. The Society may also give recognition to those who have contributed to the saving or attempted saving of life, though they may not have put their own life at risk. In these instances a Certificate of Commendation may be granted. In addition, Resuscitation Certificates may be granted to those who, though not professionally trained to do so, carry out a successful resuscitation.

By the Victorian era, the sporting tradition remained but after the establishment of The Kennel Club in the UK in 1873 and the American Kennel Club in 1884, dog portraits soared in popularity mainly because of newly introduced breed standards or world pictures. There were differences between the British and European style of depiction. William Secord, founding director of The Dog Museum of America and a world expert on canine art, described it by stating: "Belgian, Dutch, Flemish and German artists were more influenced by realism, depicting the dog the way it really looked, with dirt on its coat and slobber and that kind of thing whereas the British depictions were more idealized as they want it pretty.

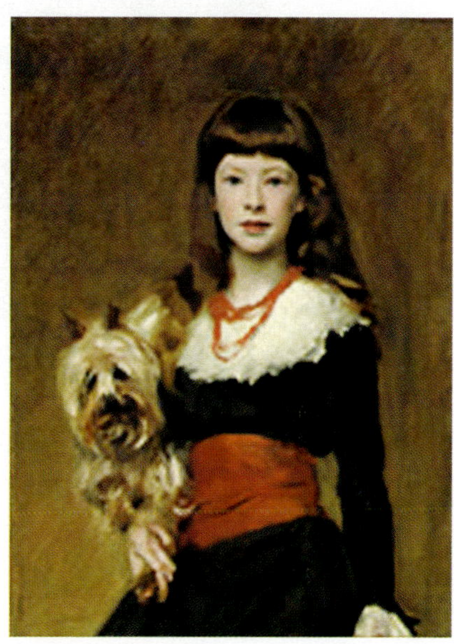

Miss Beatrice Townsend with her pet by John Singer Sargent

The prices achieved for canine art increased in the 1980–90s and started to gain popularity in established art circles rather than antique markets. Buyers could generally be divided into three dominant categories, hunters, breeders and exhibitors of pedigree dogs and owners of companion animals. Pablo Picasso, a Spanish painter, sculptor, printmaker, ceramicist, stage designer, poet and playwright who spent most of his adult life in France, frequently included his canine companions in his paintings. He was one of the greatest and most influential artists of the 20th century and a Dachshund, named "Lump" featured often in his work. Lump, was a male Dachshund born in 1956 in Stuttgart, Germany and named after the German word for "rascal". He was purchased by David Douglas Duncan, an American photographer from a German family. David with Lump, first met Picasso on 19th April, 1957 at La Californie, Picasso's hillside mansion in Cannes, France. Picasso enquired if the dog had ever had a plate of his own. When Duncan responded no, Picasso picked up a brush and painted a portrait of Lump on his own dinner plate with the work dated and inscribed to Lump. He handed over the plate to Duncan as a gift. The dog felt immediately at home and stayed with Picasso for the next six years at La Californie living with Picasso's Boxer Yan and a goat named Esmeralda. Duncan often spoke of Lump and Picasso, "This was a love affair. Picasso would take Lump in his arms and feed him from his hand. Duncan photographed Picasso with Lump on several occasions along with his children, while Picasso preferred to work alone, he would often be seen accompanied by Lump.

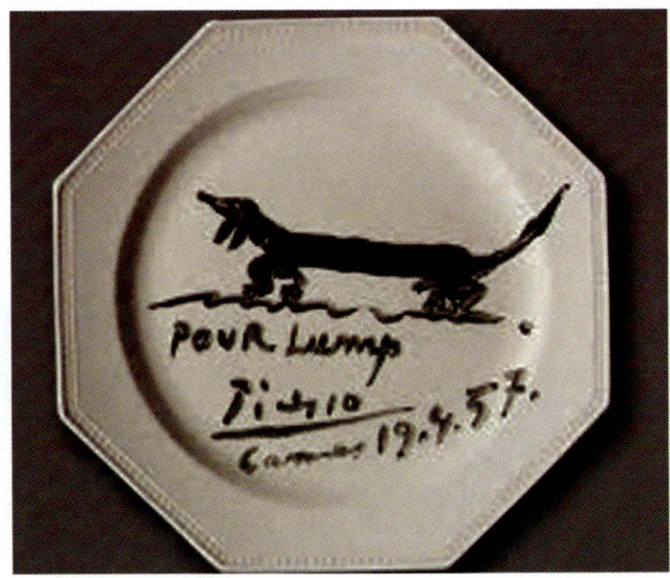

Picasso once said, 'Lump, he's not a dog, he's not a little man, he's somebody else.'

Bibliography

Aaron HS (2011): Empire of Dogs: Canines, Japan and the Making of the Modern World. Cornell University Press, USA.

Ambros B (2009): Vengeful Spirits or Loving Spiritual Companions? Changing Views of Animal Spirits in Contemporary Japan. Asian Ethnology, 69(1), 35–67.

Ambros B (2010): The Necrogeography of Pet Memorial Spaces: Pets as Liminal Family Members in Contemporary Japan. Material Religion: The Journal of Objects, Art and Belief, 6(3), 304–335.

Anthony CY (1977): The Journey to the West. Chicago and London: The University of Chicago Press.

Arthur FD (1993): A Complete Guide to Heraldry. Gramercy Books, New York.

Bansum A (2014): Stubby: the War Dog, The True Story of World War I's Bravest Dog. National Geographic Stores, Margate FL, USA.

Behan JM (1946): Dogs of War, Scribner's, New York, USA.

Bertha WS (2205): Only A Dog: The True Story of a Dog's Devotion to His Master During World War I, 2nd ed. Diggory Press, Cornwall, UK.

Brookes JA (1991): Ghosts and Legends of Wales. Jarrold Publishing.

Bruchac J (1991): Native American Stories. Fulcrum Publising, Golden, Colorado, USA.

Bruchac J (1995): Dog People: Native Dog Stories. Fulcrum Publishing, Golden, Colorado, USA.

Bulu Imam (2003): The Santhal Hound. Sanskriti Publishing, Hazaribagh, India.

Bulu Imam (2006): The Manjhi Santhals of Hazaribagh—Hunt Rules, Songs, Lifestyle and Folklore. Sanskriti Publishing, Hazaribagh, India.

Burnam JC (1999): Dog Tags of Courage: The Turmoil of War and the Rewards of Companionship. Lost Coast Press, Fort Bragg, CA, USA.

Burnam JC (2006): Dog Tags of Courage: Combat Infantrymen and War Dog Heroes in Vietnam. Lost Coast Press, Fort Bragg, CA, USA.

Case LP (1999): The Dog, Its Behaviour, Nutrition, and Health. Ames, Iowa State University Press, USA.

Chattopadhyaya KP (1970): Ancient Indian Culture Contacts and Migrations, FKL Mukhopadhyaya Publishers, Calcutta, India.

Christie A (1968): Chinese Mythology. Feltham, Hamlyn Publishing. ISBN: 0600006379.

Clayton CG (1945): Dogs at War. Macmillan Publishers, London.

Cooper J (1983): Animals in War. Heinemann Publishers, London.

Coren S (2013): Picasso's Dogs, Modern Dog Magazine. Retrieved, 23rd, November, 2013.

Currie WB (1988): Structure and Function of Domestic Animals. Butterworth Publishers, Stoneham, MA, USA.

David W (1992): Debrett's Guide to Heraldry and Regalia. Headline Books, London.

Dean CL (2005): Soldiers and Sled Dogs. University of Nebraska Press, USA.

Dorothee B (2007): The Domestication of Empire: Human-Animal Relations at the Intersection of Civilization, Evolution, and Acclimatization in the Nineteenth Century. In: A Cultural History of Animals in the Age of Empire, Oxford: Berg Publishers, UK.

Dorothy HP (2012): Dogs on Duty, Soldier's Best Friends on the Battle Field and Beyond. Walker Books, London.

Douglas K (2001): Buddies Men, Dogs and World War II. Zenith Press, USA.

Dowling MC (2011): Sergeant Rex, the Unbreakable Bond between a Marine and His Military Working Dog. Atria Books, USA.

Duncan DD (2006): Picasso and Lump, A Dachshund's Odyssey. Bulfinch Press, New York, USA.

Dyer WA (2006): Pierrot the Carabinier: Dog of Belgium. Meadow Book, UK.

Ernest B (1927): Animal Heroes of the Great War. The Macmillan Company, London.

Evans WY (1981): The Fairy Faith in Celtic Countries. Billings & Sons Ltd.

Flood J (1983): Archaeology of the Dreamtime. Collins Publishers.

Goldstraw L (1991): The Paratrooper and his Dog, After the Battle, No. 74.

Grambo RL (2005): Wolf: Legend, Enemy, Icon. Firefly Books, USA.

Hammer B (2006): Dogs at War. Carlton Books, London.

Haran P (2000): Trackers: The Untold Story of the Australian Dogs of War. New Holland Publishers, Australia.

Harbison C (1990): 270 Sexuality and Social Standing in Jan Van Eyck's Arnolfini Double Portrait. Renaissance Quarterly, 43 (2) pp. 270.

Harbison C (1991): Jan Van Eyck, The Play of Realism. Reaktion Books, London, 1991.

Hill A (2005): Animal Heroes. Penguin Australia, Melbourne.

Jack C (2005): A Humorous Guide to Heraldry, Black Knight Books, Boston, USA.

Jager TF (1910): Ambulance Dogs, The British Medical Journal, 2 (2293), 1589–1590.

Jager TF (1917): Scout, Red Cross and Army Dogs. Arrow Printing Co., New York.

Jessica W (2012): Dogs and the Making of the American State: Voluntary Association, State Power, and the Politics of Animal Control in New York City, 1850–1920, The Journal of American History, 98 (4), 1001–1002.

John CB (1999): Dogs Tags of Courage: The Turmoil of War and the Rewards of Companionship. Lost Coast Press, Fort Bragg, CA, USA

John GC (2001): The Hound and the Hawk, the Art of Medieval Hunting. St Martin Press, New York, USA.

John CB (2009): A Soldier's Best Friend: Scout Dogs and their Handlers in the Vietnam War. Lost Coast Press, Fort Bragg, CA, USA.

Juliet CB (1995): Origin of the Dog, Domestication and Early History. In: the Domestic Dog: Its Evolution, Behavior, and Interactions with People. Cambridge University Press, USA.

Keister D (2004): Stories in Stone: A Field Guide to Cemetery Symbolism and Iconography. Salt Lake City, Gibbs Smith, Utah, USA.

Katherine CG (2006): Pets in America: A History, Chapel Hill, North Carolina, University Press, 161–166.

Kathleen K (2007): Introduction: Animals and Human Empire. In: A Cultural History of Animals in the Age of Empire. Berg Publishers, Oxford, UK.

Kleiner FS (2009): Gardner's Art through the Ages: The Western Perspective. Wadsworth Publishing Company, Belmont, CA, USA.

Kolig E (1978). Aboriginal Dogmatics: Canines in Theory, Myth and Dogma. Brill Publishers, Leiden, USA.

Kveldulf HG (1992): The Folklore of the Wild Hunt and the Furious Host, Mountain Thunder, Celtic Myth Podshow 7th Issue. Winter 1992: First presented as lecture to the Cambridge Folklore Society at the house of Dr HR Ellis-Davidson.

Lisa R (2011): The Dogs of War, the Courage, Love and Loyalty of Military Working Dogs. St Martin's Griffin Press, New York.

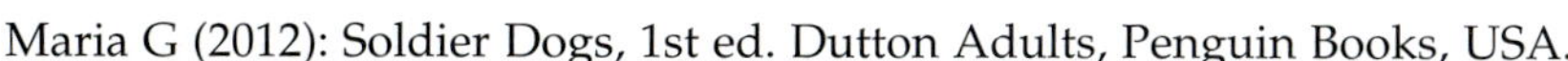

Maria G (2012): Soldier Dogs, 1st ed. Dutton Adults, Penguin Books, USA.

Martin CL (1845): The History of the Dog. Knight's Weekly Vol. Xliv. London, Excerpted in the Electric Review, New Series vol. XX.

McCarthy C (2014): K-9 Comfort Dog Arrives on CUW's Campus. Concordia University Wisconsin, USA.

Michael GL (1999): War Dogs: A History of Loyalty and Heroism. Potomac Books, Inc. Dulles, Virginia, USA.

Michael GL (2009): Forever Forward, K9 Operations in Vietnam. Schiffer Publishing, Pennsylvania, USA.

Michel R and Gary B (2013): Trident K9 Warriors, my tales from the training ground to the battle with the elite Navy Seal canines, Re ed. St Martin's Griffin Press, New York.

Michael JR (1999): The Dog Who Walked with God. Illustrated by Stan Fellows. Candlewick Press, Cambridge, MA, USA.

Mike D (2012): Seargent Rex, The Unbreakable Bond between a Marine and His Military Working Dog, Re ed. Atria Books, New York, USA.

Military Working Dogs (2005): Field Manual No. 3–19.17, Published by Headquarters, Department of the Army, Washington DC, USA.

Morgan P (1999): K-9 Soldiers, Vietnam and After. Hellgate Press, London.

Nancy MW (2007): Chips: A Hometown Hero. Based on the True Life Adventures of the World War II K9 hero. Off Lead Publications, New York.

Nigel A (2014): Smoky: The War Dog. New Holland Publications, Chatswood, NSW, Australia.

Nigel A (2012): Cry Havoc: The History of War Dogs. New Holland Publications, Chatswood, NSW, Australia.

Nigel A (2012): Australian War Dogs: The Story of Four-legged Diggers. New Holland Publications, Chatswood, NSW, Australia.

Rannels K (1945): War Dogs in Morotai Island, Mil Rev. 25, pp 44–45.

Raymond C and Richard S (1995): Evolution of Working Dogs. In: The Domestic Dog: Its Evolution, Behavior, and Interactions with People. Cambridge University Press, USA.

Rice D (1996): The Complete Book of Dog Breeding. Barron's Educational Series, Hauppauge, New York (USA).

Richardson EH (1910): War, Police and Watch Dogs. William Blackwood and Sons, London.

Richardson EH (1920): British War Dogs: Their training and Psychology. Skeffington and Sons Ltd. London.

Robart R (2011): US Military Dogs in World War II. Schiffer Publishing Ltd, USA.

Ronald P (2013): Horrie the War Dog, Allen and Unwin, Sydney, Australia.

Rose DB (1992): Dingo Makes us Human, Life and Land in an Aboriginal Australian Culture. Cambridge University Press, USA.

Shiu H and Stokes L (2008): Buddhist Animal Release Practices: Historic, Environmental, Public health and Economic Concerns, Contemporary Buddhism. Roultledge, London.

Silberman V (2001): Who Let the Dog Out. Art Business News 28(5). Retrieved 24th September, 2013.

Squibb G (1953): The Law of Arms in England. The Coat of Arms II(15), 244.

Susan O (2012): Rin Tin Tin: The Life and the Legend, Reprint ed. Simon and Schuster, New York, USA.

Waters N (2010): History of the Talbot Tiles, Dog World, Archived from the original on 18th January, 2014.

Terri C and Cynthia H (2011): No Body Left Behind, Bringing US troops' Dogs and Cats Safely Home from the Combat Zone. Lyons Press, 1st ed, Guilford, USA.

Thurston ME (1994): Jack, Stubby, Ebony, Zucha, Bub—all were soldiers of a sort, all were Dogs. Mil. History, February issue, pp 26, 28 and 87–88.

The Army Dogs (2002): The Silent Warrior and Saviour, Published by Addl Dte Gen RVS, QMG's Br. Army HQ, New Delhi.

US Military Working Dog Training Handbook (2012): Department of Defence, USA. Lyons Press, Guilford, USA.

Varner JG and Varner JJ (1983): Dogs of Conquest, Norman OK. University of Oklahoma Press.USA.

Veldkamp E (2009): The Emergence of Pets as Family and the Socio-Historical Development of Pet Funerals in Japan. Anthrozoos: A Multidisciplinary Journal of the Interactions of People & Animals, 22(4), 333.

Whitehead S (1999): Dog: The Complete Guide, Team Media, Ltd. London, UK.

William CP (2003): Always Faithful: A Memoir of the Dogs of World War II. Potomac Books Inc. Dulles,Virginia, USA.

Yang, Lihui *et al.* (2005). Handbook of Chinese Mythology. Oxford University Press, New York, USA. ISBN: 978-0-19-5332633-6.

Index

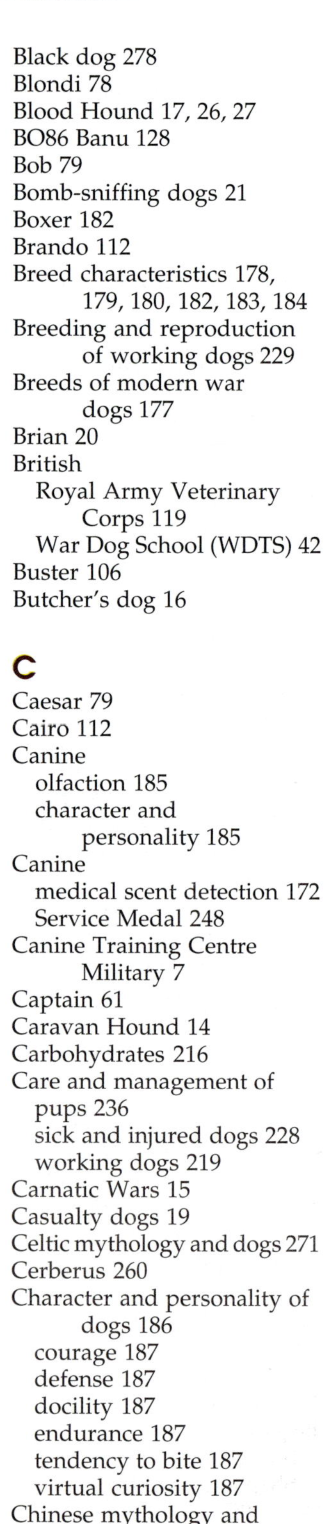

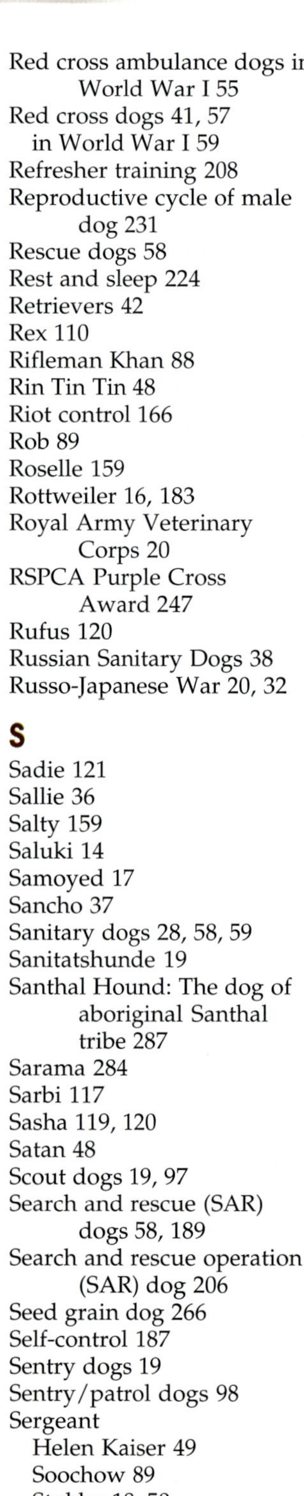